Current Clinical Oncology

Maurie Markman, MD, Series Editor

For further volumes:
http://www.springer.com/series/7631

James C. Yao · Paulo M. Hoff · Ana O. Hoff
Editors

Neuroendocrine Tumors

Humana Press

Editors
James C. Yao, MD
Department of Gastrointestinal
Medical Oncology
The University of Texas
M.D. Anderson Cancer Center
Houston, TX, USA
jyao@mdanderson.org

Paulo M. Hoff, MD
Instituto do Cancer do Estado de
São Paulo, Faculdade de Medicina da
Universidade de São Paulo, and
Hospital Sirio Libanes
São Paulo, Brazil
paulo.hoff@icesp.org.br

Ana O. Hoff, MD
Endocrine Neoplasia Unit
Instituto do Cancer do Estado de
São Paulo, Faculdade de Medicina da
Universidade de São Paulo,
São Paulo, Brazil
Department of Endocrinology,
Fleury Group,
São Paulo, Brazil
ana.hoff@icesp.org.br

ISBN 978-1-61779-756-9 ISBN 978-1-60327-997-0 (eBook)
DOI 10.1007/978-1-60327-997-0
Springer New York Dordrecht Heidelberg London

Printed on acid-free paper

Humana Press is part of Springer Science+Business Media (www.springer.com)

Preface

Neuroendocrine tumors arise from cells dispersed throughout the body. Historically, they have been thought to be a group of very rare and indolent diseases capable of causing a variety of esoteric hormonal syndromes. Over the past decade, a number of major advances were made in our understanding of the epidemiology and molecular biology of these not-so-rare tumors. Although several studies have demonstrated a significant heterogeneity among neuroendocrine tumors by primary site and proliferative rate, recent analyses of the population-based registries confirm a consistent and continuing rise in its incidence. Further, because of the relative longer survival enjoyed by patients with this disease, it is now recognized that the prevalence of neuroendocrine tumors exceeds 100,000 individuals in the United States alone.

Neuroendocrine tumors are often well differentiated and associated with an indolent clinical course, but they can also present in much more aggressive forms. Due to their ability to produce hormones, their clinical presentations can be rather unusual and dramatic, requiring prompt expert treatment. Some neuroendocrine tumors are associated with genetic syndromes, which should be suspected particularly when the tumors arise at an early age or in family clusters.

While early stage neuroendocrine tumors can be cured by surgery, the disease is generally incurable when presenting with metastases. Despite the reputation of being indolent, most patients with advanced disease will eventually succumb to the disease. Successful management requires an understanding of the disease process as a whole and a multi-modality approach. Depending on the case, the inputs from medical oncology, surgery, endocrinology, gastroenterology, pathology, radiology, genetics, and nuclear medicine are required.

While our understanding of the molecular pathogenesis of neuroendocrine tumors remains incomplete, progress has been made. Studies of the MEN1 gene function have led to our understanding of its role in epigenetic regulation and control of endocrine cell proliferation. More recent studies have also demonstrated the importance of angiogenesis and the activation of the mammalian target of rapamycin (m-TOR) pathway in the genesis and progression of neuroendocrine tumors.

These advances have generated a renewed interest in the development of novel therapeutic options for neuroendocrine tumors using the novel molecular targeted agents. During the last few years, three of those targeted agents have been evaluated in pivotal randomized phase III studies for neuroendocrine tumors. Octreotide, sunitinib, and everolimus have successfully demonstrated significant antitumor activity against neuroendocrine tumors. These studies not only demonstrated that rigorous evaluation of antitumor agents in what was thought to be a rare disease is feasible, but also demonstrated that the integration of molecular targeted agents can lead to critical advances in the management of those patients.

In this volume, we have gathered an impressive array of thought leaders in the field from around the world. They have generously undertaken a comprehensive review of the epidemiology, biology, and management of neuroendocrine tumors. Recent advances in our understanding of molecular biology and emerging therapeutic options are emphasized.

We, as all the participating authors, hope that this work will help demystify some important misconceptions regarding neuroendocrine tumors, and that it may help to improve the treatment of patients and families affected by this diseases.

Good reading!

Houston, TX — James C. Yao
São Paulo, Brazil — Paulo M. Hoff
São Paulo, Brazil — Ana O. Hoff

Contents

Contributors

Mohamed Khalaf Aly Asran, MD Department of Diagnostic Radiology, The University of Texas M.D. Anderson Cancer Center, Houston, TX, USA

Joao E. Bezerra, MD Department of Medical Oncology, Cancer Institute of São Paulo, São Paulo, Brazil

Piyaporn Boonsirikamchai, MD Department of Diagnostic Radiology, The University of Texas M.D. Anderson Cancer Center, Houston, TX, USA

Glenda G. Callender, MD Department of Surgical Oncology, The University of Texas M.D. Anderson Cancer Center, Houston, TX, USA

Cleber Camacho, MD Department of Endocrinology, Federal University of São Paulo, São Paulo, Brazil

Chusilp Charnsangavej, MD Department of Diagnostic Radiology, Division of Diagnostic Imaging, The University of Texas M.D. Anderson Cancer Center, Houston, TX, USA

Barbro Eriksson, MD, PhD Department of Medical Sciences, Uppsala University Hospital, Uppsala, Sweden

Jason B. Fleming, MD Department of Surgical Oncology, The University of Texas M.D. Anderson Cancer Center, Houston, TX, USA

Bernardo Garicochea, MD, PhD Department of Oncology, Hospital São Lucas, Pontifical Catholic University, Porto Alegre, RS, Brazil

Elizabeth G. Grubbs, MD Department of Surgical Oncology, The University of Texas M.D. Anderson Cancer Center, Houston, TX, USA

Manal M. Hassan, MD Department of Gastrointestinal Medical Oncology, The University of Texas M.D. Anderson Cancer Center, Houston, TX, USA

Ana O. Hoff, MD Endocrine Neoplasia Unit, Instituto do Cancer do Estado de São Paulo, Faculdade de Medicina da Universidade de São Paulo, São Paulo, Brazil Department of Endocrinology, Fleury Group, São Paulo, Brazil

Paulo M. Hoff, MD, FACP Instituto do Cancer do Estado de São Paulo, Faculdade de Medicina da Universidade de São Paulo, Hospital Sirio Libanes, São Paulo, Brazil

Leonid Izikson, MD Department of Dermatology, Roswell Park Cancer Institute, and University of Buffalo, Buffalo, NY, USA

Camilo Jimenez, MD Department of Endocrine Neoplasia and Hormonal Disorders, The University of Texas M.D. Anderson Cancer Center, Houston, TX, USA

Neda Kalhor, MD Department of Pathology, The University of Texas M.D. Anderson Cancer Center, Houston, TX, USA

Matthew H. Kulke, MD, MMSc Medical Oncology, Dana-Farber Cancer Institute, Harvard Medical School, Boston, MA, USA

Christine S. Landry, MD Department of Surgical Oncology, The University of Texas M.D. Anderson Cancer Center, Houston, TX, USA

Jeffrey E. Lee, MD Department of Surgical Oncology, The University of Texas M.D. Anderson Cancer Center, Houston, TX, USA

Rui M.B. Maciel Section of Endocrinology, Fleury Group, São Paulo, Brazil Department of Endocrinology, Federal University of São Paulo, São Paulo, Brazil

Cesar A. Moran, MD Department of Pathology, The University of Texas M.D. Anderson Cancer Center, Houston, TX, USA

Nancy D. Perrier, MD Department of Surgical Oncology, Section of Surgical Endocrinology, The University of Texas M.D. Anderson Cancer Center, Houston, TX, USA

Alexandria T. Phan, MD Department of Gastrointestinal Medical Oncology, The University of Texas M.D. Anderson Cancer Center, Houston, TX, USA

Thereasa Rich, MS Department of Surgical Oncology/Clinical Cancer Genetics Program, The University of Texas M.D. Anderson Cancer Center, Houston, TX, USA

Rachel P. Riechelmann, MD, PhD Department of Medical Oncology, Gastrointestinal Tumors, Cancer Institute of São Paulo, São Paulo, Brazil

Jonathan Strosberg, MD Department of Gastrointestinal Oncology, H. Lee Moffitt Cancer Center and Research Institute, Tampa, FL, USA

Saul Suster, MD Department of Pathology and Laboratory Medicine, Medical College of Wisconsin, Milwaukee, WI, USA

James C. Yao, MD Department of Gastrointestinal Medical Oncology, The University of Texas M.D. Anderson Cancer Center, Houston, TX, USA

Nathalie C. Zeitouni, MDCM, FRCPC Department of Dermatology, Roswell Park Cancer Institute and University of Buffalo, Buffalo, NY, USA

Chapter 1
Global Epidemiology of Neuroendocrine Tumors

Manal M. Hassan and James C. Yao

Abstract A significant increase in the annual age-adjusted incidence of neuroendocrine tumors (NETs) was observed in the United States over the last three decades. The underlying reason for such increase has not been explained by epidemiological studies. However, there is strong evidence that NETs occur sporadically, regardless of disease site and that positive family history of cancer is associated with risk of developing NETs that did not arise in the context of other hereditary syndromes.

The role of prior history of chronic medical conditions needs to be addressed by epidemiological studies where detailed history about these diseases and their duration prior to NETs diagnosis should be documented. The impact of environmental and genetic factors needs to be well studied in different populations, different ethnicity, and in men and women separately.

Keywords Carcinoids • Anatomic origination of NETs • Tumor histology • Age-adjusted incidence of NETs

Introduction

Carcinoids are rare well-differentiated neuroendocrine tumors (NETs) that are capable of producing biogenic amines and polypeptide hormones [1–3]. NETs may develop at many locations and can be classified according to anatomic origination, tumor histology, and biological activity.

M.M. Hassan (✉)
Department of Gastrointestinal Medical Oncology,
The University of Texas M.D. Anderson Cancer Center,
1515 Holcombe Boulevard, Box 426, Houston, TX 77030, USA
e-mail: mhassan@mdanderson.org

J.C. Yao et al. (eds.), *Neuroendocrine Tumors*, Current Clinical Oncology,
DOI 10.1007/978-1-60327-997-0_1, © Springer Science+Business Media, LLC 2011

A significant increase in the annual age-adjusted incidence of NETs was observed from 1973 (1.09/100,000) to 2004 (5.25/100,000) [4]. Of the 35,618 patients with NETs identified in the SEER database, 7,004 (48%) were men. Eighty-one percent of the patients were white, 12% were African American, 5% were Asian/Pacific Islander, and 1% was American Indian/Alaskan native. Moreover, the most common primary tumor site varied by race, with the lung being the most common in white patients, and the rectum is the most common in Asian/Pacific Islander, American Indian/Alaskan Native, and African American patients [4].

The same report [4] indicated that survival duration varied by histologic grade. In multivariate analysis of patients with well-differentiated to moderately differentiated NETs, disease stage, primary tumor site, histologic grade, sex, race, age, and year of diagnosis were predictors of outcome ($P<0.001$).

Very little is known about the risk factors associated with NETs which is probably due to the rarity of this cancer and to the lack of large epidemiologic studies to examine several risk factors simultaneously while making proper adjustments for potential confounders.

This chapter reviews the available data on these risk factors and generally discusses the pathogenesis of HCC development.

Risk Factors

Cigarette Smoking

There is very limited information about the association between cigarette smoking and NETs. A recent US case-control study of 740 patients with different NETs and 924 healthy controls indicated no association between cigarette smoking and NETs at lung, stomach, pancreatic, colon, and small bowel in men and women separately [5]. Moreover, compared with nonsmokers, cigarette smokers had no significant trend in risk of NETs development by duration of smoking neither by number of smoked cigarettes per day. Ex-smokers were at a nonsignificantly increased risk of NETs development at all studied sites of disease (lung, gastric, small bowel, pancreas, and rectum), relative to nonsmokers. In addition to this US study, three studies have explored the role of smoking in small intestine NETs [6–8]. The first study by Chow et al. [7] also found no increase in risk for smokers; however, the study did not include any histologic classification of small intestinal cancer to discriminate NETs from other tumor types. The second study by Chen et al. [6] was limited to 17 patients with small intestine carcinoids and 52 controls and found only nonsignificant increases in odds ratio (OR) due to cigarette smoking [OR=4.2; 95% confidence interval (CI), 0.8–22.4]. Moreover, the estimated ORs were not adjusted for important confounders such as race or family history of cancer. The third study by Kaerlev et al. [8] is the largest European population-based case-control study to date, analyzing 84 patients with small intestine carcinoids and 2,070 controls. The authors reported a moderate risk increase for small bowel carcinoids among ever smokers; however,

Table 1.1 Single and pooled odds ratios for association between cigarette smoking and small bowel neuroendocrine tumors (NETs): case-control studies

Study	Type	Site	Year	Cases	Controls	SOR (95% CI)[a]	POR (95% CI)[b]	*P*
Hassan et al.	Hospital-based case-control	USA	2008	325	924	1.3 (0.9–1.8)	–	
Chow et al.	Population-based	USA	1993	260	570	0.9 (0.8–1.3)	–	
Kaerlev et al.	Population-based	Europe	2002	84	2,070	1.9 (1.1–3.2)	–	
Chen et al.	Hospital-based	USA	1994	17	52	4.2 (0.8–22.4)	–	
Summary	–	–	–	–	–	–	1.2 (0.8–1.6)	0.2

[a]*SOR* Single odds ratio reported by each study
[b]*POR* Pooled odds ratio from all studies

Table 1.2 Single and pooled odds ratios for association between alcohol consumption and small bowel NETs: case-control studies

Study	Type	Site	Year	Cases	Controls	SOR (95% CI)[a]	POR (95% CI)[b]	*P*
Hassan et al.	Hospital-based case-control	USA	2008	325	924	1 (0.7–1.4)	–	
Chow et al.	Population-based	USA	1993	260	570	1.1 (0.8–1.5)	–	
Kaerlev et al.	Population-based	Europe	2002	84	2,070	1.1 (0.6–2)	–	
Chen et al.	Hospital-based	USA	1994	17	52	3.1 (0.7–13.9)	–	
Summary	–	–	–	–	–	–	1.1 (0.8–1.4)	0.9

[a]*SOR* Single odds ratio reported by each study
[b]*POR* Pooled odds ratio from all studies

the increase was significantly observed among ex-smokers only, not among current smokers. Table 1.1 presents the summary OR of 4 studies for the association between cigarette smoking and small bowel NETs. The estimated overall OR = 1.12 (95% CI, 0.76–1.58). No significant heterogenicity between studies; $P = 0.145$.

Unlike risk association with NETs development, smoking was shown to be a significant prognostic factor for poor survival of early stage cervical NET [9]. These disparate findings indicate that the effects of smoking on the clinical outcome of patients with NETs need to be explored further.

Alcohol Consumption

Except for small bowel NETs, the association between alcohol consumption and NETs has not been well investigated. Table 1.2 showed that four studies presented no significant association between alcohol use and small bowel NET. The overall estimated OR of all four studies is 1.08 (95% CI; 0.80–1.35). The difficulty in determining the association between alcohol use and NETs is very common in cancer research in general. It is mainly attributable to difficulty of assessing the cumulative intake of alcohol and ethanol intake from all types of alcoholic beverages prior to cancer development over the lifetime of individual. In addition, the association between alcohol intake and cancer development may vary between men and women. A recent review by Mancinelli et al. [10] suggested that women may experience a more rapid progression of alcohol damage than men. The lower body mass index (BMI) and body fluid content in women than men may contribute to lowered ethanol diffusion and high blood concentration in women [11]. Moreover, the activity of gastric alcohol dehydrogenase, which is responsible for the first-pass metabolism of ethanol in the stomach, is significantly lower in women than in men, which implies that large amounts of alcohol will be metabolized by hepatic alcohol dehydrogenase [12, 13]. It is also possible that genetic variations in carcinogen metabolism, inflammatory response, DNA repair, and cell-cycle regulation play a role in determining individual susceptibility to alcohol carcinogenesis for specific cancers like NETs.

Family History of Cancer

A genetic etiology of NETs has been suggested and may occur as part of hereditary syndromes, such as multiple endocrine neoplasia type 1 (MEN-1) [14, 15], von Hippel–Lindau syndrome [15, 16], neurofibromatosis type 1 [17, 18], tuberous sclerosis [19–21], and nonpolyposis colon cancer [22]. Of these, MEN-1 syndrome, an autosomal dominant disorder characterized by parathyroid hyperplasia, pituitary adenomas, and pancreatic tumors, is the one in which NETs most frequently occur. The occurrence of familial NETs not associated with hereditary syndromes is rare as most NETs occur as nonfamilial (sporadic) tumors [14], regardless of disease site. However, there is evidence for a positive association between family history of cancer and risk of developing NETs that did not arise in the context of other hereditary syndromes. It is highly believed that having a first-degree relative with any cancer is a risk factor for the subject's development of small intestinal, gastric, pulmonary, or pancreatic NETs. However, familial clusterings of NETs are rarely reported.

The association of parental NETs was supported by several anecdotal reports of familial NETs of the small intestine [23–25], stomach [26], rectum [22], and lung [27], and by 5 epidemiologic studies, two conducted in the USA [28, 29] and one in Sweden [30, 31]. The Swedish population-based study estimated a fourfold increase in risk of developing NETs in the offspring of affected parents. Their results were later confirmed by US site. The study from Mayo Clinic hospital-based study [28] in which the authors reported that 3.7% of 245 patients diagnosed with NETs had ≥1 first-degree relative with the same malignancy. The prevalence of a positive family history of cancer among first-degree relatives in the second US study was conducted at MD Anderson Cancer Center [29] and was comparable to that of the Mayo study.

The elevated risk of developing NETs extended to individuals with a family history of other cancers (not NETs) like colorectal prostate cancers [29] among first-degree relatives. Such association could be attributed to common genetic abnormalities (e.g., point mutation, chromosomal loss or gain, and DNA methylation) or environmental factors that may cause genetic alterations in members of the same family and may later predispose healthy family members to develop malignancies.

The presence of NETs and other cancers in first-degree relatives may be consistent with several inherited cancer syndromes in which genetic mutations are associated with both NETs and cancers of other types, such as hereditary nonpolyposis colorectal cancer and small intestinal NETs [23]. Moreover, the risk of patients with small intestinal NETs to later develop colorectal carcinoma is 3 times higher than what would be expected in the general population [28].

Several studies indicated an increase in the risk of small intestinal NET development in relation to the presence of a family history of prostate cancer among a patient's first-degree relatives. This observation is supported by the findings of subsequent development of prostate cancer among patients with small intestinal NETs [30, 32]. In addition, the coexistence of prostatic adenocarcinoma and a small intestinal NET was previously described [33, 34]. It is not clear why patients with small intestinal NETs have a high tendency for developing prostate cancer. One explanation is the high tendency of patients with NETs to have a positive family history of cancer as compared to healthy individuals. Thus, a possible positive family history of prostate cancer among patients with NETs may increase their likelihood for developing prostate cancer during their lifetime [35–37]. This hypothesis may be supported by the results of the Swedish familial study [30] in which a significant risk of developing prostate cancer was observed during long-term follow-up of subjects. Even though such link between a positive family history of colorectal or prostate cancer and the development of small intestinal NETs was not supported by other investigations [28].

Nutritional Factors

Assessment for the potential impact of nutritional factors indicated a significant association between high intake of saturated fat and NETs of the small intestine [38]. The estimated hazard ratio and 95% CI was 3.72 (1.79–7.74) for each 10-g increase in intake per 1,000 kcal. On the other hand, intake of fiber from grains was associated with 40% reduction in risk of small bowel NETs [39].

Occupational Factors

The association between occupational histories and the risk of NETs was evaluated by European investigators in a population-based case-control study in Denmark and

Germany [40] where 84 patients with small bowel NETs and 2,070 control subjects who were interviewed for industrial and occupational histories. For industries, authors reported that small bowel risk is associated with whole sale of food and beverages for women. However, in men the highest risk of industries was observed for footwear and metal structure. The association was more significant for long-term exposure of 25 years time lag after exposure was estimated. On the other hand, a significant association between specific occupation and risk of small bowel NETs was observed for bookkeepers, shoe makers, machine filters, and construction painters. The estimated OR (95% CI) were 3.1 (1.1–8.7), 4.7 (1.1–20.6), 2.3 (1.0–5.3), and 3.6 (1.0–13.1), respectively. Exposure to sandblasting, lead, and organic solvents was suggested as common denominators in the reported exposures with high risk of small bowel carcinoids. Nevertheless, the conclusion by this study should be cautiously undertaken because of the small number of patients in the exposed category which may lack precise estimation for the measurement of the association between these factors and risk of NETs development.

Chronic Medical Conditions

The relationship between recent onset diabetes and NETs could be a consequence of the tumor itself or attributable to a malignancy-associated impairment in glucose metabolism such as the presence of a large hepatic metastasis [41]. In fact, the relationship between diabetes and active carcinoid tumors was reported in a study by Feldman et al. [42] who assayed glucose tolerance and insulin secretion in 17 patients with "active" or "inactive" metastatic carcinoid tumors, depending on whether or not carcinoid syndrome was present. The study showed a high incidence of glucose intolerance (80%), elevated serum serotonin, and impaired insulin secretion in patients with carcinoid syndrome, suggesting that serotonin plays a role in producing these alterations.

Alternatively, the association between prior history of diabetes mellitus and NETs has not been well investigated. For pancreatic NETs, it has been postulated to be related to consequence of therapy or and the presence of a glucagon-producing tumor originating from the alpha cells of the pancreas [43, 44].

A recent case-control study in the USA reported significant association between gastric NETs and diabetes mellitus [5]. The study compared 55 patients with gastric NETs and 924 healthy controls yielding a significant fivefold increase in risk of gastric NETs; the estimated OR (95% CI) is 5.6 (2.1–14.5). The mechanisms by which diabetes mellitus induce gastric NETs are unknown. It is possible that long-term diabetes mellitus may act as a mediator for chronic inflammation and may increase individual susceptibility to chronic atrophic gastritis and enhanced oxidative stress inside the cell, which may lead to DNA mutation and the development of gastric NETs [45].

The observation of positive association between gastric NETs and diabetes was supported by two case reports of the development of gastric carcinoids in two diabetic patients [46, 47]. One report described the clinical outcome of a 48-year-old woman with type 2 diabetes [46] and the other a 45-year-old man with type 1 diabetes [47]. During their clinical follow-up, both patients developed autoimmune hepatitis, cirrhosis, type 1 gastritis, and later gastric carcinoids. The authors of the second report [47] indicated that the patient's serum was positive for parietal-cell antibodies (PCAs). In addition to these reports, a clinical study of 93 patients with type 1 diabetes showed that 33% of the diabetic patients were positive for PCA. Those with PCA+ serum were at significant risk of autoimmune gastritis (OR = 17) and enterochromaffin-like (ECL) cell hyper-dysplasia (OR = 23) compared with PCA− patients [48]. Both outcomes are predisposing factors for gastric carcinoid [49].

Adult-onset diabetes is highly correlated with obesity, and obesity may be associated with insulin resistance and type 2 diabetes development in patients with NETs; therefore, the effect of obesity on the risk of NETs cannot be excluded. Baseline BMI at the time of diagnosis may be subject to bias in determining the impact of prior history of obesity on NETs because some NETs patients experienced disease-related weight loss, therefore the baseline BMI may not have accurately reflected these patients' obesity history.

Prior history of cholecystectomy and peptic ulcer were significantly reported in patients with small bowel NET (3/17) as compared to controls [6]. The association between gallstones and NETs was supported by a follow-up Danish study of 42,098 patients with gallstones; the estimated relative risk for carcinoid development was 4.1 (95% CI, 2.3–6.7). However, another European study failed to detect such significant association between gallstones and small bowel NETs specially after taken into consideration the duration of cholecystectomy prior to cancer diagnosis [8]. There is no association between prior history of hepatitis, cirrhosis, Crohn's disease, or ovarian diseases and the risk of small bowel development [6, 8].

Molecular Epidemiology of NETs

Several genetic pathways may be implicated in neuroendocrine carcinogenesis. Polymorphisms of genes involved in these pathways may have significant impact on NETs susceptibility. Moreover, they may act on disease risk only in the presence of environmental risk factors. Therefore, they can be considered as modifying factors on the pathway from exposure to cancer. Examples of these pathways are carcinogen metabolism, oxidative stress, inflammatory, methylation, and DNA repair pathways.

For NETs, there is strong evidence that immune response plays important role in tumor growth [50, 51]. Cytokines may facilitate cross talking between immune and NET growth. Interleukin 2 (IL-2) deficiency was correlated with lower value of gastrointestinal neuroendocrine peptides in a mice model [52] susceptible to gastrointestinal inflammatory conditions. In Croatia, a recent small-scale case control study of 46 cases and 150 controls indicated a significant difference in *G*-allele distribution of IL-2 −330 polymorphisms between patients with NETs and control subjects. The estimated ORs (95% CI) were 6.3 (1.9–20.3), 4.9 (1.3–19.1), and 7.9

(2.1–28.8) for gastroenteropancreatic, gastrointestinal, and pancreatic NETs, respectively [53]. Moreover, *G*-allele at −330 position in the IL-2 promoter was found to be significantly correlated with high serum level of IL-2 ($P=0.03$). However, such finding needs to be confirmed in large-scale studies and in different populations.

Another small-scale case-control study conducted in Italy included 50 patients with gastroenteropancreatic NETs and 100 healthy controls. The study examined the prevalence of nuclear factor-kappaB (NF-kappaB) −94 insertion (I)/deletion (D) ATTG promoter polymorphism. Authors reported no significant difference of deletion/deletion (DD) or insertion/insertion (II) genotypes of NFKB1 −94 I/D between cases and controls [54].

Summary

A significant increase in the annual age-adjusted incidence of NETs was observed in the USA over the last three decades. The underlying reason for such increase has not been explained by epidemiological studies. However, there is strong evidence that NETs occur sporadically, regardless of disease site and that positive family history of cancer is associated with risk of developing NETs that did not arise in the context of other hereditary syndromes.

The role of prior history of chronic medical conditions needs to be addressed by epidemiological studies where detailed history about these diseases and their duration prior to NETs diagnosis should be documented. The impact of environmental and genetic factors needs to be well studied in different populations, different ethnicity, and in men and women separately.

References

1. Kulke MH, Mayer RJ. Carcinoid tumors. N Engl J Med. 1999;340:858–68.
2. Robertson RG, Geiger WJ, Davis NB. Carcinoid tumors. Am Fam Physician. 2006;74:429–34.
3. Schnirer II, Yao JC, Ajani JA. Carcinoid – a comprehensive review. Acta Oncol. 2003;42:672–92.
4. Yao JC, Hassan M, Phan A, et al. One hundred years after "carcinoid": epidemiology of and prognostic factors for neuroendocrine tumors in 35,825 cases in the United States. J Clin Oncol. 2008;26:3063–72.
5. Hassan MM, Phan A, Li D, Dagohoy CG, Leary C, Yao JC. Risk factors associated with neuroendocrine tumors: a U.S.-based case-control study. Int J Cancer. 2008;123:867–73.
6. Chen CC, Neugut AI, Rotterdam H. Risk factors for adenocarcinomas and malignant carcinoids of the small intestine: preliminary findings. Cancer Epidemiol Biomarkers Prev. 1994;3:205–7.
7. Chow WH, Linet MS, McLaughlin JK, Hsing AW, Chien HT, Blot WJ. Risk factors for small intestine cancer. Cancer Causes Control. 1993;4:163–9.
8. Kaerlev L, Teglbjaerg PS, Sabroe S, et al. The importance of smoking and medical history for development of small bowel carcinoid tumor: a European population-based case-control study. Cancer Causes Control. 2002;13:27–34.

9. Chan JK, Loizzi V, Burger RA, Rutgers J, Monk BJ. Prognostic factors in neuroendocrine small cell cervical carcinoma: a multivariate analysis. Cancer. 2003;97:568–74.
10. Mancinelli R, Binetti R, Ceccanti M. Woman, alcohol and environment: emerging risks for health. Neurosci Biobehav Rev. 2007;31:246–53.
11. Ely M, Hardy R, Longford NT, Wadsworth ME. Gender differences in the relationship between alcohol consumption and drink problems are largely accounted for by body water. Alcohol Alcohol. 1999;34:894–902.
12. Baraona E, Abittan CS, Dohmen K, et al. Gender differences in pharmacokinetics of alcohol. Alcohol Clin Exp Res. 2001;25:502–7.
13. Frezza M, di Padova C, Pozzato G, Terpin M, Baraona E, Lieber CS. High blood alcohol levels in women. The role of decreased gastric alcohol dehydrogenase activity and first-pass metabolism. N Engl J Med. 1990;322:95–9.
14. Debelenko LV, Zhuang Z, Emmert-Buck MR, et al. Allelic deletions on chromosome 11q13 in multiple endocrine neoplasia type 1-associated and sporadic gastrinomas and pancreatic endocrine tumors. Cancer Res. 1997;57:2238–43.
15. Hammel PR, Vilgrain V, Terris B, et al. Pancreatic involvement in von Hippel-Lindau disease. The Groupe Francophone d'Etude de la Maladie de von Hippel-Lindau. Gastroenterology. 2000;119:1087–95.
16. Lubensky IA, Pack S, Ault D, et al. Multiple neuroendocrine tumors of the pancreas in von Hippel-Lindau disease patients: histopathological and molecular genetic analysis. Am J Pathol. 1998;153:223–31.
17. Cappelli C, Agosti B, Braga M, et al. Von Recklinghausen's neurofibromatosis associated with duodenal somatostatinoma. A case report and review of the literature. Minerva Endocrinol. 2004;29:19–24.
18. Mayoral W, Salcedo J, Al-Kawas F. Ampullary carcinoid tumor presenting as acute pancreatitis in a patient with von Recklinghausen's disease: case report and review of the literature. Endoscopy. 2003;35:854–7.
19. Yao JC. Neuroendocrine tumors. Molecular targeted therapy for carcinoid and islet-cell carcinoma. Best Pract Res Clin Endocrinol Metab. 2007;21:163–72.
20. Verhoef S, van Diemen-Steenvoorde R, Akkersdijk WL, et al. Malignant pancreatic tumour within the spectrum of tuberous sclerosis complex in childhood. Eur J Pediatr. 1999;158:284–7.
21. Eledrisi MS, Stuart CA, Alshanti M. Insulinoma in a patient with tuberous sclerosis: is there an association? Endocr Pract. 2002;8:109–12.
22. Katdare MV, Fichera A, Heimann TM. Familial rectal carcinoid: report of two first-degree relatives with rectal carcinoid and review of the literature. Tech Coloproctol. 2006;10:143–6.
23. Yeatman TJ, Sharp JV, Kimura AK. Can susceptibility to carcinoid tumors be inherited? Cancer. 1989;63:390–3.
24. Wale RJ, Williams JA, Beeley AH, Hughes ES. Familial occurrence in carcinoid tumours. Aust N Z J Surg. 1983;53:325–8.
25. Anderson RE. A familial instance of appendiceal carcinoid. Am J Surg. 1966;111:738–40.
26. Yoshikane H, Nishimura K, Hidano H, et al. Familial occurrence of gastric carcinoid tumors associated with type A chronic atrophic gastritis. Am J Gastroenterol. 1998;93:833–4.
27. Oliveira AM, Tazelaar HD, Wentzlaff KA, et al. Familial pulmonary carcinoid tumors. Cancer. 2001;91:2104–9.
28. Babovic-Vuksanovic D, Constantinou CL, Rubin J, Rowland CM, Schaid DJ, Karnes PS. Familial occurrence of carcinoid tumors and association with other malignant neoplasms. Cancer Epidemiol Biomarkers Prev. 1999;8:715–9.
29. Hassan MM, Phan A, Li D, Dagohoy CG, Leary C, Yao JC. Family history of cancer and associated risk of developing neuroendocrine tumors: a case-control study. Cancer Epidemiol Biomarkers Prev. 2008;17:959–65.
30. Hemminki K, Li X. Familial carcinoid tumors and subsequent cancers: a nation-wide epidemiologic study from Sweden. Int J Cancer. 2001;94:444–8.
31. Hiripi E, Bermejo JL, Sundquist J, Hemminki K. Familial gastrointestinal carcinoid tumours and associated cancers. Ann Oncol. 2009;20:950–4.

32. Neugut AI, Santos J. The association between cancers of the small and large bowel. Cancer Epidemiol Biomarkers Prev. 1993;2:551–3.
33. Llanes GL, Romero CI, Llorente AC, et al. [Prostatic adenocarcinoma associated with incidental intestinal carcinoid]. Actas Urol Esp. 1998;22:699–701.
34. Adams Jr JR, Culkin DJ, Mata JA, Venable DD. Incidental ileal carcinoid associated with multiple urologic malignancies. J La State Med Soc. 1991;143:27–9.
35. Herkommer K, Paiss T, Merz M, Gschwend JE, Kron M. [Association of a positive family history with histopathology and clinical course in early-onset prostate cancer]. Urologe A. 2006;45:1532–9.
36. Ponder BA. Inherited predisposition to cancer. Trends Genet. 1990;6:213–8.
37. Lynch HT, Brodkey FD, Lynch P, et al. Familial risk and cancer control. JAMA. 1976;236:582–4.
38. Cross AJ, Leitzmann MF, Subar AF, Thompson FE, Hollenbeck AR, Schatzkin A. A prospective study of meat and fat intake in relation to small intestinal cancer. Cancer Res. 2008;68:9274–9.
39. Schatzkin A, Park Y, Leitzmann MF, Hollenbeck AR, Cross AJ. Prospective study of dietary fiber, whole grain foods, and small intestinal cancer. Gastroenterology. 2008;135:1163–7.
40. Kaerlev L, Teglbjaerg PS, Sabroe S, et al. Occupational risk factors for small bowel carcinoid tumor: a European population-based case-control study. J Occup Environ Med. 2002;44:516–22.
41. Leichter SB. Clinical and metabolic aspects of glucagonoma. Medicine (Baltimore). 1980;59:100–13.
42. Feldman JM, Plonk JW, Bivens CH, Lebovitz HE. Glucose intolerance in the carcinoid syndrome. Diabetes. 1975;24:664–71.
43. Teh BT, Grimmond S, Shepherd J, Larsson C, Hayward N. Multiple endocrine neoplasia type I: clinical syndrome to molecular genetics. Aust N Z J Surg. 1995;65:708–13.
44. Wermers RA, Fatourechi V, Kvols LK. Clinical spectrum of hyperglucagonemia associated with malignant neuroendocrine tumors. Mayo Clin Proc. 1996;71:1030–8.
45. Bartsch H, Nair J. Chronic inflammation and oxidative stress in the genesis and perpetuation of cancer: role of lipid peroxidation, DNA damage, and repair. Langenbecks Arch Surg. 2006;391:499–510.
46. Ormann W. [Autoimmune hepatitis, autoimmune gastritis, hypergastrinemia and stomach carcinoid]. Dtsch Med Wochenschr. 1995;120:361–5.
47. De Block CE, De Leeuw I, Pelckmans PA, et al. Autoimmune hepatitis, autoimmune gastritis, and gastric carcinoid in a type 1 diabetic patient: a case report. J Diabetes Complications. 2000;14:116–20.
48. De Block CE, Colpin G, Thielemans K, et al. Neuroendocrine tumor markers and enterochromaffin-like cell hyper/dysplasia in type 1 diabetes. Diabetes Care. 2004;27:1387–93.
49. Modlin IM, Lye KD, Kidd M. Carcinoid tumors of the stomach. Surg Oncol. 2003;12:153–72.
50. Calender A. Molecular genetics of neuroendocrine tumors. Digestion. 2000;62 Suppl 1:3–18.
51. Mocellin S, Wang E, Marincola FM. Cytokines and immune response in the tumor microenvironment. J Immunother. 2001;24:392–407.
52. Garrelds IM, van Meeteren ME, Meijssen MA, Zijlstra FJ. Interleukin-2-deficient mice: effect on cytokines and inflammatory cells in chronic colonic disease. Dig Dis Sci. 2002;47:503–10.
53. Berkovic MC, Jokic M, Marout J, Radosevic S, Zjacic-Rotkvic V, Kapitanovic S. IL-2 −330 T/G SNP and serum values-potential new tumor markers in neuroendocrine tumors of the gastrointestinal tract and pancreas (GEP-NETs). J Mol Med. 2010;88:423–9.
54. Burnik FS, Yalcin S. NFKB1 −94 insertion/deletion ATTG polymorphism in gastroenteropancreatic neuroendocrine tumors. Chemotherapy. 2009;55:381–5.

Chapter 2
Pathology

Neda Kalhor, Saul Suster, and Cesar A. Moran

Abstract Neuroendocrine tumors are ubiquitous neoplasms that may occur anywhere in the human body. Although these tumors have been recognized for more than 100 years, a unifying concept regarding classification has been controversial, and concepts introduced a century ago are still kept in use in today's nomenclature. In addition, some of the current entities encompassed in the rubric of neuroendocrine carcinomas still require better definition and proper study. Interestingly, even though it is known that the great majority of neuroendocrine neoplasms occur in the gastrointestinal tract, most of the current concepts regarding classification and nomenclature are being driven by studies in thoracic tumors. Nevertheless, one of the issues that has been put forward to keep separate nomenclatures for these tumors in different organ systems is the supposed different clinical behavior of these neoplasms in the different systems.

The emphasis in this chapter will be the morphological approach with the idea of unifying histological criteria for the diagnosis of the spectrum of these tumors whether they are in the genitourinary, gynecological, thoracic, or gastrointestinal system. The use of ancillary methods such as immunohistochemistry or electron microscopy although important will be included as a manner to refine the diagnosis.

Keywords Carcinoid • Atypical carcinoid • Neuroendocrine carcinoma • Gastrointestinal tract • Thoracic tumors • Classification of tumors

C.A. Moran (✉)
Department of Pathology, The University of Texas M.D. Anderson Cancer Center,
1515 Holcombe Boulevard, Houston, TX 77030, USA
e-mail: cesarmoran@mdanderson.org

J.C. Yao et al. (eds.), *Neuroendocrine Tumors*, Current Clinical Oncology,
DOI 10.1007/978-1-60327-997-0_2, © Springer Science+Business Media, LLC 2011

Introduction

Neuroendocrine tumors are ubiquitous neoplasms that may occur anywhere in the human body. Although these tumors have been recognized for more than 100 years, a unifying concept regarding classification has been controversial, and concepts introduced a century ago are still kept in use in today's nomenclature. In addition, some of the current entities encompassed in the rubric of neuroendocrine carcinomas still require better definition and proper study. Interestingly, even though it is known that the great majority of neuroendocrine neoplasms occur in the gastrointestinal tract, most of the current concepts regarding classification and nomenclature are being driven by studies in thoracic tumors. Nevertheless, one of the issues that has been put forward to keep separate nomenclatures for these tumors in different organ systems is the supposed different clinical behavior of these neoplasms in the different systems. All the same, it is important to note that whether a conventional schema or a new classification is used in the definition of these tumors, it is likely that there is still going to be some controversy about the best way to classify neuroendocrine neoplasms. The most important aspect regarding this group of tumors is the fact that they should be considered neoplasms capable of local recurrence and distant metastasis. Close clinical correlation and appropriate treatment is important in order to improve survival rate in this group of patients. Because of the wide spectrum of tumors that can be categorized as "neuroendocrine," the emphasis in this chapter will be predominantly with the spectrum of epithelial neoplasms that correspond to the low, intermediate, and high-grade neuroendocrine carcinomas (so-called carcinoid, atypical carcinoid, and small and large cell neuroendocrine carcinoma). We will keep in the differential diagnosis other neuroendocrine tumors that may pose a problem in the differential diagnosis, thus contrasting when appropriate such other tumoral conditions.

As stated before, the ubiquitous distribution of these tumors in the human body is a well-known fact, and tumors with similar histological features as those seen in the gastrointestinal tract or in the thoracic area have also been described in other anatomic areas, including the male and female genitourinary system [1, 2]. Although "carcinoids" in some anatomic areas are believed to represent "benign tumors," the experience with these neoplasms in general does not reflect such consideration. Unfortunately, the use of different nomenclature and classifications has obscured the fact that "carcinoids" and "atypical carcinoids" metastasize in approximately 15% of the cases for the former while the survival rate for the latter has been estimated to be 56 and 35% at 5 and 10 years, respectively [3–18]. On the other hand, the distribution of these neoplasms is of importance as primary thymic neuroendocrine carcinomas (carcinoids), although not very common tumors representing no more than 5% of all mediastinal tumors appear to behave more aggressively in approximately 80% of the cases [19–21] while the opposite may be true for the incidental appendiceal "carcinoid tumor." In addition, depending on the anatomic location, some of these tumors may be associated with clinical conditions that may play a role in the survival of these patients. For instance, when these neoplasms occur in the mediastinal region, they may be associated with the multiple endocrine neoplasia (MEN) syndrome. Because of these clinical associations they have been the subject to numerous reports, some emphasizing clinical aspects while others emphasizing more histopathological aspects [22–76]. The diverse clinical conditions as well as classification schema for primary thymic neuroendocrine tumors have been reported in only a few large series in the literature, with the largest series comprising 80 thymic primary neuroendocrine carcinomas (carcinoid and atypical carcinoid) [77, 78]. On the contrary, similar tumors with almost identical histopathological features occurring in the gastrointestinal tract are divided differently assuming that some of them are benign. In addition, their classification involves not only the morphology of the neoplasm but also the endocrine activity of the tumor as well as the use of immunohistochemistry, namely Ki-67, which is a proliferating marker [79]. Needless to say, the emphasis in this chapter will be the morphological approach with the idea of unifying histological criteria for the diagnosis of the spectrum of these tumors whether they are in the genitourinary, gynecological, thoracic, or gastrointestinal system. The use of ancillary methods such as immunohistochemistry or electron microscopy although important will be included as a manner to refine the diagnosis.

Clinical Aspects

The clinical features of neuroendocrine tumors are wide and to some extent will depend on the anatomic area in which these tumors may be located. For instance, thymic neuroendocrine tumors are more commonly associated to the MEN, type I endocrinopathy [21], which in some authors view, may alter the prognosis of these tumors [19]. In that regard, it is possible that previous cases of thymomas associated with endocrinopathies such as Cushing's syndrome may in fact represent thymic neuroendocrine carcinomas as has been reported in other occasions [36, 38, 47, 80–82]. Nevertheless, thymic neuroendocrine carcinomas may also be associated to other conditions including polyarthropathy, proximal myopathy, and peripheral neuropathy [24]; hyperparathyroidism [30, 39]; incomplete Sipple syndrome (MEN-II) [31]; ADH secretion; Eaton–Lambert syndrome; hypertrophic osteoarthropathy [83]; secretion of ACTH [36]; and secretion of parathyroid hormone, calcitonin, beta-lipoprotein, and serotonin [84]. It has been estimated that about half of all neuroendocrine carcinomas in the thymus are functionally active or associated to MEN while about 30% are malignant on the basis of local invasion, metastasis, or both [33]. Interestingly thymic carcinoids have not been associated with myasthenia gravis, carcinoid syndrome, or hypogammaglobulinemia. On the other hand, it is exactly the concept of hormonal functionality that has been the driving force for the classification of these tumors, when they occur in the gastrointestinal tract [79].

Gross Features

Regardless of the anatomic location, these tumors may be well circumscribed or may be infiltrative including extension into adjacent organs. Those occurring primarily within the lung may have a central location, namely endobronchial location, or may be peripheral tumors. Primary pulmonary neuroendocrine tumors regardless of their histological grade may present with lymph node involvement or extra-thoracic spread. Those occurring in the gastrointestinal area may show similar features regarding well circumscription or infiltrative pattern similarly to those in the genitorurinary system. Also, the size of these tumors may vary, as some tumors may be as small as 0.5 cm in diameters while other tumors may show a larger size of more than 10 cm in greatest dimension. It is important to mention that the size of these tumors plays an important role in the current nomenclature as those tumors under 0.5 cm in diameter are coined as "carcinoid tumorlet" when they occur in the lung parenchyma. This so-called carcinoid tumorlet may be analogous to the small incidental "carcinoid tumor" found in the appendix.

At cut surface they may show a tan color with a homogeneous surface while other tumors may show areas of hemorrhage and/or necrosis. These latter features are commonly used in the grading and classification of these tumors and its presence or absence may upgrade or downgrade a particular tumor.

Histopathological Features

Neuroendocrine carcinomas (carcinoids, atypical carcinoids, small or large cell neuroendocrine carcinoma) share similar histopathological features regardless of the anatomic site (Figs. 2.1–2.3). More recently, a more expanded view of the different histopathologic growth patterns that may be observed in these tumors has been presented [85–89]. Nevertheless, the basic concept of cell morphology is applicable to these tumors regardless of the anatomic distribution. In some cases, certain growth patterns may be seen more often in some anatomic areas but in general the basic histopathology is similar.

These tumors are characterized at low magnification view by a prominent nesting and a homogenous growth pattern. The nests are separated by thin fibrocollagenous tissue while in other areas the growth pattern is that of ribbons of cells exhibiting similar cytological features. The characteristic cytology is that of small or medium size cells with moderate amounts of light eosinophilic or pale cytoplasm, round to oval nuclei, and inconspicuous nucleoli. The tumors in occasions may show a prominent oncocytic differentiation in which the tumor cells appear slightly larger than those of the conventional growth pattern. In this setting, the cells show moderate amounts of eosinophilic cytoplasm and the nuclei appears to be more prominent. However, the nucleoli are still inconspicuous. Tumors with prominent spindle cell features also may be seen and in these cases the cells adopt a fusiform shape mimicking a mesenchymal tumor. In some cases, melanin pigment may be observed

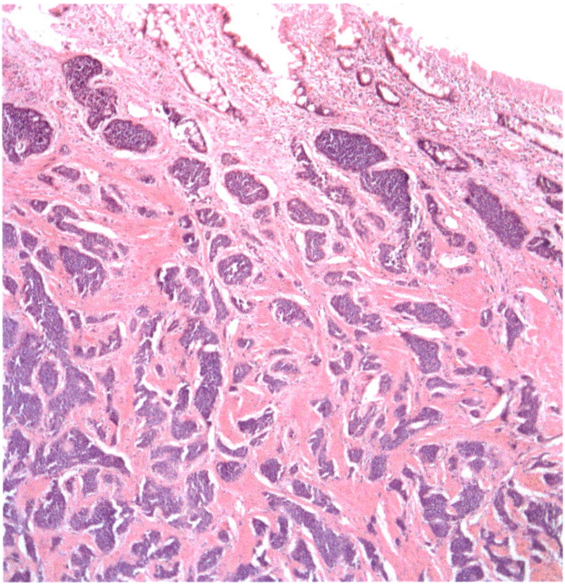

Fig. 2.1 Well-differentiated neuroendocrine carcinoma (low grade, Grade I) involving the colonic mucosa. Note the well-organized nesting pattern

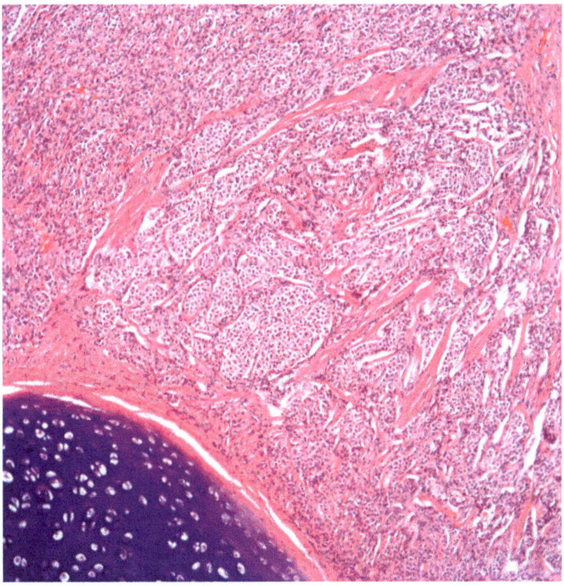

Fig. 2.2 Similar type of tumor involving the lung. Once again, note the well-organized nested pattern. A portion of the bronchial cartilage is also present

in any of the growth patterns and these tumors are regarded as pigmented neuroendocrine carcinomas (carcinoids). In very unusual circumstances, the tumor may display a characteristic angiectatic growth pattern similar to that observed in vascular tumors. In these tumors, the presence of large ectatic areas filled with red cells may

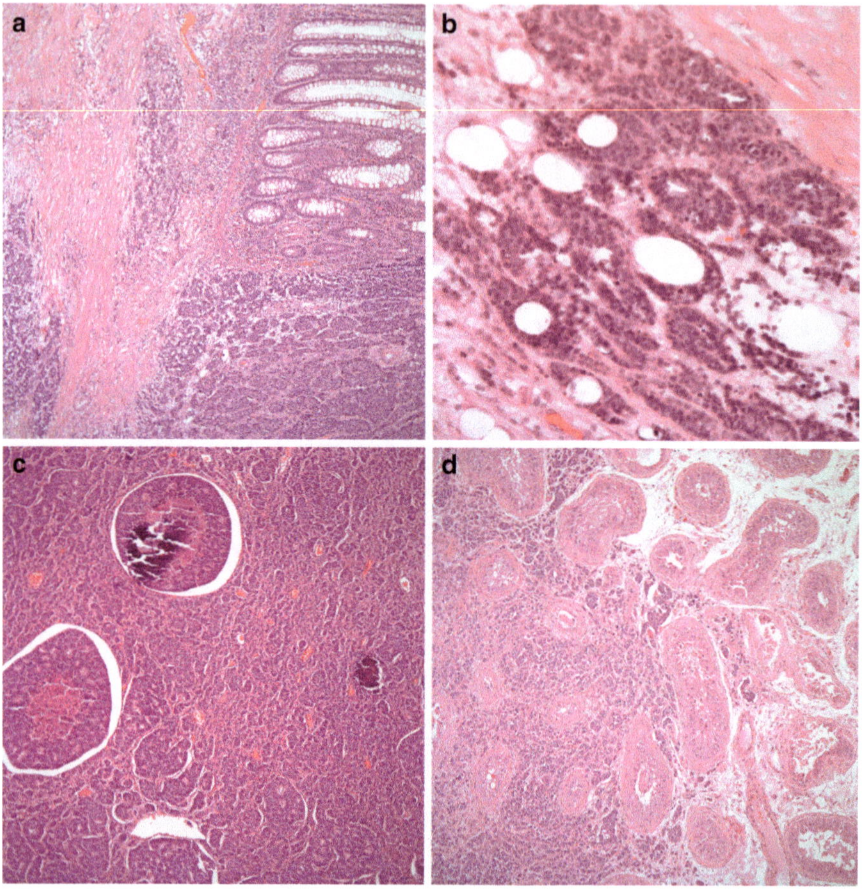

Fig. 2.3 Moderately differentiated neuroendocrine carcinoma (intermediate grade, Grade II) displaying similar characteristics in different anatomic areas. (**a**) Moderately differentiated neuroendocrine carcinoma involving the mucosa and muscular layer of the colon; (**b**) same tumor infiltrating deeply and involving the serosa and adipose tissue; (**c**) similar tumor in the mediastinal compartment showing the classical come-like necrosis; (**d**) similar tumor involving the testis, note the presence of seminiferous tubules

be confused with a vascular tumor. However, the areas in which these ectatic areas are seen show the typical cytological features of a neuroendocrine tumor. Also important to note is the presence of tumors in which the neoplastic cells are embedded in an acellular eosinophilic amyloid-like stroma. Tumors showing this type of growth pattern may be confused with tumors of different origin such as thyroid medullary carcinoma.

Other unusual variants that are important to be recognized include mucinous neuroendocrine carcinoma (carcinoid) [90], signet ring cell, goblet cell (Figs. 2.4 and 2.5), and tumors that share combined features of low- and high-grade differentiation [85]. In the mucinous variant, the tumor cells may be scant and embedded in

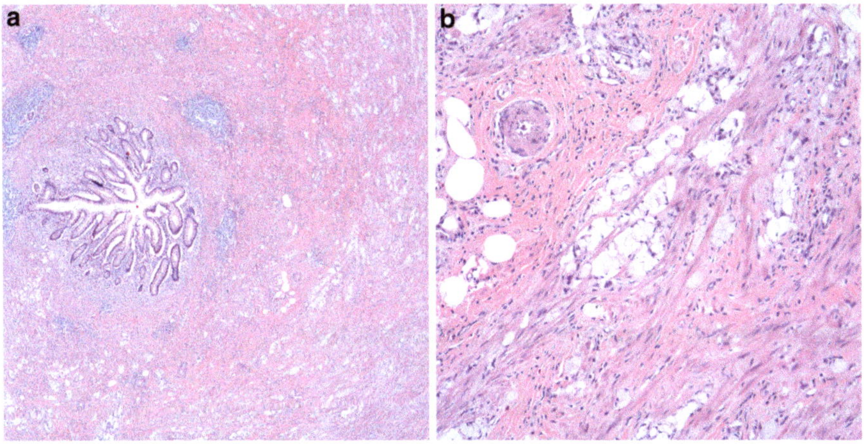

Fig. 2.4 (**a**) So-called Goblet cell carcinoid tumor involving the appendix; (**b**) higher magnification showing the presence of "goblet-like cells" splitting fibromuscular fibers

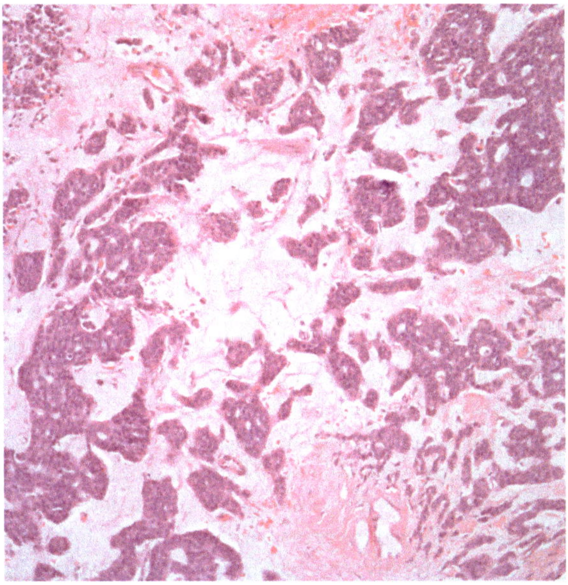

Fig. 2.5 Mediastinal mucinous neuroendocrine carcinoma, note the presence of clusters of neoplastic cells embedded in a mucinous stroma. This type of tumors is more commonly seen in the gastrointestinal area

large pools of mucin, which may be confused with a primary mucinous adenocarcinoma. Similar problem may arise when the morphology of the tumor is that of goblet cells or signet ring cells in which the tumor may be confused with a conventional adenocarcinoma. On the other hand, there are some tumors that may show alternating areas of conventional "carcinoid" admixed with other areas more in keeping with conventional "small cell carcinoma." It is important to keep these histopathological growth patterns in mind, namely in the setting of limited mediastinoscopic biopsies.

In this context, it is also important to mention that neuroendocrine carcinomas (carcinoids) may also be associated or admixed with other neoplasms such as thymic carcinoma or mesenchymal tumors [60, 90].

Since most of these histopathological growth patterns are recognized in complete surgical resection, a practical approach to the diagnosis of these tumors has been put forward when dealing with small limited biopsy material [91]. Although not a complete full proof schema, it provides important information for the treating physician to outline a treatment approach.

Immunohistochemistry and Ultrastructure

In general, the use of neuroendocrine markers including chromogranin, synaptophysin, and Leu-7 are important markers in the evaluation of neuroendocrine neoplasms. More recently, a study of 40 cases of primary thymic neuroendocrine carcinomas [76] using a panel of antibodies including CAM 5.2 low molecular weight keratin, broad spectrum keratin cocktail, chromogranin, synaptophysin, and Leu-7 was performed showing strong positive reaction for CAM 5.2 in all cases while broad-spectrum keratin was positive in approximately 88% of the cases studied. Of the neuroendocrine markers tested, chromogranin was seen positive in 75%; synaptophysin in 73%, and Leu-7 in 68%. In only 60% of the cases a dual staining with chromogranin and synaptophysin was observed. Interestingly, in our experience, p53 was seen only focally positive in less than 5% of the cases studied. More recently, a new antibody CD56 has become available as a new neuroendocrine marker. This panel of immunohistochemical markers is commonly used for the diagnostic evaluation of neuroendocrine carcinomas. Nevertheless, when these tumors occur in the gastrointestinal tract, other immunohistochemical antibodies directed against hormonal antigens are also used. In addition, in gastrointestinal tumors, the use of Ki-67 has been used to measure the proliferating index of these tumors. Assessments of more than or less than 2% have been drawn to determine whether the tumor is benign or of low-grade malignancy. Interestingly, it is not clear whether that 2% is assessed in a biopsy material or in a resected tumor. Obviously, that percentage will fluctuate depending on the size of the material studied. Also of questionable value will be the use of a proliferative marker Ki-67 in a resected specimen in which the pathologist is able to determine the presence of mitotic activity, nuclear atypia, and the presence of necrosis by light microscopy alone.

Ultrastructurally, the finding of neurosecretory granules in tumor cells is the most important feature. However, the presence of neurosecretory granules is more readily seen in better-differentiated neoplasms.

Classification

Since the original description by Oberndorfer and Frankfurt [92] of carcinoid tumor, there have been numerous attempts to correlate specific features of these tumors with clinical behavior, which in due process have given rise to the several classification schemas presented over the last decades. Although none of those schemas has been universally accepted, numerous important contributions to our understanding of these tumors have been presented. For instance, the introduction of the term "atypical carcinoid" by Arrigoni et al. [8] who separated tumors which today are considered to behave more aggressively than the conventional "carcinoid tumor." However, it is important to recognize that because of this terminology, some authors have considered that the conventional "carcinoid tumor" represents a benign neoplasm. Other authors have advanced the field by highlighting the necessity for a more expanded classification system. This expanded view of neuroendocrine tumor has generated some gain but also some confusion as the histopathological evaluation of these tumors has been joined with the immunohistochemical results; thus, the reluctance of some authors to completely endorse those schemas. Nevertheless, important issues including recognition of the Kultchistky cell as the origin of these tumors, expanding the classification system from three to four different categories, and proposing that these tumors are part of a spectrum of differentiation ranging from low- to high-grade neoplasms are among the important gains and contributions to our understanding of these tumors [3–18]. However, each one of those systems has brought some controversy. Table 2.1 depicts the conventional, modern/practical, and World Health Organization (WHO) histopathological classification of neuroendocrine tumors [93]. However, it is important to also note that the American Joint Committee on Cancer (AJCC) [94] also has established a staging system for these tumors, which for the most part uses the conventional TNM. That system applies mainly to tumors of the gastrointestinal tract and also subdivides tumors into well-differentiated neuroendocrine tumor and well-differentiated neuroendocrine carcinoma, making an exact correlation with other nomenclatures difficult. In addition, it is important to note that even in the last publication of the WHO for thoracic tumors, which includes lung and mediastinum, there is still some inconsistency in the approach for primary lung tumors as opposed to mediastinal neoplasms. While mediastinal tumors that have been proved to be more aggressive depending on their histological grade, according to the WHO, these tumors are separated into well and poorly differentiated tumors. On the contrary, similar pulmonary tumors that are considered less aggressive than their mediastinal counterparts are separated into four different categories. Needless to say, this very exact issue denotes the obscurity that different authors and classifications systems have embedded in the literature. On the other hand, there are some other issues that remain unsolved, such as the diagnostic criteria for the so-called large cell neuroendocrine carcinoma. The diagnostic criteria for the latter tumor does not depend on light microscopic diagnosis but one that requires positive immunohistochemical neuroendocrine markers or presence of neurosecretory granules by electron microscopy in addition to the "neuroendocrine pattern." As currently defined, the diagnosis cannot be made on a small biopsy due to the possible lack of "neuroendocrine pattern." Additionally, any given nonsmall cell carcinoma may show neuroendocrine differentiation by immunohistochemistry, thus, creating a problem on when to separate large cell neuroendocrine carcinoma from the nonsmall cell carcinoma with neuroendocrine differentiation. Furthermore, the controversy deepens when one encounters a tumor that has a "reasonable neuroendocrine pattern" but yet the

Table 2.1 Different classifications schemas for neuroendocrine carcinomas

Conventional	Moran and Suster	WHO (thymus)	WHO (lung)	WHO (gastrointestinal)
Carcinoid tumor	Low grade neuroendocrine Ca	Well-differentiated neuroendocrine Ca	Carcinoid	Well-differentiated tumor
Atypical carcinoid	Intermediate grade neuroendocrine Ca	Well-differentiated neuroendocrine Ca	Atypical carcinoid	Well-differentiated neuroendocrine Ca
Small cell carcinoma	High grade neuroendocrine Ca[a] Small cell type	Poorly differentiated neuroendocrine Ca	Small cell carcinoma	Poorly differentiated neuroendocrine Ca
	High grade neuroendocrine Ca[a] Large cell type	Poorly differentiated neuroendocrine Ca	Large cell neuroendocrine Ca	Poorly differentiated neuroendocrine Ca

[a] In the Moran and Suster approach both small and large cell neuroendocrine carcinomas belong to the high-grade category

immunohistochemical neuroendocrine markers are negative. Then the diagnosis of large cell neuroendocrine carcinoma (LCNECa) cannot be made, leaving the diagnosis of large cell carcinoma with neuroendocrine pattern. In this regard, the pathologist is left with three possibilities to assess such problem:

- *Large Cell Neuroendocrine Carcinoma*: neuroendocrine pattern plus positive neuroendocrine markers.
- *Large Cell Carcinoma with Neuroendocrine Pattern*: neuroendocrine pattern is present but immunohistochemical markers are negative.
- *Large Cell Carcinoma with Neuroendocrine differentiation*: positive neuroendocrine markers by immunohistochemistry in a tumor that does not show neuroendocrine histological growth pattern.

Although histologically speaking thoracic neuroendocrine carcinomas are similar to those seen in other areas such as the gastrointestinal tract, great care must be exercised in their classification since the prognosis for these tumors in the thymus appears to be different than those in the lung or gastrointestinal tract. Thus, a modified approach and nomenclature of these tumors when they occur in the thymus has been argued [76, 77] following the notion already presented by others [61, 82] that these tumors represent a spectrum of differentiation. In addition, we currently use similar histological criteria for those tumors occurring in the lung parenchyma [95], and consider that similar histopathological approach should also be extended to similar tumors regardless of their anatomic location. Nevertheless, it must be understood that the classification scheme takes into account not only the presence of necrosis, cellular atypia, and mitotic count but also takes into account that in order to provide a more precise classification, a surgical resection of the tumor must take place. The use of this classification based on limited biopsies may prove limited.

The working schema that has been proposed in the evaluation of neuroendocrine carcinomas is as follows:

Biopsy Material

- Low or intermediate grade neuroendocrine carcinoma – for those tumors that follow in the range of low or intermediate grade tumors (carcinoid or atypical carcinoid) and the tumor is more than 5 mm in greatest diameter (the pathologist must specify the possibilities of this diagnosis).
- Small cell carcinoma.
- Other types of conventional carcinomas, nonneuroendocrine or possibly a large cell neuroendocrine carcinoma.

Surgical Resections

1. Well-differentiated (low grade, Grade I) neuroendocrine carcinoma (conventional carcinoid)
    - Mild cellular atypia
    - 0–3 mitotic figures/10 hpf
    - Small focus of punctuate comedonecrosis may be allowed

2. Moderately differentiated (intermediate grade, Grade II) neuroendocrine carcinoma (atypical carcinoid)
   - Moderate cellular atypia
   - 4–10 mitotic figures/10 hpf
   - More extensive foci of necrosis
3. Poorly differentiated (high grade, Grade III) neuroendocrine carcinoma (small cell carcinoma or large cell neuroendocrine carcinoma – because of the restricted diagnostic parameters imposed on the diagnosis of large cell neuroendocrine carcinoma, it has been considered that such designation may be given for those tumor that show the conventional light microscopic features with or without positive immunohistochemical markers.)
   - Severe or prominent cellular atypia
   - More than 10 mitotic figures/10 hpf
   - Extensive areas of necrosis

It is important to note that some of these tumors may show overlap of features and mix histologies [66]. Therefore, careful interpretation of the different histological grades is necessary.

Differential Diagnosis

The most important consideration regarding primary neuroendocrine carcinomas is to establish the site of origin. Since all these tumors share similar histopathological features, the diagnosis of primary tumor will depend largely on clinical evaluation and proper exclusion of the most common sites, i.e., gastrointestinal and lung. In this particular setting, the use of TTF-1 and CDX2 immunohistochemical studies may provide help as tumors of lung origin will likely express TTF-1 and not CDX2 while those of gastrointestinal origin would do the opposite. Other tumors that may be easily confused with neuroendocrine carcinomas include paragangliomas and/or ectopic parathyroid adenoma. Both of these tumors may pose considerable difficulty since both tumors are by definition neuroendocrine in nature. In paragangliomas, the histopathologic characteristic is that these tumors will show a similar growth pattern as neuroendocrine carcinomas. However, they are also characterized by the presence of large "megalic" cell with bizarre forms and shapes but very few mitotic figures if any. In addition, paragangliomas will display negative staining for keratin while neuroendocrine carcinomas show for the most part positive staining [96]. In cases of ectopic parathyroid adenomas, the presence of prominent clear cells (chief cells) admixed with oncocytic cells may lead in the correct interpretation. In addition, the use of periodic acid-Schiff to determine the presence of glycogen and the use of immunohistochemical studies for parathyroid hormone will also be helpful in this setting. In the gastrointestinal tract, one other tumor that may pose a problem in diagnosis mainly with limited biopsy material is glomus tumor. However, the use of immunohistochemical studies will show glomus tumor positive for smooth muscle actin and negative for neuroendocrine markers, leading to a more accurate interpretation.

Prognosis

Based on our experience, we consider that the prognosis of neuroendocrine tumors is linked to the size of the tumor, degree of differentiation, and proliferative activity [76]. For instance, in tumors occurring in the thymus and showing better-differentiated features, it is expected that the survival rate be around 50% at 5 years; those showing moderately differentiated features 20% at 5 years; and those showing poorly differentiated features 0% at 5 years. On the other hand, "carcinoid" of lung origin has 15% rate of lymph node metastasis and 90% 5-year survival, while the rates for "atypical carcinoid" are 25 and 56%, respectively [16]. Therefore, we consider that every attempt should be made to properly classify these tumors according to the degree of differentiation and extent of infiltration. However, it is also important to mention that those tumors that have been coined as "carcinoid tumorlets," which by definition measure less than 5 mm in diameter, may observe a much better survival rate of possible 100% at 5 years. Similar analogy may be seen with the incidental microscopic "carcinoid tumor" of the appendix.

Conclusion

It has been more 100 years since the term "carcinoid" was introduced in the literature [92] in order to separate a group of tumors in the small intestine that behave better than conventional carcinomas. Currently, similar tumors have also been described in other anatomic areas and in some of them time has proven that the behavior is not necessarily of a benign tumor. Thus, we have proposed to abandon the term "carcinoid" for a more appropriate term, neuroendocrine carcinoma. It is hoped that by providing this "more meaningful" approach, more research can be done in terms of better therapeutic panels to improve the life expectancy of these patients. We also consider that the term neuroendocrine carcinoma with their different grades of differentiation denotes the spectrum of differentiation that these tumors may show.

References

1. Conner MG, Richter H, Moran CA, et al. Small cell carcinoma of the cervix: a clinicopathologic and immunohistochemical study of 23 cases. Ann Diagn Pathol. 2002;6(6):345–8.
2. Reyes A, Moran CA, Suster S, et al. Neuroendocrine carcinomas (carcinoid tumor) of the testis: a clinicopathologic and immunohistochemical study of 10 cases. Am J Clin Pathol. 2003;120(2):182–7.
3. Reyes A, Moran CA. Low-grade neuroendocrine carcinoma (carcinoid) of the prostate. Arch Pathol Lab Med. 2004;128(12):166–8.
4. Gosset A, Masson P. Tumeurs endocrines de l'appendice. Presse Med. 1914;22:37–40.
5. Goodner JT, Berg JW, Watson WL. The non-benign nature of bronchial carcinoids and cylindromas. Cancer. 1961;14:539–45.

6. Markel SE, Abell MR, Haight C, et al. Neoplasms of bronchus commonly designated as adenomas. Cancer. 1964;17:590–605.
7. Smith RA. Bronchial carcinoid tumors. Thorax. 1969;24:43–7.
8. Arrigoni MG, Woolner LB, Bernatz PE. Atypical carcinoid tumors of the lung. J Thorac Cardiovasc Surg. 1972;64:413–21.
9. Mills SE, Walker AN, Cooper PH, et al. Atypical carcinoid tumor of the lung: a clinicopathologic study of 17 cases. Am J Surg Pathol. 1982;6:643–54.
10. Gould VE, Linnoila RI, Memoli VA, et al. Neuroendocrine cells and neuroendocrine neoplasms of the lung. Pathol Annu. 1983;18:287–330.
11. Warren WH, Gould VE, Faber PL, et al. Neuroendocrine neoplasms of the bronchopulmonary tract. J Thorac Cardiovasc Surg. 1985;89:819–25.
12. Paladugu RR, Benfield JR, Pak HY, et al. Bronchopulmonary Kultchitsky cell carcinoma: a new classification scheme for typical and atypical carcinoids. Cancer. 1985;55:1303–11.
13. Grote TH, Macon WR, Davis B, et al. Atypical carcinoid of the lung: a distinct clinicopathologic entity. Chest. 1988;93:370–5.
14. Valli M, Fabris GA, Dewart A, et al. Atypical carcinoid tumour of the lung: a study of 33 cases with prognostic features. Histopathology. 1994;24:363–9.
15. Dressler CM, Ritter JH, Patterson GA, Wick M. Clinical-pathologic analysis of 40 patients with large cell neuroendocrine carcinoma of the lung. Ann Thorac Surg. 1997;63:180–5.
16. Travis WD, Rush W, Flieder DB, et al. Survival analysis of 200 pulmonary neuroendocrine tumors with classification of criteria of atypical carcinoid and its separation from typical carcinoid. Am J Surg Pathol. 1998;22:934–44.
17. Huang Q, Muzitansky A, Mark EJ. Pulmonary neuroendocrine carcinomas: a review of 234 cases and a statistical analysis of 50 cases treated at one institution using a simple clinicopathologic classification. Arch Pathol Lab Med. 2002;126:545–53.
18. Schreurs JM, Westermann JJ, van den Bosch JMM, et al. A twenty-five year follow-up of ninety-three resected typical carcinoid tumors of the lung. J Thorac Cardiovasc Surg. 1992;104:1470–5.
19. Duh QY, Hybarger CP, Geist R, Gamsu G, Goodman PC, Gooding GAW, et al. Carcinoids associated with multiple endocrine neoplasia syndromes. Am J Surg. 1987;154:142–8.
20. Rosai J, Higa E. Mediastinal endocrine neoplasm of probable thymic origin related to carcinoid tumor. Cancer. 1972;29:1061–74.
21. Rosai J, Higa E, Davie J. Mediastinal endocrine neoplasm in patients with multiple endocrine adenomatosis: a previously unrecognized association. Cancer. 1972;29:1075–83.
22. Manes JL, Taylor HB. Thymic carcinoid in familial multiple endocrine adenomatosis. Arch Pathol. 1973;95:252–5.
23. Tanaka T, Tanaka S, Kimura H, Ito J. Mediastinal tumor of thymic origin and related to carcinoid tumor. Acta Pathol Jpn. 1974;24:413–26.
24. Lowenthal RM, Gumpel JM, Kreel L, McLaughlin JE, Skeggs BL. Carcinoid tumour of the thymus with systemic manifestations: a radiological and pathological study. Thorax. 1974;92:553–8.
25. Hughes JP, Ancalmo N, Leonard GL, Ochsner JL. Carcinoid tumour of the thymus gland: report of a case. Thorax. 1975;30:470–5.
26. Sundstrom C, Wilander E. Thymic carcinoid: a case report. Acta Pathol Microbiol Scand. 1976;84:311–6.
27. DeLellis RA, Wolfe HJ. Calcitonin in spindle cell thymic carcinoid tumors. Arch Pathol Lab Med. 1976;100:340.
28. Chalk S, Donald KJ. Carcinoid tumour of the thymus. Virchows Arch A. 1977;377:91–6.
29. Ho FCS, Ho JCI. Pigmented carcinoid tumour of the thymus. Histopathology. 1977;I:363–9.
30. Lokich JJ, Li F. Carcinoid of the thymus with hereditary hyperparathyroidism. Ann Intern Med. 1978;89:364–5.
31. Marchevsky AM, Dikman SH. Mediastinal carcinoid with an incomplete Sipple's syndrome. Cancer. 1979;43:2497–501.
32. Stewart CA, Kingston CW. Carcinoid tumour of the thymus with Cushing's syndrome. Pathology. 1980;12:487–94.

33. Wick MR, Scott RE, Li YC, Carney JA. Carcinoid tumor of the thymus: a clinicopathologic report of seven cases with a review of the literature. Mayo Clin Proc. 1980;55:246–54.
34. Gelfand ET, Basualdo CA, Callaghan JC. Carcinoid tumor of the thymus associated with recurrent pericarditis. Chest. 1981;79:350–1.
35. Floros D, Dosios T, Tsourdis A, Yiatromanolakis N. Carcinoid tumor of the thymus with multiple endocrine adenomatosis. Pathol Res Pract. 1982;175:404–9.
36. Brown LR, Aughenbaugh GL, Wick MR, Baker BA, Salassa RM. Roentgenologic diagnosis of primary corticotropin-producing carcinoid tumors of the mediastinum. Radiology. 1982;142:143–8.
37. Fetissof F, Boivin F. Microfilamentous carcinoid of the thymus: correlation of ultrastructural study with Grimelius stain. Ultrastruct Pathol. 1982;3:9–15.
38. Thorner MO, Martin WH, Ragan GE, MacLeod RM, Feldman PS, Bruni C, et al. A case of ectopic ACTH syndrome: diagnostic difficulties caused by intermittent secretion. Acta Endocrinol. 1982;99:364–70.
39. Birnberg FA, Webb WR, Selch MT, Gamsu G, Goodman PC. Thymic carcinoid tumors with hyperparathyroidism. Am J Radiol. 1982;139:1001–4.
40. Vener JD, Zuckerbraun L, Goodman D. Carcinoid tumor of the thymus associated with a parathyroid adenoma. Arch Otolaryngol. 1982;108:324–6.
41. Blom P, Johannessen JV. Mediastinal mass in a young man. Ultrastruct Pathol. 1983;4:391–5.
42. Miettinen M, Partanen S, Lehto VP, Virtanen I. Mediastinal tumors: ultrastructural and immunohistochemical evaluation of intermediate filaments as diagnostic aids. Ultrastruct Pathol. 1983;4:337–47.
43. Wick MR, Scheithauer BW, Kovacs K. Neuron-specific enolase in neuroendocrine tumors of the thymus, bronchus, and skin. Am J Clin Pathol. 1983;79:703–7.
44. Adkins RB, Maples MD, Haisworth JD. Primary malignant mediastinal tumors. Ann Thorac Surg. 1984;38:648–59.
45. Kogan J. Carcinoid tumor of the thymus. Postgrad Med. 1984;75:291–6.
46. Wick MR, Scheithauer BW. Thymic carcinoid. Cancer. 1984;53:475–84.
47. Huntrakoon M, Lin F, Heitz PU, Tomita T. Thymic carcinoid tumor with Cushing's syndrome: report of a case with electron microscopic and immunoperoxidase studies for neuron-specific enolase and corticotropin. Arch Pathol Lab Med. 1984;108:551–4.
48. Lieske TR, Kincaid J, Sunderrajan JV. Thymic carcinoid with cutaneous hyperpigmentation. Arch Intern Med. 1985;145:361–3.
49. Otto HF. Letters to the case. Pathol Res Pract. 1985;180:448–9.
50. Herbst WM, Kummer W, Hofmann W, Otto H, Heym C. Carcinoid tumors of the thymus: an immunohistochemical study. Cancer. 1987;60:2465–70.
51. Lagrange W, Dham HH, Karstens J, Feichtinger J, Mittermayer C. Melanocytic neuroendocrine carcinoma of the thymus. Cancer. 1987;59:484–8.
52. Economopoulos GC, Lewis JW, Lee MW, Silverman NA. Carcinoid tumors of the thymus. Ann Thorac Surg. 1990;50:58–61.
53. Steen RE, Kapelrud H, Haug E, Frey H. In vivo and in vitro inhibition by ketoconazole of ACTH secretion from a human thymic carcinoid tumour. Acta Endocrinol. 1991;125:331–4.
54. Paties C, Zangrandi A, Vasallo G, Rindi G, Solcia E. Multidirectional carcinoma of the thymus with neuroendocrine and sarcomatoid components and carcinoid syndrome. Pathol Res Pract. 1991;187:170–7.
55. Miura K, Sasaki C, Katsushima I, Ohtomo T, Sato S, Demura H, et al. Pituitary-adrenocortical studies in a patient with Cushing's syndrome induced by thymoma. J Clin Endocrinol Metab. 1967;27:631–7.
56. Gartner LA, Voorhess ML. Adrenocorticotropin hormone-producing thymic carcinoid in a teenager. Cancer. 1993;71:106–11.
57. Valli M, Fabris GA, Dewar A, Chikte S, Fisher C, Corrin B, et al. Atypical carcinoid tumour of the thymus: a study of eight cases. Histopathology. 1994;24:371–5.
58. Wang DY, Chang DB, Kuo SH, Yang PC, Lee YC, Hsu HC, et al. Carcinoid tumours of the thymus. Thorax. 1994;49:357–60.

59. Llaverias S, Valls C, Picas E. Carcinoid tumor of the thymus. Am J Roentgenol. 1994;163:478.
60. Kuo TT. Carcinoid tumor of the thymus with divergent sarcomatoid differentiation: report of a case with histogenetic consideration. Hum Pathol. 1994;25:319–23.
61. Montpreville VT, Macchiarini P, Dulmet E. Thymic neuroendocrine carcinoma (carcinoid): a clinicopathologic study of fourteen cases. J Thorac Cardiovasc Surg. 1996;111:134–41.
62. Kimura N, Ishikawa T, Sasaki Y, Sasano N, Onodera K, Shimizu Y, et al. Expression of prohormone convertase, PC2, in adrenocorticotropin-producing thymic carcinoid with elevated plasma corticotropin-releasing hormone. J Clin Endrocrinol Metab. 1996;81:390–5.
63. Rao U, Takita H. Carcinoid tumour of possible thymic origin: a case report. Thorax. 1977;32:771–6.
64. Salyer WR, Salyer DC, Eggleston JC. Carcinoid tumors of the thymus. Cancer. 1976;37:958–73.
65. Fishman ML, Rosenthal S. Optic nerve metastasis from a mediastinal carcinoid tumour. Br J Ophthalmol. 1976;60:583–8.
66. Wick MR, Carney JA, Bernatz PE, Brown LR. Primary mediastinal carcinoid tumors. Am J Surg Pathol. 1982;6:195–205.
67. Baker J, Holdaway IM, Jagush M, Kerr AR, Donald RA, Pullan PT. Ectopic secretion of ACTH and met-enkephalin from a thymic carcinoid. J Endocrinol Invest. 1982;5:33–8.
68. Yamaji I, Iimura O, Mito T, Yoshida S, Shimamoto K, Minase T. An ectopic ACTH producing oncocytic carcinoid tumor of the thymus: report of a case. Jpn J Med. 1984;23:62–6.
69. Loon G, Schiby G, Milo S. Lesions of the thymus. A study of 53 cases. Isr J Med Sci. 1980;16:433–9.
70. Asbun HJ, Calabria RP, Calmes S, Lang AG, Bloch JH. Thymic carcinoid. Am Surg. 1991;57:442–5.
71. Zeiger MA, Swartz SE, MacGillivray DC, Linnoila I, Shakir M. Thymic carcinoid in association with MEN syndromes. Am Surg. 1992;58:430–4.
72. Wollensak G, Herbst EW, Beck A, Schaefer HE. Primary thymic carcinoid with Cushing's syndrome. Virchows Arch A Pathol Anat. 1992;420:191–5.
73. John LC, Hornick P, Lang S, Wallis J, Edmonson SJ. Giant thymic carcinoid. Postgrad Med. 1991;67:462–5.
74. Dusmet ME, McKneally MF. Pulmonary and thymic carcinoid tumors. World J Surg. 1996;20:189–95.
75. Zahner J, Borchard F, Schmitz U, Scheneider W. Thymus carcinoid in multiple endocrine neoplasms type I. Dtsch Med Wochenschr. 1994;119:135–40.
76. Moran CA, Suster S. Neuroendocrine carcinomas (carcinoid tumor) of the thymus: a clinicopathological analysis of 80 cases. Am J Clin Pathol. 2000;113(1):100–10.
77. Klemm KM, Moran CA. Primary neuroendocrine carcinomas of the thymus. Semin Diagn Pathol. 1999;16:32–41.
78. Kay S, Willson MA. Ultrastructural studies of an ACTH-secreting thymic tumor. Cancer. 1970;26:445–52.
79. Kloppel G, Perren A, Heitz PU. The gastroenteropancreatic neuroendocrine cell system and its tumors. The WHO classification. Ann N Y Acad Sci. 2004;1014:13–27.
80. Duguid JB, Kennedy AM. Oat-cell tumours of mediastinal glands. J Pathol. 1932;23:93–9.
81. Pimstone BL, Uys CJ, Vogelpoel L. Studies in a case of Cushing's syndrome due to an ACTH-producing thymic tumour. Am J Med. 1972;53:521–8.
82. Wick MR, Rosai J. Neuroendocrine neoplasms of the thymus. Pathol Res Pract. 1988;183:188–99.
83. Viebahn R, Hiddemann W, Klinke F, Bassewitz DB. Thymus carcinoid. Pathol Res Pract. 1985;180:445–8.
84. Moran CA, Suster S. Thymic neuroendocrine carcinomas with combined features ranging from well-differentiated (carcinoid) to small cell carcinoma. Am J Clin Pathol. 2000;113:345–50.
85. Moran CA, Suster S. Spindle cell neuroendocrine carcinomas of the thymus (spindle-cell thymic carcinoid): a clinicopathologic and immunohistochemical study of seven cases. Mod Pathol. 1999;12:587–91.

86. Moran CA, Suster S. Angiomatoid neuroendocrine carcinoma of the thymus: report of a distinctive morphological variant of neuroendocrine tumor of the thymus resembling a vascular neoplasm. Hum Pathol. 1999;30:635–9.
87. Moran CA, Suster S. Primary neuroendocrine Carcinoma (thymic carcinoid) of the thymus with prominent oncocytic features: a clinicopathological study of 22 cases. Mod Pathol. 2000;13(5):489–94.
88. Klemm KM, Moran CA, Suster S. Pigmented thymic carcinoids: a clinicopathological and immunohistochemical study of two cases. Mod Pathol. 1999;12:946–8.
89. Suster S, Moran CA. Thymic carcinoid with prominent mucinous stroma: report of a distinctive morphologic variant of thymic neuroendocrine neoplasm. Am J Surg Pathol. 1995;19:1277–85.
90. Sensaki K, Aida S, Takagi K, Shibata H, Ogata T, Tanaka S, et al. Coexisting undifferentiated thymic carcinoma and thymic carcinoid tumor. Respiration. 1993;60:247–9.
91. Moran CA, Suster S, Coppola D, Wick MR. Neuroendocrine carcinomas of the lung: a critical review. Am J Clin Pathol. 2009;131:206–21.
92. Oberndorfer S, Frankfurt Z. Karzinoide tumoren des Duenndarms. Pathology. 1907;1:426–30.
93. Travis WD, Brambilla E, Muller-Hermelink K, Harris CC, editors. World Health Organization (WHO). Pathology and genetics of tumours of the lung, pleura, thymus, and heart. Lyon: IARC Press; 2004.
94. American Joint Committee on Cancer (AJCC). AJCC cancer staging manual. Neuroendocrine tumors. 7th ed. New York: Springer; 2010. p. 181–5.
95. Moran CA, Suster S. Tumors of the lung/pleura. In: Fletcher CD, editor. Diagnostic histopathology of tumors. 2nd ed. Philadelphia: Churchill Livingstone; 2000.
96. Moran CA, Suster S, Fishback N, Koss MN. Mediastinal paragangliomas: a clinicopathologic and immunohistochemical study of 16 cases. Cancer. 1993;72:2358–64.

Chapter 3
Multiple Endocrine Neoplasia

Christine S. Landry, Thereasa Rich, Camilo Jimenez, Elizabeth G. Grubbs, Jeffrey E. Lee, and Nancy D. Perrier

Abstract The term "multiple endocrine neoplasia" was first used by Steiner in the late 1960s when he described three distinct endocrine disorders. The first disorder, multiple endocrine neoplasia type I (MEN 1) (also known as Wermer syndrome), described patients with familial pituitary, parathyroid, and pancreatic islet cell tumors. The second syndrome, multiple endocrine neoplasia type II (MEN 2) (also known as Sipple syndrome), was associated with familial pheochromocytomas, medullary thyroid carcinoma (MTC), and hyperparathyroidism. The third syndrome, called multiple endocrine neoplasia type III (MEN 3), included patients with papillary thyroid carcinomas and nonfamilial parathyroid tumors.

Today, the term "multiple endocrine neoplasia" refers to three autosomal dominant disorders: MEN 1, MEN 2A, and MEN 2B. In addition, the most recent guidelines from the American Thyroid Association (ATA) in 2009 concluded that familial medullary thyroid carcinoma (FMTC) should be considered a subset of MEN 2A. This chapter discusses the clinical manifestations, diagnosis, genetic testing, treatments, and prognosis of each syndrome.

Keywords Pancreatic islet cell tumors • Wermer syndrome • Sipple syndrome • Pheochromocytoma • Medullary thyroid carcinoma • Hyperparathyroidism • Pancreatic neuroendocrine tumor • Pituitary adenoma • MEN 1 • MEN 2A • MEN 2B

Introduction

In 1903, Jacob Erdheim described one of the first accounts of a patient with two endocrine tumors: a pituitary and a parathyroid tumor [1]. Over the next 70 years, the contributions of multiple case reports led to the description of various familial

N.D. Perrier (✉)
Department of Surgical Oncology, Section of Surgical Endocrinology,
The University of Texas M.D. Anderson Cancer Center, Houston, TX, USA
e-mail: nperrier@mdanderson.org

J.C. Yao et al. (eds.), *Neuroendocrine Tumors*, Current Clinical Oncology,
DOI 10.1007/978-1-60327-997-0_3, © Springer Science+Business Media, LLC 2011

endocrine syndromes. In 1954, Paul Wermer, an internist at Columbia University, recognized the autosomal dominant transmission of a syndrome initially described by Underdahl in 1953 [1, 2]. This disorder, referred to as Wermer syndrome, was characterized by adenomas of the anterior pituitary gland, parathyroid gland, and islet cells of the pancreas. Similarly, in 1962 John Sipple, a pulmonologist at the State University of New York Upstate Medical Center in Syracuse, reported an association with carcinoma of the thyroid gland and pheochromocytoma, later referred to as Sipple syndrome [1].

The term "multiple endocrine neoplasia" was first used by Steiner in the late 1960s when he described three distinct endocrine disorders [1]. The first disorder, multiple endocrine neoplasia type I (MEN 1) (also known as Wermer syndrome), described patients with familial pituitary, parathyroid, and pancreatic islet cell tumors [1]. The second syndrome, multiple endocrine neoplasia type II (MEN 2) (also known as Sipple syndrome), was associated with familial pheochromocytomas, medullary thyroid carcinoma (MTC), and hyperparathyroidism [1]. The third syndrome, called multiple endocrine neoplasia type III (MEN 3), included patients with papillary thyroid carcinomas and nonfamilial parathyroid tumors [1].

During the 1970, Sizemore and Chong further classified patients with MEN 2 into two groups: MEN 2A and MEN 2B [1]. MEN 2A patients had MTC, pheochromocytoma, and hyperparathyroidism with a normal physical appearance. MEN 2B patients had MTC, pheochromocytoma, no evidence of hyperparathyroidism, and an abnormal physical appearance including neuromas of the tongue and oral mucosa, thickened and everted eyelids, and other mesodermal irregularities.

Today, the term "multiple endocrine neoplasia" refers to three autosomal dominant disorders: MEN 1, MEN 2A, and MEN 2B. In addition, the most recent guidelines from the American Thyroid Association (ATA) in 2009 concluded that familial medullary thyroid carcinoma (FMTC) should be considered a subset of MEN 2A [3]. This chapter discusses the clinical manifestations, diagnosis, genetic testing, treatments, and prognosis of each syndrome (Table 3.1).

Multiple Endocrine Neoplasia Type I

Overview

MEN 1 is an autosomal dominant disorder caused by germline mutations of the *MEN1* gene, a tumor suppressor gene located on chromosome 11q13 that encodes the protein menin. The exact function of menin is unknown, but it is involved in DNA replication and repair, transcription, and chromatin modification [4]. Affected individuals are predisposed to develop tumors primarily of the anterior pituitary, parathyroid, and endocrine pancreas. However, combinations of over 20 various endocrine and nonendocrine tumors have been described in patients with MEN 1 [5]. Other clearly associated endocrine tumors include foregut carcinoids (thymic,

Table 3.1 Comparison of multiple endocrine neoplasia syndromes

	MEN 1	MEN 2A	MEN 2B
Gene	*MEN1*	*RET*	*RET*
Gene location	11q13	10q11.2	10q11.2
Gene product	Menin	Tyrosine kinase	Tyrosine kinase
Genotype–phenotype correlation	No	Yes	Yes
Classical endocrine tumors	• Pituitary adenoma • Primary hyperparathyroidism • Pancreas/duodenum	• Medullary thyroid carcinoma • Pheochromocytoma • Primary hyperparathyroidism	• Medullary thyroid carcinoma • Pheochromocytoma
Other endocrine tumors	• Foregut carcinoid • Adrenocortical abnormalities		
Distinguishing features	• Facial angiofibromas • Lipoma	• Cutaneous lichen amyloidosis	• Marfanoid habitus • Nodular lips • Thickened eyelids • Neuromas of the GI tract

bronchial, gastric, and duodenal) and adrenocortical lesions. Associated nonendocrine tumors include facial angiofibromas and collagenomas. Thyroid nodules, meningiomas, ependymomas, leiomyomas, and lipomas have been reported to occur with increased frequency in MEN 1 patients. However, whether there is a true association versus fortuitous increased detection is unclear.

The initial manifestation of individuals with MEN 1 usually occurs during late adolescence or early adulthood. The specific endocrine gland involved and the age of onset is variable among individuals and families, but primary hyperparathyroidism (PHPT) is commonly the initial endocrinopathy [4–6]. The youngest reported MEN 1 related tumor was a pituitary adenoma in a child 5 years of age [5, 7]. The high penetrance of MEN 1 is evident in that half of affected patients show biochemical manifestations of the disease by 20 years of age [8]. By 50 years of age, 80% of affected individuals show manifestations of the syndrome, and nearly 100% of patients are symptomatic by age 60 years [8].

Parathyroid tumors

PHPT is the most common endocrinopathy associated with MEN 1, and it is often the first clinical manifestation [5]. The typical age of onset of PHPT ranges from 20 to 25 years, which is approximately 30 years earlier than sporadic PHPT [4]. Nearly 100% of MEN 1 patients develop PHPT by 50 years of age [5]. Because PHPT in MEN 1 patients develops at a young age and is typically associated with four gland hyperplasia, in patients younger than 40 years with multiglandular PHPT should be considered for genetic counseling and/or testing for MEN 1. PHPT may be completely asymptomatic or present as nephrolithiasis, osteopenia or osteoporosis, fatigue, peptic ulcer disease, myopathy, and neurocognitive deficits including depression and problems with sleep [9, 10].

High-risk patients or patients who are identified with a *MEN1* mutation may be screened for PHPT starting at age 8 years with annual serum calcium and parathyroid hormone (PTH) levels [5]. The diagnosis is rendered with elevated or high normal serum calcium and a concomitant inappropriate elevation of PTH. Once PHPT is diagnosed, surgical intervention is indicated when there is objective evidence of disease (i.e., kidney stones, osteoporosis, pancreatitis), or for patients with a serum calcium greater than 1 mg/dL of the upper limit of normal, calculated creatinine clearance less than 60 mL/min, glomerular filtration rate (GFR) greater than 30% below normal, bone mineral density with a *t*-score less than −2.5 at any site, age less than 40 years, or any previous fracture fragility [11]. After biochemical confirmation of disease, we recommend obtaining an ultrasonographic examination of the cervical region to identify concomitant thyroid disease before proceeding to operative intervention.

Because MEN 1 patients have multiglandular disease, surgical treatment of PHPT is different than for sporadic PHPT cases. According to the 2009 NCCN guidelines, patients with MEN 1 are recommended to undergo one of two different surgical approaches for PHPT [12]. One surgical approach is subtotal parathyroidectomy, bilateral upper thymectomy, and possible cryopreservation of the parathyroid glands. This surgery is associated with a 30–40% rate of recurrent hyperparathyroidism [13–15]. The second operative approach is a total parathyroidectomy with autotransplantation, bilateral upper thymectomy, and possible cryopreservation of the parathyroid glands [12]. This surgery carries a risk of permanent hypoparathyroidism in up to one third of patients secondary to autograft failure [14–16]. Bilateral thymectomy is recommended for MEN 1 patients with PHPT because they are at a higher risk of developing a thymic carcinoid tumor. Also, resection of the thymus removes supranumerary parathyroid glands.

The decision to pursue subtotal or total parathyroidectomy in MEN 1 patients is controversial. At the University of Texas MD Anderson Cancer Center (MDACC), we recommend three and a half gland parathyroidectomy, transcervical thymectomy, and parathyroid cryopreservation as insurance in the event of aparathyroidism. If hyperparathyroidism recurs, we then recommend completion total parathyroidectomy with autografting and cryopreservation of the remaining parathyroid tissue [15].

Pituitary tumors

Ten to 60% of patients with MEN 1 are diagnosed with anterior pituitary adenomas [8, 17, 18]. Approximately 10% of patients with MEN 1 present with pituitary adenomas as the initial manifestation [5, 8]. The average age of onset is around

35 years of age, which is no different than the sporadic counterpart [4]. Moreover, women are more likely than men to develop pituitary adenomas [18].

Because pituitary tumors are twice as likely to be macroadenomas (>10 mm) in MEN 1 when compared to sporadic disease (85 vs. 42%), patients with MEN 1 more frequently present with symptoms of local compression [17, 18]. Compressive symptoms include headache, visual field deficits, hypopituitarism, cranial nerve dysfunction (cranial nerves III or VI), temporal lobe epilepsy, and mild hyperprolactinemia from stalk compression [19]. The preferred imaging modality for diagnosing pituitary adenomas is magnetic resonance imaging (MRI) with and without gadolinium at 3 mm intervals [19]. One millimeter intervals are advantageous for patients with Cushing's disease [19]. Functional status is determined by measuring pretreatment basal hormonal levels; the most common being prolactinomas (60%) followed by nonfunctional (15%), somatotropinomas (10–15%), and corticotrophin-secreting tumors (5%) [8, 18].

Symptoms associated with prolactinomas include amenorrhea or galactorrhea in women, or signs of hypogonadism in men (sexual dysfunction or gynecomastia). The biochemical diagnosis of prolactinoma is confirmed when the serum prolactin level is greater than 200 ng/mL and a concomitant adenoma is identified on MRI [19]. MEN 1-associated prolactinomas have a worse response to treatment when compared to sporadic counterparts [8, 17, 18]. Prolactinomas are initially treated with cabergoline or bromocriptine, which are long acting dopamine agonists [20]. Surgical resection is indicated when patients are unresponsive or intolerant to medical therapy [19].

Patients with somatotroph adenomas produce an excess of insulin growth-like factor (IGF-1) and/or growth hormone (GH). If the adenoma develops before puberty, the patient develops gigantism, whereas adult-onset tumors result in acromegaly. Patients with acromegaly may develop frontal bossing, coarse facial features, and enlargement of the hands, feet, and lower jaw. Other clinical manifestations include sweating, dental malocclusion, carpal tunnel syndrome, osteoarthritis, diabetes, hypertension, nephrolithiasis, skin tags, and colon polyps [19]. Somatotropinomas are confirmed with an elevated IGF-1 and a lesion on MRI. Serum GH may or may not be elevated in this setting. The most definitive test for a somatotropinoma is failure to suppress GH levels to less than 5 ng/dL after administering 1.75 g/kg (max 100 g) of oral glucose [19]. Surgical resection is typically the first treatment for somatotropinomas [19]. Focused irradiation after surgical debulking may be beneficial in some cases. Patients who are high risk for operative resection may be considered for medical therapy using a dopamine agonist, somatostatin analog, or the GH receptor blocker pegvisomant [19].

Corticotropin-secreting tumors result in Cushing's disease. Symptoms include central weight gain, mood changes, thinning of the skin, easy bruising, diabetes, hypertension, and osteoporosis [19]. Urinary free cortisol measurement is the most reliable test to identify excess cortisol production. Other screening tests include plasma ACTH level, dexamethasone suppression test, and midnight salivary cortisol levels [19]. The most definitive test to confirm pituitary-dependent Cushing's disease is inferior petrosal sinus sampling, but the procedure has associated risks [19].

The treatment of choice for corticotropin secreting tumors is surgical resection. If unsuccessful, other options include focused irradiation or bilateral adrenalectomy. Ketoconazole and metyrapone, drugs that inhibit adrenal steroid production, may be used on a short-term basis for symptom control. However, these drugs should not be used long term due to the side effects such as liver toxicity with ketoconazole [19].

Approximately 15% of pituitary tumors in patients with MEN 1 are nonfunctioning, and tumors are either diagnosed incidentally on imaging or from symptoms of compression [18]. If the prolactin level is elevated, but less than 100 ng/mL and there is an adenoma on MRI, the tumor is likely nonfunctioning. In this case, the elevated prolactin level is secondary to stalk compression. Surgical resection is indicated for growing tumors or if symptomatic [12].

Patients who are determined to be high risk or have an *MEN1* mutation should be screened with annual serum prolactin and IGF-1 levels beginning as early as age 5 years. Also, MRI of the brain should be considered every 2–3 years [5, 8].

Pancreatic Neuroendocrine Tumors

Neuroendocrine tumors of the pancreas (Also may be referred to as pancreatic endocrine tumors) develop in 50–75% of patients with MEN 1 and are the most common cause of MEN 1-specific death [21]. MEN 1 patients develop pancreatic neuroendocrine tumors (PNET) earlier than their sporadic counterparts [22]. The majority of PNETs will develop malignant progression over time [23]. PNETs typically become symptomatic in the fourth or fifth decade of life, but hormonal symptoms may be apparent earlier [24]. Often, the ambiguity of the symptoms from excess hormones produced by PNETs results in a delay in diagnosis [25]. Asymptomatic MEN 1 patients have occasionally been identified with nonfunctioning tumors of the pancreas before 20 years of age [26]. Grossly, these tumors may be solitary or multifocal, functional (most commonly gastrinoma or insulinoma) or nonfunctional, and solid or cystic [8]. Pathologically, the pancreas is often found to have multiple microadenomas, islet cell hypertrophy, hyperplasia, and dysplasia [8]. The majority of these neoplasms stain positive for chromogranin A, synaptophysin, and neuron-specific enolase with immunohistochemistry [8].

Success rates in localizing PNETs depend on tumor size and imaging modality. Twenty percent of PNETs smaller than 1 cm, 30–40% of tumors 1–3 cm, and 75% of tumors greater than 3 cm will be identified on computed tomography (CT), MRI, or ultrasound [25]. Endoscopic ultrasound, the most sensitive technique for identifying PNETs, has detected neoplasms as small as 0.3 cm in size [27]. In addition, octreotide imaging may be beneficial for the localization of PNETs [25].

More than 50% of MEN 1 associated PNETs are nonfunctional [24] even though 69–100% of patients have an elevated serum chromogranin A, and 50–100% of patients have an elevated pancreatic polypeptide (PP) level [25]. PP levels should be obtained when patients are fasting. Hormone overproduction does not result in symptoms for nonfunctional tumors [28]. In addition, clinicians must be aware that chromogranin A may be falsely elevated among patients on proton-pump inhibitors. Similarly, PP may also be elevated in patients with older age, alcoholism, renal failure, and inflammatory conditions [25].

Nonfunctional PNETs are often diagnosed late in the course of the disease because symptoms are not apparent until the tumor grows large enough to produce compression of adjacent structures. Clinical manifestations include abdominal pain, weight loss, and jaundice. According to the 2009 NCCN guidelines, patients with nonfunctional PNETS should undergo surgical resection with regional lymph node dissection for localized disease [12]. Patients with distant metastasis should undergo surgical intervention if a complete resection can be achieved [12].

Functional PNETs oversecrete specific hormones resulting in a distinct pattern of clinical symptoms often referred to as a specific "syndrome" (i.e., Zollinger–Ellison syndrome). While several types of functional PNETs can occur within the same patient, usually one hormonal syndrome dominates (Table 3.2). The most common functional PNET or duodenal tumor in MEN 1 patients is a gastrinoma. More than 80% of gastrinomas in patients with MEN 1 are located in the duodenum [8]. Gastrinomas are often multifocal and can be located anywhere within the pancreas, duodenum, or the gastrinoma triangle [28]. The gastrinoma triangle includes the duodenum, the pancreatic head, and the hepatoduodenal ligament [29]. Patients with MEN 1 develop gastrinomas approximately 10 years younger than their sporadic counterparts (35 vs. 45 years) [4].

Gastrinomas secrete gastrin, a hormone which induces hyperchlorhydria. Patients present with abdominal pain (75–100%), diarrhea (35–73%), heartburn (44–64%), duodenal and prepyloric ulcers (71–91%), and complications associated with ulcer disease [25, 29]. Patients with a suspected gastrinoma should be screened with a fasting gastrin level 2 weeks after discontinuing antisecretory medications such as proton pump inhibitors (PPIs) if feasible [25]. Withdrawal of PPI among patients with gastrinoma should, however, be done with caution as perforation can occur if not carefully monitored. Clinicians should be aware that other causes of hypergastrinemia include PPI use, autoimmune pernicious anemia, *Helicobacter pylori* gastritis with atrophy, vagotomy, fundectomy, gastric outlet obstruction, large intestinal resection, or chronic renal failure [25]. If the fasting gastrin level is greater than 1,000 pg/mL with a concurrently low gastric pH, then the diagnosis is highly suggestive of a gastrinoma [25]. To confirm the diagnosis in the setting of occult disease where an obvious tumor is not found, a basal acid output greater than 15 mEq/h and a positive secretin stimulation test is required [25].

The surgical management of a gastrinoma in patients is controversial because the symptoms associated with gastric acid hypersecretion can be controlled with medications and recurrence is likely after surgical resection [23]. Patients with concomitant hyperparathyroidism should undergo parathyroidectomy first, since correcting hypercalcemia can decrease serum gastrin levels [8]. According to the 2009 NCCN guidelines, patients with a gastrinoma should first be treated with a PPI or a histamine (H2) antagonist. If a tumor can be identified on imaging, enucleation or resection is recommended with a regional lymph node dissection [12]. Thirty to 50% of

Table 3.2 Pancreatic neuroendocrine tumors associated with MEN-1

Neoplasm	Hormone	Clinical manifestations	Laboratory testing	Treatment
Gastrinoma	Gastrin	Abdominal pain, diarrhea, GERD, ulcers	Fasting gastrin >1,000 pg/mL Basal acid output >15 mEq/h Positive secretin stimulation test	Parathyroidectomy (if HPT exists) PPI Surgical resection with regional lymphadenectomy
Insulinoma	Insulin	Hypoglycemic episodes, sweating, weakness, tremors, palpitations	72 h fasting with monitoring of insulin:glucose ratio every 4–6 h	Frequent small meals Diazoxide Surgical resection
Glucagonoma	Glucagon	Glucose intolerance, weight loss, migratory necrolytic erythema	Glucagon >500–1,000 pg/mL	Surgical resection with regional lymphadenectomy
VIPoma	Vasoactive intestinal peptide (VIP)	Large volume diarrhea, electrolyte imbalance, dehydration, hyperglycemia, flushing	Fasting plasma VIP >500 pg/mL	Hydration Correction of electrolytes Octreotide Surgical resection with regional lymphadenectomy
Somatostatinoma	Somatostatin	Diabetes mellitus, cholelithiasis, steatorrhea, weight loss, anemia, diarrhea	Somatostatin >100 pg/mL	Surgical resection with regional lymphadenectomy

patients who undergo surgical resection have regional lymph node metastasis [8]. One analysis of 81 patients with MEN 1 and gastrinomas demonstrated that patients with locally advanced gastrinomas who have surgical resection have a similar survival as patients with localized tumors [30].

Approximately 10% of patients with MEN 1 are diagnosed with an insulinoma [28]. The hypersecretion of insulin associated with these tumors results in hypoglycemic episodes especially during periods of fasting or exercise. Neuroglycopenic symptoms may occur such as confusion, visual changes, altered consciousness, or convulsions [25]. Also, patients may develop a sympathetic overdrive during an insulin surge manifested by sweating, weakness, tremors, hyperphasia, and palpitations [25]. Insulinomas are diagnosed with a monitored 72 h fast where plasma glucose and insulin levels are measured every 4–6 h. An insulin-to-glucose ratio of 0.4 or greater is diagnostic of an insulinoma. One third of patients will become symptomatic within 12 h, 80% at 24 h, 90% at 48 h, and 100% at 72 h [25]. Depending on the size, these tumors may be identified by CT, MRI, or endoscopic ultrasound. Octreotide scanning is of limited benefit since some insulinomas (especially smaller localized ones) may not express somatostatin receptor-2 [5].

As with other PNETs, insulinomas can be multifocal and may be located throughout the pancreas. The primary treatment is surgical resection since medical therapy is not effective. Even though insulinomas have a higher recurrence rate after surgical resection in MEN 1 patients when compared to sporadic counterparts, they are usually benign (85–95%) [8, 25]. Prior to surgery, glucose levels should be controlled with frequent small meals and diazoxide, a drug that inhibits insulin release and promotes glycogenolysis [12, 25]. Distal pancreatectomy with enucleation of pancreatic head tumors using intraoperative ultrasound is the most common operative approach [8, 12, 14].

As many as 5% of MEN 1 patients with PNETs have other functional tumors such as glucagonomas, vasoactive intestinal peptide tumors (VIPomas), and somatostatinomas [14, 28]. Glucagonomas are characterized by excess secretion of glucagon resulting in glucose intolerance, weight loss, and necrolytic migratory erythema. Inappropriately elevated glucagon levels greater than 500–1,000 pg/mL is diagnostic for a glucagonoma. However, clinicians should be aware that elevated glucagon levels may also be present in patients with cirrhosis, pancreatitis, diabetes mellitus, prolonged fasting, renal failure, burns, sepsis, familial glucagonemia, and acromegaly [25]. Treatment usually entails surgical resection with regional lymph node dissection [12].

VIPomas are characterized by large volume diarrhea, electrolyte imbalances, dehydration, hyperglycemia, hypercalcemia, and flushing [25]. Fasting plasma VIP levels greater than 500 pg/mL along with high volume diarrhea is highly suggestive of a VIPoma even if not visualized on imaging [25]. These tumors may be identified on CT, MRI, endoscopic ultrasound, or octreotide scanning. Prior to operative intervention, patients should be hydrated, electrolytes should be normalized, and octreotide should be administered [12]. The operative approach involves resection with regional lymph node dissection as these tumors do have malignant potential [5, 12, 14].

Somatostatinomas may be located in the pancreas or duodenum. Affected patients develop diabetes mellitus, cholelithiasis, steatorrhea, weight loss, anemia, and diarrhea. The diagnosis is obtained with a somatostatin level greater than 100 pg/mL and a tumor on imaging (CT, MRI, octreotide scan, endoscopic ultrasound). Surgical resection with regional lymph node dissection is appropriate for these patients [12].

Recommended screening for high-risk patients or patients identified with an MEN 1 mutation is to obtain annual serum fasting glucose, insulin, gastrin, chromogranin-A, glucagon, and proinsulin levels. CT or MRI is recommended every 1–3 years to evaluate for nonfunctioning pancreatic tumors [5].

Other Manifestations of MEN 1

As many as 55% of MEN 1 patients have adrenocortical abnormalities [31]. The majority of these abnormalities include nonfunctional nodular hyperplasia or adenomas [31]. Adrenal lesions in MEN 1 patients are usually small, benign, and nonfunctional. However, there have been reports of patients with functioning tumors such as aldosterone-secreting tumors, cortisol-secreting tumors, and rarely, pheochromocytomas or adrenocortical carcinomas [8, 31, 32]. The diagnosis and treatment of adrenal disease is the same as the sporadic counterparts.

Foregut carcinoid tumors (bronchial, thymic, gastric, duodenal) may be identified in 5–10% of MEN 1 patients, and represent the second most common MEN 1-specific cause of death [8, 14]. The average age of onset is 35 years, which is no different than the sporadic counterpart [4]. Thymic carcinoids are the most aggressive and carry a poor prognosis [33]. Even prophylactic thymic resection as part of a surgery for PHPT does not eliminate the risk of future development of thymic carcinoids [8]. Carcinoid tumors of the stomach and duodenum are often multiple and have malignant potential. Gastric carcinoids may be a result of hypergastrinemia from MEN 1 related gastrinoma [8]. In these cases, suppression of gastrin may lead to regression of gastric carcinoid [34]. The management of the hepatic metastasis of carcinoid tumors achieves the best survival with surgical resection, but other modalities such as radiofrequency ablation and chemoembolization can safely be performed [35].

Diagnosis of MEN 1 and the Role of Genetic Testing

MEN 1 is diagnosed clinically for patients who develop two or more of the classic tumors associated with the disease (pituitary, parathyroid, or endocrine tumors of the pancreas or duodenum), or for patients who have one of the classic tumors and at least one close relative with a clinical diagnosis of MEN 1 [5]. The early recognition of patients with MEN 1 can be challenging because MEN 1 is rare and accounts for only a small percentage of all patients presenting with hyperparathyroidism, a pituitary adenoma, or a pancreatic endocrine tumor. Moreover, the diagnosis may be missed and not considered until after the patient has developed a second or third tumor.

On the other hand, MEN 1 may be diagnosed prior to the development of the clinical manifestations using genetic testing if a deleterious germline mutation of the *MEN1* gene is identified. Approximately 90% of patients with classic, familial MEN 1 have an identifiable mutation [36]. The remainder of patients with classic MEN 1 may have a mutation not detected by the methodology used (i.e., large gene deletion or duplication which accounts for another 1–4% of *MEN1* mutations), or a mutation may not be identifiable because the patient has somatic mosaicism [36]. In addition, some patients with features of MEN 1 may actually represent phenocopies (coincidental occurrence of MEN 1-related tumors in a person without a germline *MEN1* mutation), particularly those that are nonfamilial with older-onset hyperparathyroidism.

Germline *MEN1* mutations have been found at lower rates in patients presenting with nonclassic MEN 1 [36]. For example, 15–20% of patients with apparently isolated familial PHPT have been found to have a germline *MEN1* mutation, mainly in patients with young onset and multiglandular disease. It is not clear whether familial isolated hyperparathyroidism is a distinct subtype of MEN 1, whether some of the families with *MEN1* mutations might have had other clinically occult disease, or whether additional diseases can develop in the future.

New genetic mutations have been recognized among individual families. For example, recently a germline *CDKN1B* mutation was identified in a patient who had a pituitary macroadenoma and PHPT, but she did not have a mutation in the *MEN1* gene [37]. Her father, diagnosed with acromegaly, and her sister, found to have renal angiomyolipoma (nonendocrine tumor associated with MEN 1), both had mutations in *CDKN1B*. The *CDKN1B* gene encodes the protein, p27, which is a cyclin-dependent kinase inhibitor involved in cell cycle progression [38]. Interestingly, a similar mutation in *CDKN1B* in rats leads to the development of endocrine tumors seen in MEN disease [37]. Even though mutations in the *CDKN1B* gene have not been identified in any other family, this phenotype may represent a rare form of MEN 1 [39, 40].

There is a wide range of mutation types within the *MEN1* gene and often specific mutations are unique to each family. To date, no genotype–phenotype correlations have been established [34]. Even so, genetic testing for MEN 1 is still beneficial for some patients. The two main benefits of genetic testing are to: (1) confirm or decrease the likelihood of a diagnosis of MEN 1 in a patient with a suspicious clinical or family history so that appropriate medical management recommendations can be made and (2) to identify the disease-causing mutation in a known MEN 1 patient so that the patient's relatives can be offered predictive genetic testing. Moreover, affected patients may use this information to consider reproductive planning options such as preimplantation genetic diagnosis or prenatal genetic testing. Once the disease-causing mutation is identified, at-risk relatives can be tested for the mutation such that mutation-negative relatives can be identified and spared from tumor screening tests.

An accurate family history is the most important tool to identify MEN 1 patients. However, as many as 10% of patients are found to have a de novo mutation of the *MEN1* gene, in which case the family history is noncontributory [41]. Genetic counseling/testing should be offered to all patients with a clinical diagnosis of MEN 1, patients with one classic feature and a nonclassic tumor such as a foregut carcinoid or lipoma, and individuals with one of the classic tumors plus a family history of a classic tumor.

Before proceeding with genetic testing, patients should be counseled about the purpose of genetic testing, the likelihood of a positive result, and implications of a positive/negative result to them and their relatives. In addition, the patient can be provided with anticipatory guidance and counseling about reproductive risks and prenatal genetic testing options, should they wish to use the information in planning a pregnancy. Also, the cost of the test as well as the psychological consequences should be discussed [36].

In the past, clinicians did not find genetic testing for the early diagnosis of high risk individuals to be beneficial. However, biochemical evidence of tumor development may be found as early as 10 years before the patient becomes symptomatically apparent [22]. Prompt recognition and treatment of functioning neoplasms may help prevent complications associated with long-term hormonal excess. Monitoring and early intervention of pancreatic and duodenal tumors may help to prevent the development of advanced malignancies. It is recommended that screening of children at risk for inheriting MEN disease should begin as early as age 5 years, given that this is the youngest diagnosis of an MEN 1-related tumor. However, it is not clear that screening children, as opposed to waiting to begin screening until early adulthood, will reduce morbidity and mortality. Life-threatening manifestations of MEN 1 are rare in young children, and testing in childhood has potential to cause psychosocial harm. Therefore, patients should be carefully counseled regarding the timing of genetic testing in their children [36].

Multiple Endocrine Neoplasia Type 2

Overview

MEN 2 is an autosomal dominant disorder caused by germline activating missense mutations of the *RET* (rearranged during transfection) proto-oncogene. Approximately 95% of MEN 2 patients have an identifiable *RET* mutation [3]. The *RET* gene, located on chromosome 10q11.2, contains 21 exons and encodes a tyrosine kinase that is primarily expressed in neuroendocrine and neural cells [42]. Patients with MEN 2 are at risk to develop medullary thyroid cancer (MTC), pheochromocytomas, and PHPT. In addition, inactivating germline mutations of the RET proto-oncogene have been implicated in 10–40% of patients with Hirschsprung disease, a condition defined by the loss of enteric innervation [3]. MEN 2 is unique in that the specific *RET* mutation predicts the MEN 2 subtype and the aggressiveness of

MTC [42]. MEN 2 has been classified into three subtypes: MEN 2A, FMTC, and MEN 2B. All three subtypes are associated with a high risk for MTC. Individuals with MEN 2A have a relatively high risk for pheochromocytoma and PHPT, whereas patients with FMTC have a low risk for pheochromocytoma and PHPT. MEN 2B patients are at risk for pheochromocytoma and have specific physical characteristics not apparent in MEN 2A or FMTC patients.

MEN 2A

At least 75% of MEN 2 patients are classified as having MEN 2A [5]. MEN 2A is characterized by the presence of MTC (90%), PHPT (up to 20–30%), and pheochromocytoma (up to 50%) [5]. The age of onset of MTC can range from children less than 10 years old to the fourth decade of life [3]. MTC is usually the first manifestation of MEN 2 [5, 42]. The majority of MEN 2A patients have mutations affecting cysteine residues in exons 10 and 11 most commonly in codon 634, but also in codons 618 and 620, and less commonly in others [3]. A small percentage of patients with mutations in codon 634 exhibit cutaneous lichen amyloidosis, a pruritic skin rash that develops on the dorsal torso [3, 27].

The diagnosis of MEN 2A is established by identifying a germline *RET* mutation [3]. Over 95% of MEN 2A patients are found to have a specific *RET* mutation; rarely, MEN 2 families do not have an identifiable mutation [3, 43]. In the absence of a RET mutation, the diagnosis of MEN 2A requires a high index of suspicion and the presence of at least two of the classic features of the disease (MTC, pheochromocytoma, PHPT) [3].

Familial medullary thyroid cancer (FMTC) may be thought of as a clinical variant of MEN 2A where MTC is usually the only manifestation, and the risk for pheochromocytoma and PHPT is low [3]. For instance, mutations in codons 609, 611, 630, 768, 790, 804, and 891 are associated with low risks for pheochromocytoma and PHPT [3]. However, families once thought to have FMTC have later developed clinical manifestations of MEN 2A [3].

MEN 2B

MEN 2B is less common than MEN 2A, but is associated with an aggressive form of MTC. The American Thyroid Association (ATA) defines MEN 2B as a condition with the "presence of MTC, marfanoid habitus, medullated corneal nerve fibers, ganglioneuromatosis of the gut and oral mucosa, and pheochromocytoma associated with a germline *RET* mutation [3]." Greater than 95% of MEN 2B patients have the mutation M918T in exon 16, and 2–3% of patients have the mutation A883F in exon 15 [3]. MEN 2B patients do not have an increased risk of developing PHPT. The age of onset of MTC in MEN 2B patients is approximately 10 years earlier than patients with MEN 2A [3, 44]. Approximately 50% of patients

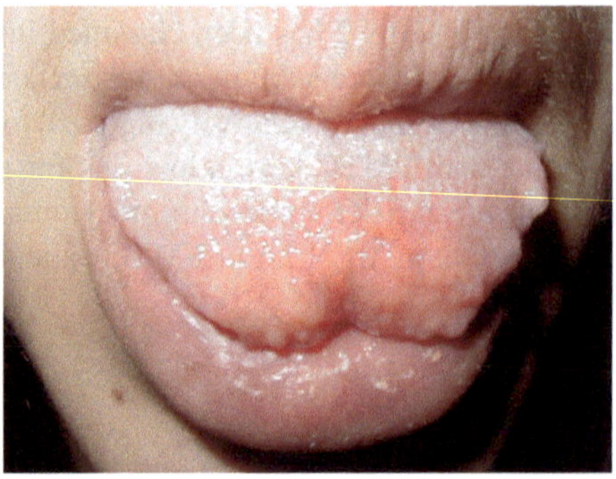

Fig. 3.1 Mucosal neuromas of the tongue in a patient with MEN 2B: the physical characteristics of MEN 2B patients include an elongated face with enlarged and nodular lips, thickened and everted eyelids, and neuromas of the tongue and oral mucosa

with MEN 2B develop pheochromocytomas. The physical characteristics of MEN 2B patients include an elongated face with enlarged and nodular lips, thickened and everted eyelids, and neuromas of the tongue and oral mucosa (Fig. 3.1) [44]. Skeletal abnormalities include genu valgum, pes cavus, club foot, and kyphoscoliosis [44]. The majority of neuromas are found in the gastrointestinal tract, but they may also be identified in any organ with a submucosa, such as the bronchi and bladder [44]. Ganglioneuromatosis of the GI tract may cause abdominal distention, megacolon, constipation, and diarrhea [44].

Medullary Thyroid Carcinoma in MEN 2

MTC develops from the parafollicular cells (C-cells) of the thyroid gland which produce calcitonin. Calcitonin works to lower plasma calcium by inhibiting osteoclastic bone absorption and inducing urinary excretion of calcium and phosphate. In contrast to sporadic MTC, tumors in patients with familial MTC are often bilateral and multicentric [44]. In the familial form, the development of MTC is preceded by C-cell hyperplasia which can increase the serum calcitonin. C-cells are concentrated in the superior one third of the thyroid gland which is where the majority of MTC is identified [44]. The C-cells in MTC secrete increased amounts of calcitonin, and the presence of calcitonin after total thyroidectomy is an indicator of residual or persistent disease. A serum level of calcitonin greater than 1,000 pg/mL with an elevated carcinoembryonic antigen (CEA) is highly suggestive of MTC. The diagnosis may be confirmed with a pentagastrin stimulation test, identification of a thyroid mass, and positive cytologic evidence of MTC on ultrasound guided fine needle aspiration [44].

Patients with MTC often present with neck pain, a palpable neck mass, or diarrhea from the elevated serum calcitonin level. Patients with dysphagia and hoarseness frequently have advanced disease. MTC is known for being an aggressive form of thyroid cancer. Likewise, the aggressiveness of MTC depends on the *RET* mutation. Initially, metastasis occurs in cervical or mediastinal lymph nodes, and later to the lung, liver, and bone [44].

Table 3.3 Aggressiveness of MTC according to *RET* mutation

ATA level	Codons	Aggressiveness of MTC	Age of prophylactic thyroidectomy
A	768, 790, 791, 804, 891	Lowest	After 5 years[a]
B	609, 611, 618, 620, 630	Low	Before 5 years[a]
C	634	High	Before 5 years
D	883, 918	Highest	Within first year of life

[a]Surgery may be delayed until 5 years of age if serum calcitonin and cervical ultrasound are normal

Over 90% of MEN 2A patients and almost all MEN 2B patients develop MTC, and it is usually the first clinical manifestation of MEN 2 [5]. Because MTC is resistant to chemotherapeutic or radioactive iodine therapies, surgical resection is the primary method of treatment. Also, since the biologic behavior of MEN 2 can be predicted by the specific *RET* mutation, the timing and extent of surgery can be individualized to achieve the best overall outcome [42]. In 2009, the ATA guidelines task force published recommendations for screening and treatment for patients with hereditary MTC according to the specific *RET* mutation (Table 3.3) [3].

Initial evaluation for MTC includes a cervical neck ultrasound, serum CEA, serum calcium, and a serum calcitonin level. Patients who have no evidence of local invasion and no lymph node metastasis should undergo total thyroidectomy with prophylactic central neck dissection. However, patients with an elevated calcitonin level greater than 400 pg/mL or evidence of lymph node metastasis should obtain neck, chest, and three-phase liver CT or MRI to rule out distant metastasis. If distant metastatic disease is evident, less aggressive surgery may be considered in order to preserve speech and swallowing function [3]. Prior to operative intervention, patients should be evaluated for pheochromocytoma with serum metanephrine levels, and PHPT with serum calcium and PTH levels.

The ATA recommends total thyroidectomy with therapeutic central lymph node dissection for patients who have identified central neck disease. The necessity of a lateral neck dissection for patients without evidence of lateral neck disease is not currently established. Patients who are found to have lateral neck disease should undergo a lateral neck dissection of levels IIA, III, IV, and V on the affected side [3].

Following thyroidectomy, patients should be given thyroid hormone replacement therapy rather than thyroid hormone suppression therapy, a treatment reserved for follicular and papillary thyroid cancer. Likewise, radioactive iodine is not an effective treatment for MTC. Two to 3 months following thyroidectomy, baseline serum calcitonin and CEA levels should be obtained. These markers should initially be followed every 6–12 months, and then annually thereafter. Also, a baseline cervical ultrasound 6 months after surgical resection should be obtained. Patients with undetectable tumor markers may be followed with serial laboratory assessments. If the calcitonin level is elevated but less than 150 pg/mL, the affected individual should undergo a neck ultrasound to evaluate for persistent or recurrent disease. If the serum calcitonin is greater than 150 pg/mL, additional imaging is warranted such as neck, chest, and three phase liver CT or MRI. The role of adjuvant chemotherapy and external beam radiation is unclear in patients with unresectable disease, and the use of these treatments should be individualized [3].

Genetic testing: Genetic counseling should be encouraged for all patients who undergo genetic testing in order to understand the purpose of testing, the natural history of the disease, the pattern of inheritance, and the psychological consequences. Patients who are diagnosed with MTC, primary C-cell hyperplasia, cutaneous lichen amyloidosis, early onset adrenergic pheochromocytoma, or MEN 2 should be offered genetic testing for RET mutations. Likewise, individuals with a positive family history of MEN 2 or FMTC should be offered RET testing because of an autosomal dominant inheritance pattern. Testing should begin before 5 years of age in MEN 2A, and shortly after birth in MEN 2B [3]. If a specific RET mutation is identified within a family, all first-degree relatives should be offered testing before the age of recommended prophylactic thyroidectomy if possible.

Prophylactic thyroidectomy: The ATA developed a classification system of specific *RET* genetic mutations according to the aggressiveness of MTC. By knowing the biological behavior of each *RET* mutation, the timing of prophylactic thyroidectomy can be determined to improve overall survival. ATA level A *RET* mutations represent the least aggressive form of MTC, and include codons 768, 790, 791, 804, and 891. ATA level B *RET* mutations are slightly more aggressive and include codons 609, 611, 618, 620, and 630. Both ATA levels A and B *RET* mutations have been identified in MEN 2A patients. The timing of prophylactic thyroidectomy for ATA levels A and B may be delayed beyond 5 years of age if serum calcitonin and neck ultrasound are normal, and the family history of MTC is not particularly aggressive. These patients must be screened with annual serum calcitonin levels and cervical ultrasonography. If the ultrasound or calcitonin is abnormal, then surgical resection is indicated at that time. Because patients with ATA level B mutations have slightly more aggressive disease, prophylactic thyroidectomy in a tertiary care setting may be considered prior to 5 years of age [3].

ATA level C disease has a higher risk of aggressive MTC, and includes codon 634 which is found in most MEN 2A kindreds. These patients should undergo prophylactic thyroidectomy at an experienced tertiary care center before 5 years of age [3].

The most aggressive form of MTC is found in patients with ATA level D mutations. Patients in this category have MEN 2B and have mutations in codon 883 or 918. They have the youngest age of onset and the highest risk of metastatic disease. Prophylactic total thyroidectomy is recommended within the first year of life in an experienced tertiary care setting [3].

Primary Hyperparathyroidism in MEN 2A

Ten to 35% of patients with MEN 2A develop PHPT [42]. It is most commonly associated with a mutation of codon 634. PHPT has also been identified at lower rates in patients with mutations in codons 609, 611, 618, 620, 790, and 791 [42]. Patients with MEN 2B are not at an increased risk for PHPT. MEN 2A patients with PHPT are often asymptomatic, but may present with nephrolithiasis and hypercalcemia like their sporadic counterparts [5]. PHPT in MEN 2A is milder than patients with MEN 1 [5]. However unlike MEN 1, PHPT in MEN 2A patients ranges from a single adenoma to four gland hyperplasia [5]. The diagnosis and indications for surgery in MEN 2A patients with PHPT is the same as for MEN 1 individuals and patients with sporadic disease as described previously in this chapter.

Surgical options for the management of MEN 2A patients who have evidence of PHPT at the time of initial thyroidectomy include resection of visibly enlarged glands with possible forearm autograft, subtotal parathyroidectomy leaving one or a piece of one gland in situ, or total parathyroidectomy with forearm autograft [3]. Due to the risk of permanent hypoparathyroidism, most surgeons avoid total parathyroidectomy unless all four glands are abnormal [3]. Patients who develop PHPT after their initial thyroidectomy should undergo surgical resection of abnormal glands with forearm autografting based on preoperative imaging [3].

The ATA guidelines task force has also made recommendations regarding the management of devascularized normal parathyroid glands in MEN 2 patients. For instance, devascularized parathyroid glands in MEN 2B patients may be reimplanted in the sternocleidomastoid muscle. However, MEN 2A patients with a strong family history of PHPT should have devascularized normal glands implanted into the forearm. MEN 2A patients with a low risk of developing PHPT based on family history and their RET mutation may have devascularized parathyroid glands implanted into the sternocleidomastoid muscle or the forearm [3]. The risk of possible devascularization at a future dissection for recurrent MTC should be taken into consideration.

Pheochromocytoma

Up to half of MEN 2A patients will develop pheochromocytoma, a catecholamine-secreting tumor of the adrenal medulla. Patients present with headache, sweating, heart palpitations, hypertension, and anxiety. Prior to developing a pheochromocytoma which is typically benign, MEN 2 patients may have hyperplasia of the adrenal medulla [44]. Pheochromocytomas in MEN 2 patients may be unilateral or bilateral (synchronous or metachronous), and are mostly associated with codons 634 and 918 [5, 42]. However, these tumors have been identified in patients with most of the other *RET* mutations associated with MEN 2 [42]. Unlike other hereditary forms of pheochromocytoma (i.e., von Hippel–Lindau syndrome), tumors in MEN 2 patients tend to secrete higher amounts of epinephrine and lower levels of norepinephrine [45]. As a result, MEN 2 patients more often present with heart palpitations, tremor, anxiety, and paroxysmal hypertension than patients with other forms of pheochromocytoma who have higher levels of norepinephrine [45].

Pheochromocytomas tend to develop 10–20 years earlier in MEN 2 patients when compared to sporadic counterparts. Diagnosis is achieved by obtaining plasma free metanephrines and normetanephrine or urine metanephrines [12]. After a biochemical diagnosis is confirmed, imaging with CT or MRI should be performed to identify an adrenal tumor. Meta-iodobenzyl guanidine scanning (MIBG) can also be helpful with preoperative localization [5]. Surgical resection is the primary treatment of choice for pheochromocytomas. Patients with MEN 2 who are also diagnosed with MTC should have the pheochromocytoma resected first to avoid a hypertensive crisis.

In order to minimize complications associated with hypertension and heart rate during surgery, patients should be hydrated and treated with an alpha antagonist at least 1–2 weeks prior to surgery [12, 46]. Phenoxybenzamine is the most common drug used and it may be started at a dose of 10 mg twice a day. The goal is to normalize blood pressure to 130/80 mm Hg while sitting and 100 mm Hg systolic when standing. Beta blockers should be used to achieve a target heart rate from 60 to 70 bpm (beats per minute) while sitting and 70–80 bpm while standing [46]. Beta-1 blockers (atenolol 12.5–25 mg 3 times per day or metoprolol 25–50 mg 2–3 times per day) are preferred and must always be used with alpha adrenergic blockade [46]. The use of beta blockers alone would worsen hypertension in pheochromocytoma patients. Moreover, a specialized team consisting of a dedicated anesthesiologist, endocrinologist, endocrine surgeon, internist, and cardiologist is imperative to minimize the risks of complications during surgical resection.

The most common operative approach for a patient with a unilateral pheochromocytoma is laparoscopic adrenalectomy. At MDACC, we prefer retroperitoneoscopic adrenalectomy as the minimally invasive approach of choice for patients with modestly sized, clinically benign pheochromocytomas [47]. This technique is beneficial because it avoids intraabdominal solid organ mobilization. Moreover, patients with bilateral tumors do not require repositioning during the procedure [47]. Patients who undergo bilateral adrenalectomy are at risk for adrenal insufficiency which requires lifelong supplemental corticosteroids. If possible, cortical sparing adrenalectomy should be performed in these patients since this procedure can avoid postoperative corticosteroid dependence in up to 65% of patients [48].

Summary

Multiple endocrine neoplasia is described by three distinct autosomal dominant syndromes: MEN 1, MEN 2A, and MEN 2B. MEN 1 is characterized by the presence of PHPT, pituitary tumors, and PNETs. MEN 2A is a syndrome associated with MTC, hyperparathyroidism, and pheochromocytoma. Patients with MEN 2B develop MTC, pheochromocytoma, and a marfanoid body habitus and multiple mucosal neuromas. The role of genetic testing has significantly impacted patients with both MEN 1 and MEN 2 to allow for better screening among families and affected individuals. Furthermore, the ability to correlate the specific *RET* genetic mutation to the phenotypic presentation in MEN 2 has allowed clinicians to optimize patient care to achieve the best clinical outcome overall survival.

References

1. Carney JA. Familial multiple endocrine neoplasia: the first 100 years. Am J Surg Pathol. 2005;29(2):254–74.
2. Wermer P. Genetic aspects of adenomatosis of endocrine glands. Am J Med. 1954;16(3):363–71.
3. Kloos RT, Eng C, Evans DB, et al. Medullary thyroid cancer: management guidelines of the American Thyroid Association. Thyroid. 2009;19(6):565–612.
4. Agarwal SK, Lee BA, Sukhodolets KE, et al. Molecular pathology of the MEN1 gene. Ann NY Acad Sci. 2004;1014:189–98.
5. Brandi ML, Gagel RF, Angeli A, et al. Guidelines for diagnosis and therapy of MEN type 1 and type 2. J Clin Endocrinol Metab. 2001;86(12):5658–71.
6. Doherty GM. Multiple endocrine neoplasia type 1. J Surg Oncol. 2005;89(3):143–50.
7. Stratakis CA, Schussheim DH, Freedman SM, et al. Pituitary macroadenoma in a 5-year-old: an early expression of multiple endocrine neoplasia type 1. J Clin Endocrinol Metab. 2000;85(12):4776–80.
8. Thompson GB, Young WF. Multiple endocrine neoplasia type 1. In: Clark OH, Duh QY, Kebebew E, editors. Textbook of endocrine surgery. 2nd ed. Philadelphia: Elsevier Saunders; 2005. p. 673–90.
9. Mittendorf EA, Wefel JS, Meyers CA, et al. Improvement of sleep disturbance and neurocognitive function after parathyroidectomy in patients with primary hyperparathyroidism. Endocr Pract. 2007;13(4):338–44.
10. Coker LH, Rorie K, Cantley L, et al. Primary hyperparathyroidism, cognition, and health-related quality of life. Ann Surg. 2005;242(5):642–50.
11. Bilezikian JP, Khan AA, Potts Jr JT. Guidelines for the management of asymptomatic primary hyperparathyroidism: summary statement from the third international workshop. J Clin Endocrinol Metab. 2009;94(2):335–9.
12. Clark OH, Ajani JA, Benson III AB, et al. NCCN clinical practice guidelines in oncology: neuroendocrine tumors. J Natl Compr Canc Netw. 2009;7(7):712–47.
13. Elaraj DM, Skarulis MC, Libutti SK, et al. Results of initial operation for hyperparathyroidism in patients with multiple endocrine neoplasia type 1. Surgery. 2003;134(6):858–64.
14. Callender GG, Rich TA, Perrier ND. Multiple endocrine neoplasia syndromes. Surg Clin North Am. 2008;88(4):863–95. viii.
15. Lambert LA, Shapiro SE, Lee JE, et al. Surgical treatment of hyperparathyroidism in patients with multiple endocrine neoplasia type 1. Arch Surg. 2005;140(4):374–82.
16. Tonelli F, Marcucci T, Fratini G, Tommasi MS, Falchetti A, Brandi ML. Is total parathyroidectomy the treatment of choice for hyperparathyroidism in multiple endocrine neoplasia type 1? Ann Surg. 2007;246(6):1075–82.
17. Beckers A, Daly AF. The clinical, pathological, and genetic features of familial isolated pituitary adenomas. Eur J Endocrinol. 2007;157(4):371–82.
18. Verges B, Boureille F, Goudet P, et al. Pituitary disease in MEN type 1 (MEN1): data from the France-Belgium MEN1 multicenter study. J Clin Endocrinol Metab. 2002;87(2):457–65.
19. Vance ML. Pituitary adenoma: a clinician's perspective. Endocr Pract. 2008;14(6):757–63.
20. Melmed S. Update in pituitary disease. J Clin Endocrinol Metab. 2008;93(2):331–8.
21. Doherty GM, Olson JA, Frisella MM, Lairmore TC, Wells Jr SA, Norton JA. Lethality of multiple endocrine neoplasia type I. World J Surg. 1998;22(6):581–6.
22. Lairmore TC, Piersall LD, DeBenedetti MK, et al. Clinical genetic testing and early surgical intervention in patients with multiple endocrine neoplasia type 1 (MEN 1). Ann Surg. 2004;239(5):637–45.
23. Hausman Jr MS, Thompson NW, Gauger PG, Doherty GM. The surgical management of MEN-1 pancreatoduodenal neuroendocrine disease. Surgery. 2004;136(6):1205–11.
24. Bartsch DK, Fendrich V, Langer P, Celik I, Kann PH, Rothmund M. Outcome of duodenopancreatic resections in patients with multiple endocrine neoplasia type 1. Ann Surg. 2005;242(6):757–64. discussion.

25. Metz DC, Jensen RT. Gastrointestinal neuroendocrine tumors: pancreatic endocrine tumors. Gastroenterology. 2008;135(5):1469–92.
26. Newey PJ, Jeyabalan J, Walls GV, et al. Asymptomatic children with multiple endocrine neoplasia type 1 (MEN1) mutations may harbour non-functioning pancreatic neuroendocrine tumors. J Clin Endocrinol Metab. 2009;94(10):3640–6.
27. Gauger PG, Scheiman JM, Wamsteker EJ, Richards ML, Doherty GM, Thompson NW. Role of endoscopic ultrasonography in screening and treatment of pancreatic endocrine tumours in asymptomatic patients with multiple endocrine neoplasia type 1. Br J Surg. 2003;90(6):748–54.
28. Doherty GM, Thompson NW. Multiple endocrine neoplasia type 1: duodenopancreatic tumours. J Intern Med. 2003;253(6):590–8.
29. Fendrich V, Langer P, Waldmann J, Bartsch DK, Rothmund M. Management of sporadic and multiple endocrine neoplasia type 1 gastrinomas. Br J Surg. 2007;94(11):1331–41.
30. Norton JA, Alexander HR, Fraker DL, Venzon DJ, Gibril F, Jensen RT. Comparison of surgical results in patients with advanced and limited disease with multiple endocrine neoplasia type 1 and Zollinger-Ellison syndrome. Ann Surg. 2001;234(4):495–505.
31. Waldmann J, Bartsch DK, Kann PH, Fendrich V, Rothmund M, Langer P. Adrenal involvement in multiple endocrine neoplasia type 1: results of 7 years prospective screening. Langenbecks Arch Surg. 2007;392(4):437–43.
32. Dackiw AP, Cote GJ, Fleming JB, et al. Screening for MEN1 mutations in patients with atypical endocrine neoplasia. Surgery. 1999;126(6):1097–103.
33. Ferolla P, Falchetti A, Filosso P, et al. Thymic neuroendocrine carcinoma (carcinoid) in multiple endocrine neoplasia type 1 syndrome: the Italian series. J Clin Endocrinol Metab. 2005;90(5):2603–9.
34. Tomassetti P, Migliori M, Caletti GC, Fusaroli P, Corinaldesi R, Gullo L. Treatment of type II gastric carcinoid tumors with somatostatin analogues. N Engl J Med. 2000;343(8):551–4.
35. Landry CS, Scoggins CR, McMasters KM, Martin RC. Management of hepatic metastasis of gastrointestinal carcinoid tumors. J Surg Oncol. 2008;97(3):253–8.
36. Rich TA, Perrier ND. Risk assessment and genetic counseling for multiple endocrine neoplasia type 1 (MEN1). Community Oncol. 2008;5(9):502–14.
37. Pellegata NS, Quintanilla-Martinez L, Siggelkow H, et al. Germ-line mutations in p27Kip1 cause a multiple endocrine neoplasia syndrome in rats and humans. Proc Natl Acad Sci USA. 2006;103(42):15558–63.
38. Georgitsi M, Raitila A, Karhu A, et al. Germline CDKN1B/p27Kip1 mutation in multiple endocrine neoplasia. J Clin Endocrinol Metab. 2007;92(8):3321–5.
39. Falchetti A, Brandi ML. Multiple endocrine neoplasia type I variants and phenocopies: more than a nosological issue? J Clin Endocrinol Metab. 2009;94(5):1518–20.
40. Igreja S, Chahal HS, Akker SA, et al. Assessment of p27 (cyclin-dependent kinase inhibitor 1B) and aryl hydrocarbon receptor-interacting protein (AIP) genes in multiple endocrine neoplasia (MEN1) syndrome patients without any detectable MEN1 gene mutations. Clin Endocrinol (Oxf). 2009;70(2):259–64.
41. Bassett JH, Forbes SA, Pannett AA, et al. Characterization of mutations in patients with multiple endocrine neoplasia type 1. Am J Hum Genet. 1998;62(2):232–44.
42. Yip L, Cote GJ, Shapiro SE, et al. Multiple endocrine neoplasia type 2: evaluation of the genotype-phenotype relationship. Arch Surg. 2003;138(4):409–16.
43. Schuffenecker I, Billaud M, Calender A, et al. RET proto-oncogene mutations in French MEN 2A and FMTC families. Hum Mol Genet. 1994;3(11):1939–43.
44. Miller CR, Ellison EC. Multiple endocrine neoplasia type 2B. In: Clark OH, Duh QY, Kebebew E, editors. Textbook of endocrine surgery. 2nd ed. Philadelphia: Elsevier Saunders; 2005. p. 757–63.
45. Eisenhofer G, Walther MM, Huynh TT, et al. Pheochromocytomas in von Hippel-Lindau syndrome and multiple endocrine neoplasia type 2 display distinct biochemical and clinical phenotypes. J Clin Endocrinol Metab. 2001;86(5):1999–2008.

46. Pacak K. Preoperative management of the pheochromocytoma patient. J Clin Endocrinol Metab. 2007;92(11):4069–79.
47. Perrier ND, Kennamer DL, Bao R, et al. Posterior retroperitoneoscopic adrenalectomy: preferred technique for removal of benign tumors and isolated metastases. Ann Surg. 2008;248(4):666–74.
48. Yip L, Lee JE, Shapiro SE, et al. Surgical management of hereditary pheochromocytoma. J Am Coll Surg. 2004;198(4):525–34.

Chapter 4
Other Genetic Syndromes (TSC, VHL, NF1, etc.)

Bernardo Garicochea

Abstract Neuroendocrine tumors (NETs) are the main feature of a few hereditary cancer syndromes, classically Multiple Endocrine Neoplasias. In this chapter, other rare cancer syndromes that may display NETs as a part of the syndrome's phenotype repertoire are reviewed. In some of them, such as pheochromocytoma-paraganglioma, the presence of NET is crucial for the syndrome diagnosis. In others, such as von Hippel Lindau or Neurofibromatosis, NETs are found in a minorirty of the cases, but their frequency is much higher than seen in the general population, which means that NETs can be the tip of the iceberg of a hereditary cancer syndrome in these families.

Therefore it is important for the physician in care of a NET patient to take a detailed family history not only for other cancers in the extended family but also for peculiar clinical findings in relatives of the patients that could lead to a diagnostic of one of these syndromes.

Keywords Neuroendocrine tumors • Multiple endocrine neoplasias 1 and 2 • von Hippel Lindau • Neurofibromatosis type 1 • Tuberous sclerosis • Carney triad • Carney–Stratakis syndrome • Pheochromocytoma-paraganglioma syndrome

Introduction

Over the past decades, neuroendocrine tumors have been described in families with heritable cancer. Most of the hereditary cancer syndromes displaying neuroendocrine tumors are multiple endocrine neoplasias 1 and 2. Some cases of neuroendocrine

B. Garicochea (✉)
Department of Oncology, Hospital São Lucas, Pontifical Catholic University,
Rua Vitor Meireles 115 AP 201 Av Ipiranga 6690 CJ 708, Porto Alegre, RS 90430160, Brazil
e-mail: bgarico@terra.com.br

J.C. Yao et al. (eds.), *Neuroendocrine Tumors*, Current Clinical Oncology,
DOI 10.1007/978-1-60327-997-0_4, © Springer Science+Business Media, LLC 2011

tumors can be observed in other hereditary syndromes, such as von Hippel Lindau (VHL), neurofibromatosis type 1 (NF1), tuberous sclerosis (TSC), Carney triad, Carney–Stratakis syndrome, and the pheochromocytoma-paraganglioma syndrome (PCC-PGL). In the present chapter, these rare syndromes will be described with emphasis to the presence of neuroendocrine tumors.

von Hippel Lindau Syndrome

VHL (OMIM 193300) is an autosomal dominant disorder resulting from germline mutations in the VHL gene. Clinically, there are two distinguishable types of VHL, based mainly on the presence or absence of pheochromocytoma. Clinical features of the VHL syndrome include the classical retinal (von Hippel) and cerebellar (Lindau) hemangioblastomas [1]. Hemangioblastomas in other neural structures can be observed, such as the brainstem and spine. The syndrome characteristically includes renal cysts, renal cell carcinomas, pancreatic cysts and islet cell tumors, cystadenomas of epididymis, and broad ligament and endolymphatic sac tumors [2]. In the pancreas, cysts are the most common disorder found in VHL (they have been described in as many as 70% of cases in one series of patients). However, endocrine pancreatic tumors can be seen in 11–17% of the cases of VHL and present malignant potential [3]. About 20–30% of VHL type 2 patients present pheochromocytoma. Typically, they are frequently multiple (bilateral adrenal and multifocal extra-adrenal), rarely become malignant, and tend to occur at a younger age than in sporadic cases [2].

Head and neck paragangliomas can be rarely associated to VHL syndrome. It is estimated that 5 in every 1,000 cases of VHL patients will present paragangliomas. Therefore, isolated cases of paraganglioma, a tumor commonly related to other hereditary cancer syndromes, as we will see ahead, should not be a indication for VHL testing unless there are other tumors in the family or in the individual which are part of VHL syndrome [4].

The VHL gene is a tumor suppressor gene located on the short arm of chromosome 3 (3p25–26). Its three exons encode the two isoforms of the VHL protein whose multiple functions are related to the control of vessel production stimulated by tissue hypoxia. The VHL protein migrates from the nucleus to the cytoplasm, where it binds to various proteins, such as elongins B and C, Cul2 and Rbx1, and degrades alpha units of hypoxia inducible factor in an oxygen-dependent manner. Lack of VHL function results in failure to regulate the hypoxia inducible factor, which leads to uncontrolled vascular production. VHL germline mutations are extremely variable, affecting almost any place of the three exons. Missense mutations seem to confer better prognosis and are more commonly detected in patients with pheochromocytoma [5].

The exact molecular mechanisms by which pheochromocytoma and gastroentero-pancreatic (GEP) tumors develop in VHL mutation bearers are unknown. Specifically for GEP neuroendocrine tumors, the analysis of allelic losses spotted genetic loci distinct from and mapping close to VHL, within 3p. It seems that 3p LOH follows VHL mutation in a stepwise manner, and that this genetic aberration may correlate to the progression of GEP neuroendocrine tumor in VHL syndrome [6].

Once the diagnosis of VHL is made, testing is extremely useful to determine which individuals are harboring the mutated allele in the family. For these individuals, the recommendations for screening are empiric. They are based on the age that tumors are observed in VHL mutation carriers and the recurrence rate seen in the ones that had a tumor diagnosed. The same program of screening is recommended for individuals of VHL family that have not been tested. The screening of pheochromocytoma and GEP include yearly clinical examination. Ultrasound of the abdomen should be initiated in childhood. After 20 years of age, CT or MRI of the abdomen should be done yearly. There seems to be no advantage in performing biochemical studies to help in finding subclinical pheochromocytoma, such as plasma or urine analysis of catecholamines and their metabolites in mutation carriers [7]. It is also unclear if surgery is necessary in clinically silent lesions found in screening tests. The wait and scan seems to be a safe option in children, but each case needs to be assessed individually. The treatment (clinical or with radionuclide) of neuroendocrine tumors in VHL syndrome does not differ from sporadic cases [2].

Neurofibromatosis Type 1

NF1 is primarily a mucocutaneous disease caused by autosomal dominant mutation with an incidence of approximately 1 in 3,000 individuals [8]. Approximately one-half of the cases are familial; the remainder are new mutations, which is the highest rate of new mutation of any known single-gene disorder [9].

The NF1 gene was mapped to chromosome 17q11.2 [10]. The gene is large, spanning over 350 kb of genomic DNA. Neurofibromin, the protein encoded by the NF1 gene, is expressed in many tissues, including brain, kidney, spleen, and thymus. So, it is no surprise to observe that mutations in the NF1 gene cause a wide spectrum of clinical findings, including NF1-associated tumors. Mutations in NF1 gene are always involved with loss of function of neurofibromin. The types of mutations include deletions, duplications, insertions, and multiple distinct point mutations, most of them producing a truncated nonfunctional protein [11].

Some phenotypic association can be found with certain types of genetic alterations in NF1. For instance, 1–5% of NF1 patients have large deletions that might include the entire NF1 gene. Such patients have a higher incidence of intellectual disability, dysmorphic facial features, and earlier appearance of neurofibromas [12]. There is no available data linking increased prevalence of malignant or neuroendocrine tumors in patients with large deletions of NF1 gene.

Neurofibromin belongs to a family of GTPase-activating proteins (GAPs) that downregulate a cellular proto-oncogene, p21-ras, an important determinant of cell growth and regulation [13]. Ras uncontrolled activation is a central feature in many human tumors. In NF1 nerve sheath tumors, neurofibromin levels are almost undetectable, suggesting that both alleles of the gene should be inactivated, a typical feature of a tumor-suppressor gene.

The clinical hallmarks of NF1 are the café-au-lait spots and the cutaneous neurofibromas. Many other findings have been related to NF1 syndrome. In 1987, a

Consensus Conference sponsored by the NIH tried to define minimal criteria for the syndrome diagnosis. These criteria have been updated 10 years later. According to this criteria, at least two of the following features must be observed for a clinical diagnosis of NF1: two or more neurofibromas or one plexiform neurofibroma; six or more café-au-lait spots >5 mm in diameter in prepubertal individual and >15 mm in postpubertal; optic glioma; two or more iris hamartomas (Lisch nodules); freckling in the inguinal or axillary regions; a distinctive bony lesion such as sphenoid dysplasia; and a first-degree relative with NF1 based on the same criteria listed [14].

Certain malignancies are typical of NF1, such as optic gliomas and malignant peripheral nerve sheath tumors (neurofibrosarcomas). Others occur more frequently than in the general population. Among those are astrocytomas, brainstem gliomas, rhabdomyosarcomas, gastrointestinal stromal tumor (GIST), nephroblastomas, and chronic myeloid leukemias of childhood.

Reports of GEP-NET in this syndrome are not frequent (they occur in about 1% of NF1 patients), but some types of this neuroendocrine tumor seem to occur in higher frequency than expected. This high frequency is the case in duodenal somatostinomas. These rare tumors display similar histological pattern as their pancreatic counterpart, but seem to be less frequently associated with metastasis at the diagnosis and is seldom related to a somatostatinoma syndrome [15, 16]. More recently, a very rare type of neuroendocrine tumor, mixed endocrine somatostatinoma, was described in association to NF1. Mixed endocrine neoplasias are tumors composed of endocrine and glandular elements [17]. These tumors may be derived from a common cell of both lineages or can arise from two lineages simultaneously. There are less than ten cases described of this disease in the literature, but the presence of a germline mutation with carcinogenic potential such as NF1 may be the explanation of at least some of the cases. Interestingly, there are six reported cases of a combination of GIST and somatostatinomas in patients with NF1, confirming that the NF1 integrity is important for many tissues, and that its deregulation may explain the presence of simultaneous malignancies in cells of distinct lineages [18].

Pheochromocytoma is much more commonly associated with syndromes like VHL or MEN 1, but it rarely presents in NF1 families. Pheochromocytoma is estimated to occur in 0.1–5.7% of patients with NF1, and in 20–50% of NF1 patients with hypertension, compared to 0.1% of all hypertensive individuals [19].

The mean age at diagnosis of pheochromocytoma in patients with NF1, 42 years, is a little earlier than in the general population, but later than the development of the majority of other types of cancer in the bearers of the mutation [20].

Tuberous Sclerosis

TSC (OMIM 191100) is an autosomal dominant disease with very high penetrance but variable phenotypes. It is estimated to affect 1 in every 10,000 individuals. The spontaneous mutation rate is expressively high, in a way that 80% of the cases of TS are sporadic. Only in 20% of the patients can another relative with TSC be found [21].

TSC is caused by mutations in TSC1 or TSC2. TSC1 gene is located in 9q34 and encodes hamartin, a protein of 140 kDa. TSC2 gene is located in 16p13 and encodes tuberin, a 200 kDa protein. These proteins tend to form heterodimers, the hamartin–tuberin complex, which ultimately target downregulating the mammalian target of rapamycin (mTOR) [22]. The complex, by its turn, is regulated negatively by Akt, which specifically phosphorylates the TSC2 protein. The serine-threonine kinase mTOR is involved in multiple cell functions. It stimulates cell growth and proliferation due to activation of *translation initiation factor 4E binding protein 1* (EIF4EBP1); mTOR is also a sensor of cellular energy status, a function that is closely mediated by the TSC1–TSC2 complex. When the cell is in a situation of energy starvation, a tumor suppressor, LKB1, activates AMPK, which in turn phosphorylates tuberin. In this situation, mTOR is downregulated and translation is inhibited, thus saving cell energetic resources. The hamartin–tuberin complex is also regulated by ras-Raf-MEK1/2-ERK1/2 pathway. This is a central signaling pathway for normal and malignant cell proliferation. Mitogen stimulation or oncogenic ras-mutation activates this pathway which phosphorylates tuberin, inactivating the complex TSC1–TSC2. Therefore, when a cell lacks a functional TSC1–TSC2 complex, the result is a continuous pro-proliferative signaling by to mTOR uncontrolled activation and a deficient energy regulation.

Mutations in TSC1 and TSC2 are widely distributed and, presently, no phenotypic correlation has been associated with any of the more than 300 mutations reported. However, it has been observed that patients with TSC1 mutations are less affected clinically than patients with TSC2 mutations [23]. In 20% of the patients who meet the criteria for TSC, no mutation has been identified, suggesting that an alternative gene might be involved [24]. As expected for tumor-suppressor genes, for TSC1 and TSC2 functional inactivation, the compromise of both alleles of either gene is necessary. Most second hits are large deletions causing LOH in the chromosomal area containing the TSC1 or TSC2 gene. These abnormalities have been found associated to angiomyolipomas and rhabdomyomas [25].

Hamartomatous lesions primarily involving the skin, CNS, kidneys, eyes, and heart and lungs are the hallmark of the syndrome, but TSC is actually a systemic disorder which includes a higher prevalence of certain malignancies. The current clinical diagnostic criteria for TSC rely on the presence of major and minor features of the disease as described in Table 4.1 [26].

The diagnosis of TSC can be complex in some cases, especially in cases in which the phenotype is not evident, or in cases of germline mosaicism, in which the parents present no feature of the disorder, but their children do. Therefore, mutational analysis of TSC genes can be provided for affected individuals, even in the case that no familial history is detected due to the possibility that the mutation might recur in future siblings. Some of the TSC features may evolve to life-threatening disorders, such as neurologic, renal, or cardiac abnormalities. Early screening for these organs may be warranted on the basis of expert opinions but, evidently, due to the rarity of the disorder, no solid evidence that frequent screening affects mortality will ever be attained.

The presence of neuroendocrine tumors in TSC is less clear than other malignancies, such as angyomyosarcomas, rhabdomyosarcomas, or renal cell carcinoma.

Table 4.1 Diagnosis of TSC: major and minor features

Major features	
	Facial angioma or forehead plaque
	Nontraumatic ungula or periungual fibroma
	Hypermelanotic macules
	Shagreen patch
	Cortical tuber
	Subependymal nodule
	Subependymal giant cell astrocytoma
	Multiple retinal nodular hamartomas
	Cardiac rhabdomyoma, single or multiple lymphangiomyomatosis
	Renal angiomyolipoma
Minor features	
	Multiple, randomly distributed pits in dental enamel
	Hamartomatous rectal polyps
	Bone cysts
	Cerebral white-matter radial migration lines
	Gengival fibromas
	Nonrectal hamartoma
	Retinal achromic patch
	"Confetti" skin lesions
	Multiple renal cysts

For the definitive diagnosis of TSC: either two major features or one major feature plus two minor
A probable case of TSC presents one major plus one minor feature
A possible case of TSC presents one major or two or more minor features
Adapted from Roach et al. [26]

However, there are several reports in the literature relating coincidental cases of these tumors and TSC. Due to the rarity of TSC and NETs, and the fact that TSC complex pathway alterations are frequently observed in NET, the possibility that NET can be part of the TSC phenotype must be considered. A recent review of the published cases in the last 50 years revealed that a broad range of different NET have been observed in TSC patients, including ACTH, prolactin and GH secreting pituitary adenomas, silent pituitary adenomas, parathyroid adenomas, pheochromocytomas, insulinomas, gastrinomas, pancreatic islet cell neoplasms, and bronchial carcinoid [27]. The most important conclusion of this review is that patients with TSC and with symptoms related to endocrine disorders might be promptly evaluated to NET, since the possibility of concomitance of both disorders is not negligible, even if their phenotypical connection is still not clear.

Hereditary Paraganglioma-Pheochromocytoma Syndromes

Hereditary paraganglioma-pheochromocytoma (PGL/PCC) OMIM 1680001 – PGL/PCC are four genetically different disorders with autosomal dominant heritance. Paragangliomas are tumors that arise from neuroendocrine tissues located in the paravertebral axis. Paragangliomas may exceptionally be found in other tissues, such as the adrenal medulla, causing pheochromocytomas. Sympathetic paragangliomas hypersecrete cathecolamines while parasympathetic are normally silent. Pheochromocytomas are typically secretory tumors in this syndrome. The clinical diagnosis of PGL/PCC syndromes should be strongly considered in individuals with multifocal or recurrent cases, young age at diagnosis (under 40 years), and with family history [28]. Nonetheless, all PGL/PCC patients should be investigated for germline mutations, since many cases present with solitary tumor and with no family history [29]. The presentation of PGL/PCC can be variable but always result from mass effects or high levels of catecholamines, which may be associated with intense sweating, palpitations, anxiety, paroxysmal elevations in blood pressure, and headache. The diagnosis relies on physical examination findings (catecholamine hypersecretion symptoms, arrhythmias, masses in neck, thorax, abdomen, or pelvis) and image exams – especially MRI and CT. MRI is very useful in discriminating between benign adrenal cortical adenomas from chromaffin neoplasms due to the high signal intensity on T2-weighted MRI displayed by the latter [30]. Both methods present equivalent sensitivity and specificity, but for certain paragangliomas, especially in carotid body, ultrasonography coupled with color Doppler might be also very useful. The use of scintigraphy with ^{123}I-metaiodobenzylguanidine (MIBG) or with octreotide may be helpful in suspicious cases in which CT or MRI are negative [31].

PGL/PCC are clinical manifestations of four different genetic syndromes: PGL1, (caused by mutations in SDHD), PGL2 (mutations in SDH5), PGL3 (mutations in SDHC), and PGL4 (mutations in SDHB). The genes SDHB, SDHC, and SDHD code the three subunits of the succinate dehydrogenase enzyme, which catalyzes the conversion of succinate to fumarate in the Krebs cycle [32–34]. The fourth, SDH5, encodes a protein that seems to be crucial for flavination of another SDH subunit, SDHA. Its function is related to the stabilization of the SDH complex [35]. Half of the cases of hereditary PGL/PCC have been associated to mutations in SDHD gene, while 20 and 4% of cases have been attributed, respectively, to SDHB and SDHC [36]. The frequency of cases with mutations in SDH5 is still unknown. Three of these four hereditary paraganglioma syndromes, types 1, 3, and 4, are associated with pheochromocytoma. Mutations in SDH5 (type 2) are extremely rare. The few families described were not reported to present pheochromocytoma [2].

Head and neck paragangliomas are more common than pheochromocytomas in families with PGL1 type. In PGL4, however, the most common tumor is pheochromocytoma, which may occur as a single, multiple, or extra-adrenal lesions. Extra-adrenal abdominal or thoracic tumors were found in 69% of this group of patients [37]. Overall, *SDHB* mutations were associated with a higher rate of malignancy than *SDHD* mutations, with 18 of 48 (37.5%) *SDHB* mutation patients reported with malignancy, as opposed to 2 of 26 (7.7%) *SDHD* mutation patients [37]. In PGL3, both forms of tumors run in the families, but the cases are almost always benign, and the age of onset is similar to the general population with sporadic pheochromocytoma and paraganglioma, differently of PGL1 and PGL4, which affect a younger population [38].

Other tumors were reported in families with paraganglioma syndromes. Renal clear cell carcinoma is related to mutations in the SDHB gene. GIST have been described in families with paragangliomas types 1, 3, and 4. The association of GIST with paraganglioma can produce two types of entities: the Carney triad and the Carney–Stratakis syndrome.

Carney triad (OMIM 604287) is the denomination of the unusual association of three tumors: paragangliomas, GIST, and pulmonary chondroma. A number of other conditions were reported to happen in these patients, such as pheochromocytoma, esophageal leiomyomas, and adrenocortical adenomas. The vast majority of the cases have been described in women. Considered by some authors as a type of multiple endocrine neoplasia, the genetic defect in this disorder is still debatable. A recent report analyzed by CGH in an international series of 37 patients and found a frequent deletion within the 1p13–q21. This region harbors the SDHC gene. Curiously, the chromosomal abnormalities in the tumors of the syndrome showed a very similar pattern revealing a probable common genetic origin [39]. A detailed analysis of the original cohort of patients which defined the Carney triad revealed that some of them presented only GIST and paragangliomas. Moreover, the distribution of the affected phenotype was similar between both sexes. These families actually presented a distinct genetic disorder that was named Carney–Stratakis syndrome (OMIM 606864) [40]. The genetic abnormalities observed so far in the Carney–Stratakis syndrome involve mutations in SDHB, SDHC, and SDHD genes, but not in c-kit and PDGFRA genes, characteristically altered in 90% of sporadic GIST patients. This finding is relevant, since it indicates a novel genetic pathway involved in GIST development beyond the almost universal c-kit and PDGFRA. Also, it indicates that in individuals with GIST with wild-type c-kit and PDGFRA, paragangliomas should be searched for with more attention. Presently, there are no guidelines for genetic counseling or genetic testing for these two diseases.

References

1. Neumann HP, Wiestler OD. Clustering of features of von Hippel-Lindau syndrome: evidence for a complex genetic locus. Lancet. 1991;337:1052–4.
2. Erlic Z, Neumann HPH. Familial pheochromocytoma. Hormones. 2009;8:29–38.
3. Corcos O, Couvelard A, Giraud S, et al. Endocrine pancreatic tumors in von Hippel-Lindau disease: clinical, histological and genetic features. Pancreas. 2008;37:85–93.
4. Boedecker CC, Erlic Z, Richard S, et al. Head and neck paragangliomas in von Hippel-Lindau disease and multiple endocrine neoplasia type 2. J Clin Endocrinol Metab. 2009;94:1938–44.
5. Maher ER, Webster AR, Richards FM, et al. Phenotypic expression in von Hippel-Lindau disease: correlation with germline VHL mutations. J Med Genet. 1996;33:328–32.
6. Lott ST, Chandler DS, Curley SA, et al. High frequency loss of heterozygosity in von Hippel-Lindau (VHL)-associated and sporadic pancreatic islet cell tumors: evidence for a stepwise mechanism for malignant conversion in VHL tumorigenesis. Cancer Res. 2002;62:1952–5.
7. Pczkowska M, Erlic Z, Hoffmann MM, et al. Impact of screening kindreds for SDHDpCys11X as a common mutation associated with paraganglioma syndrome type 1. J Clin Endocrinol Metab. 2008;93:4818–25.
8. Lammert M, Friedman JM, Kluwe L, Mautner VF. Prevalence of neurofibromatosis 1 in German children at elementary school enrollment. Arch Dermatol. 2005;141:71.
9. Theos A, Korf BR; American College of Physicians; American Physiological Society. Pathophysiology of neurofibromatosis type 1. Ann Intern Med. 2006;144:842–9.

10. Ledbetter DH, Rich DC, O'Connell P, et al. Precise localization of NF1 to 17q11.2 by balanced translocation. Am J Hum Genet. 1989;44:20.
11. Shen MH, Harper PS, Upadhyaya M. Molecular genetics of neurofibromatosis type 1 (NF1). J Med Genet. 1996;33:2–17.
12. Tonsgard JH, Yelavarthi KK, Cushner S, et al. Do NF1 gene deletions result in a characteristic phenotype? Am J Med Genet. 1997;73:80–6.
13. Weiss B, Bollag G, Shannon K. Hyperactive Ras as a therapeutic target in neurofibromatosis type 1. Am J Med Genet. 1999;89:14–22.
14. Gutmann DH, Aylsworth A, Carey JC, et al. The diagnostic evaluation and multidisciplinary management of neurofibromatosis 1 and neurofibromatosis 2. JAMA. 1997;278:51–7.
15. Mao C, Shah A, Hanson DJ, Howard JM. Von Recklinghausen's disease associated with duodenal somatostatinoma: contrast of duodenal versus pancreatic somatostatinomas. J Surg Oncol. 1995;59:67–73.
16. Anlauf M, Garbrecht N, Bauersfeld J, et al. Hereditary neuroendocrine tumors of the gastropancreatic system. Virchows Arch. 2007;451:S229–38.
17. Deschemps L, Dokmak S, Guedj N, et al. Mixed endocrine somatostatinoma of the ampulla of Vater associated with a neurofibromatosis type 1: a case report and review of the literature. J Pancreas (Online). 2010;11:64–8.
18. Chetty R, Vajpeyi R. Vasculopatic changes, a somatostatin producing neuroendocrine carcinoma and a jejuna gastrointestinal stromal tumor in a patient with type I neurofibromatosis. Endocr Pathol. 2009;20:177–81.
19. Walther MM, Herring J, Enquist E, Keiser HR, Linehan WM. Von Recklinghausen's disease and pheochromocytomas. J Urol. 1999;162:1582–6.
20. Zografos GN, Vasiliadis GK, Zagouri F, et al. Pheochromocytoma associated with neurofibromatosis type 1: concepts and current trends. World J Surg Oncol. 2010;8:14–7.
21. Rosser T, Panigrahy A, McClintock W. The diverse clinical manifestations of tuberous sclerosis complex: a review. Semin Pediatr Neurol. 2006;13:27–36.
22. Huang J, Manning BD. The TSC1-TSC2 complex: a molecular switchboard controlling cell growth. Biochem J. 2008;412:179–90.
23. Dabora SL, Jozwiak S, Franz DN, et al. Mutational analysis in a cohort of 224 tuberous sclerosis patients indicates increased severity of TSC2, compared to TSC1, disease in multiple organs. Am J Med Genet. 2001;68:64–80.
24. Sancak O, Nellist M, Goedbloed M, et al. Mutational analysis of the TSC1 and TSC2 genes in a diagnostic setting: genotype-phenotype correlations and comparison of diagnostic DNA techniques in tuberous sclerosis complex. Eur J Hum Genet. 2005;13:731–41.
25. Astrinidis A, Henske EP. Tuberous sclerosis complex: linking growth and energy signaling pathways with human disease. Oncogene. 2005;24:7475–81.
26. Roach ES, Gomez M, Rand Northrup H. Tuberous sclerosis complex consensus conference: revised clinical diagnostic criteria. J Child Neurol. 1998;13:624–8.
27. Dworakowska D, Grossman AB. Are neuroendocrine tumours a feature of tuberous sclerosis? A systematic review. Endocr Relat Cancer. 2009;16:45–58.
28. Young Jr WF, Abboud AL. Editorial: paraganglioma – all in the family. J Clin Endocrinol Metab. 2006;91:790–2.
29. Amar L, Bertherat J, Baudin E, et al. Genetic testing in pheochromocytoma and functional paraganglioma. J Clin Oncol. 2005;23:8812–8.
30. Lenders JWM, Eisenhofer G, Mannelli M, Pacak K. Phaeochromocytoma. Lancet. 2005;366: 665–75.
31. Young Jr WF. Endocrine hypertension. In: Kronenberg HM, Melmed S, Polonsky KS, Larsen PR, editors. Williams textbook of endocrinology. 11th ed. Philadelphia, PA: Saunders Elsevier; 2008. p. 505–37.
32. Baysal BE, Ferrell LE, Willett-Brozick JE, et al. Mutations in SDHD, a mitochondrial complex II gene, in hereditary paraganglioma. Science. 2000;287:848–51.
33. Niemann S, Muller U. Mutations in SDHC cause autosomal dominant paraganglioma, type 3. Nat Genet. 2000;26:268–70.

34. Astuti D, Latif F, Dallol A, et al. Gene mutations in the succinate dehydrogenase subunit SDHB cause susceptibility to familial pheochromocytoma and to familial paraganglioma. Am J Hum Genet. 2001;69:49–54.
35. Hao HX, Khalimonchuk O, Schraders M, et al. SDH5, a gene required for flavination of succinate dehydrogenase, is mutated in paraganglioma. Science. 2009;325:1139–42.
36. Baysal BE, Willett-Brozick JE, Lawrence EC, et al. Prevalence of SDHB, SDHC and SDHD germline mutations in clinical patients with head and neck paragangliomas. J Med Genet. 2002;39:178–83.
37. Benn DE, Gimenez-Roqueplo AP, Reilly JR, et al. Clinical presentation and penetrance of pheochromocytoma/paraganglioma syndromes. J Clin Endocrinol Metab. 2006;91:827–36.
38. Baysal BE, Willett-Brozick JE, Filho PA, et al. An Alu-mediated partial SDHC deletion causes familial and sporadic paraganglioma. J Med Genet. 2004;41:703–9.
39. Stratakis CA, Carney JA. The triad of paragangliomas, gastric stromal tumours and pulmonary chondromas (Carney triad), and the dyad of paragangliomas and gastric stromal sarcomas (Carney-Stratakis syndrome): molecular genetics and clinical implications. J Intern Med. 2009;266:43–52.
40. Carney JA, Stratakis CA. Familial paraganglioma and gastric stromal sarcoma: a new syndrome distinct from the Carney triad. Am J Med Genet. 2002;108:132–9.

Chapter 5
Imaging of Neuroendocrine Tumors

Piyaporn Boonsirikamchai, Mohamed Khalaf Aly Asran, and Chusilp Charnsangavej

Abstract Neuroendocrine tumors (NETs) arise from amine precursor uptake and decarboxylation (APUD) cells throughout the nervous and endocrine systems, which produce and secrete regulatory hormones. NETs commonly originate in: (1) argentaffin cells of the gut, resulting in carcinoid tumors, (2) endocrine cells in the pancreas, (3) calcitonin-producing thyroid cells, resulting in medullary thyroid carcinoma (MTC), and (4) parathyroid, adrenal, and pituitary glands. Although NETs are relatively rare and more indolent than other malignancies, occasionally they can be aggressive. Early diagnosis and accurate identification of primary tumors and metastases are necessary to appropriately treat patients before they develop complications from an aggressive disease. Imaging plays an important role in locating primary tumors, staging, and preoperative planning for resection of primary tumor and metastatic disease, and patient monitoring (follow-up). This chapter will focus on imaging modalities commonly used to diagnose and stage NETs with origins primarily in the abdomen, including gastro-intestinal (GI) carcinoids, pancreatic islet-cell tumors, pheochromocytomas, and paragangliomas.

Keywords Neuroendocrine tumors • Medullary thyroid carcinoma • Gastro-intestinal tumors • Pancreatic islet-cell tumors • Pheochromocytomas • Paragangliomas

---

C. Charnsangavej (✉)
Department of Diagnostic Radiology, Division of Diagnostic Imaging, The University of Texas M.D. Anderson Cancer Center, 1400 Pressler, Unit 1473, Houston, TX, USA
e-mail: ccharn@mdanderson.org

J.C. Yao et al. (eds.), *Neuroendocrine Tumors*, Current Clinical Oncology,
DOI 10.1007/978-1-60327-997-0_5, © Springer Science+Business Media, LLC 2011

Introduction

Neuroendocrine tumors (NETs) arise from amine precursor uptake and decarboxylation (APUD) cells throughout the nervous and endocrine systems, which produce and secrete regulatory hormones. NETs commonly originate in: (1) argentaffin cells of the gut, resulting in carcinoid tumors, (2) endocrine cells in the pancreas, (3) calcitonin-producing thyroid cells, resulting in medullary thyroid carcinoma (MTC), and (4) parathyroid, adrenal, and pituitary glands [1]. Although NETs are relatively rare and more indolent than other malignancies, occasionally they can be aggressive. Early diagnosis and accurate identification of primary tumors and metastases are necessary to appropriately treat patients before they develop complications from an aggressive disease. Imaging plays an important role in locating primary tumors, staging, and preoperative planning for resection of primary tumor and metastatic disease, and patient monitoring (follow-up). This chapter will focus on imaging modalities commonly used to diagnose and stage NETs with origins primarily in the abdomen, including gastrointestinal (GI) carcinoids, pancreatic islet-cell tumors, pheochromocytomas, and paragangliomas.

Gastrointestinal Carcinoid Tumors

Carcinoid tumors are slow-growing tumors and constitute only about 2% of all GI tumors [2]. Traditionally, GI carcinoid tumors have been classified based on their embryologic sites of origin: foregut (stomach, duodenum, thyroid, bronchus, biliary tract, and pancreas), midgut (small bowel, appendix, and ascending colon), and hindgut (transverse colon, descending colon, and rectum) [3]. In 2004, the World Health Organization (WHO) proposed a new classification system for gastroentero-pancreatic NETs, based on malignant potential, to help clinicians compare the various types of tumors and accurately predict outcomes [4].

Gastric Carcinoids

Gastric carcinoids are divided into three groups based on their clinical and histological characteristics [5, 6]. Type I is the most common subtype, accounting for 70–80% of all gastric carcinoids, and is associated with chronic atrophic gastritis. The type I tumors are usually small (<1 cm), multicentric, benign, and located predominantly in the fundus and body of the stomach. Type II is the least common subtype and accounts for 5–10% of gastric carcinoids. Type II carcinoids are associated with Zollinger-Ellison syndrome (ZES) or multiple endocrine neoplasia type 1 (MEN-1). Type III subtype occurs sporadically and accounts for 15–25% of gastric carcinoids. The tumors are usually large (>2 cm), solitary lesions with ulcerations and are not associated with hypergastrinemia. They may be aggressive and have a high incidence of metastases.

The diagnosis of type I and type II gastric carcinoids is frequently made using endoscopy and endoscopic ultrasonography (EUS) because most of these type I and II tumors are small and arise in the background of abnormal gastric mucosa. EUS is also very useful for determining layer of origin and depth of mural involvement [7]. The type I and II tumors may present as hypoechoic masses in the submucosal layer with various degrees of invasion into the muscularis propria and serosa [7]. In addition, tissue diagnosis may be made by fine-needle aspiration (FNA) biopsy.

On double-contrast upper GI studies and computed tomography (CT), type I and II gastric carcinoids may present as multiple small polyps located in the gastric fundus or body (Fig. 5.1) and thus be indistinguishable from hyperplastic or adenomatous

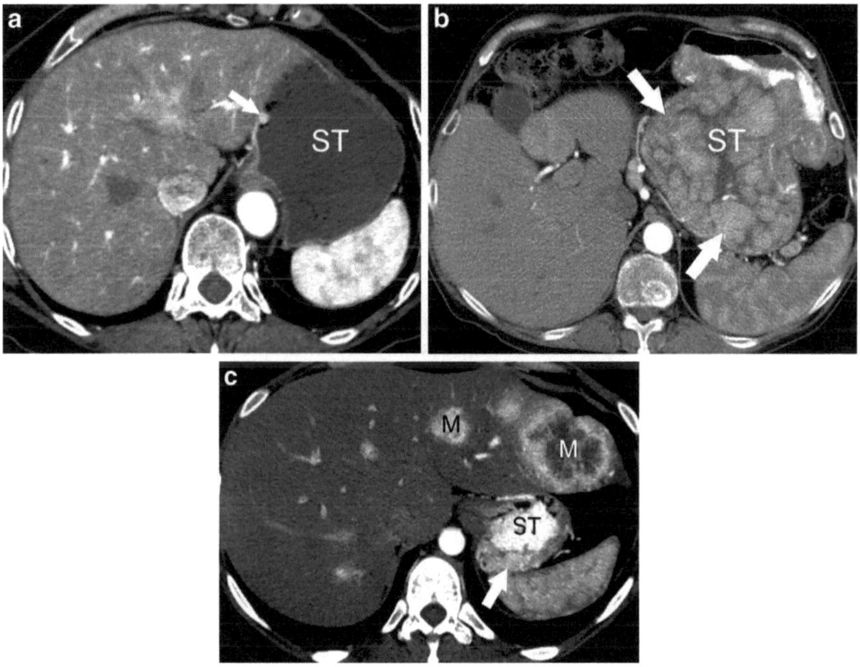

Fig. 5.1 (**a**) Type I gastric carcinoid in a 63-year-old woman who had pancreatic adeonocarcinoma and underwent preoperative CT scan. Contrast-enhanced CT during arterial phase shows a small avidly enhancing nodule (*arrow*) at the lesser curvature of the stomach (ST). Note well-distended stomach with intraluminal water. Endoscopy with biopsy of the nodule at the body of stomach was done and histopathology showed low-grade neuroendocrine tumor involving gastric mucosa with chronic atrophic gastritis. (**b**) Type II gastric carcinoid in a 51-year-old man who had gastrinoma, Zollinger-Ellison syndrome, and MEN-1 and underwent partial gastrectomy with Billroth II reconstruction. Contrast-enhanced CT obtained during arterial phase shows innumerable enhancing varying sized nodules (*arrows*) lining the thickened gastric wall. The diagnosis was made by endoscopic biopsy. (**c**) Type III gastric carcinoid with liver metastases in a 39-year-old woman who presented with abdominal pain, nausea, vomiting, and hematemesis. Contrast-enhanced CT obtaining in arterial phase shows an enhancing infiltrative lesion (*arrow*) at gastric fundus (ST) and multiple enhancing liver metastases (M). The diagnosis was made with upper endoscopic biopsy and liver biopsy

polyps [8]. Type III gastric carcinoids, however, usually appear as a submucosal gastric mass with occasional ulcerations (Fig. 5.1c). Advanced tumors can present as large polypoid masses that simulate polypoid carcinomas. Gastric carcinoids may be enhanced following administration of intravenous (IV) contrast on CT study. The enhanced gastric carcinoids are better seen when the stomach is distended, particularly when water is used as the intraluminal-contrast agent (Fig. 5.1a) [7]. In patients with ZES and MEN-1, diffusely thickened gastric folds and nodular gastric mucosal contours may be visualized and usually shows enhancement during the arterial phase of contrast-enhanced multidetector helical CT (Fig. 5.1b) [9]. Multiple gastric erosions and ulcers may be present. Hypersecretion of gastric fluids may cause flocculation of barium and poor gastric mucosal coating, impeding tumor visualization [9].

Practically, endoscopy and EUS are likely to be the first diagnostic tests performed for patients who have clinical suspicion of gastric carcinoids, particularly for types I and II. CT, magnetic resonance imaging (MRI), and nuclear imaging studies all facilitate tumor staging including nodal and hepatic metastases, which are frequently associated with type III gastric carcinoids.

Small-Bowel Carcinoids

Small-bowel carcinoids occur most commonly in the distal ileum within 60 cm of the ileocecal valve [10, 11]. Up to 30% of patients may have multiple tumors [12]. Metastases to regional lymph nodes and liver are common [13]. Primary tumors are usually small and may not be detectable by imaging studies or even found at surgery, but tumor-associated desmoplastic mesenteric or retroperitoneal fibrosis and metastatic disease frequently is the presenting findings on imaging studies, and may produce intestinal venous ischemia, partial or complete intestinal obstruction, and hydronephrosis.

CT is most commonly used for localization of primary midgut carcinoid tumors and their metastases [13]. When the carcinoid tumors are small and confined to the bowel wall, the tumors are difficult to detect on routine CT scans, particularly when barium is used as the GI contrast agent (Fig. 5.2a). Multidetector CT, which permits faster scanning and thinner beam collimation than conventional CT, can better demonstrate small carcinoid tumors as intensely enhancing submucosal lesions (Fig. 5.2b) [14]. Visualization of these small lesions may be improved by using water or negative intraluminal GI contrast agent (Volumen, E-Z-Em, Inc., Westbury, N.Y.), following a rapid IV bolus of contrast agent and multiplanar reconstruction (Fig. 5.2b) [2]. However, the value of these new CT techniques in detecting primary tumors is still under investigation.

The large tumor (>2 cm) usually invades through the intestinal wall to involve subserosa and adjacent mesentery and then metastasize via the lymphatics to regional lymph nodes (Fig. 5.2a–c) [11]. The infiltrative growth and the local release of serotonin and other substances produced by the tumor cells cause dense fibrosis or desmoplasia to form, particularly in the submucosa and adjacent mesentery. CT is an excellent modality for demonstrating the mesenteric involvement, which typically manifests as an infiltrative mass in the mesentery of the involved bowel segment with characteristic

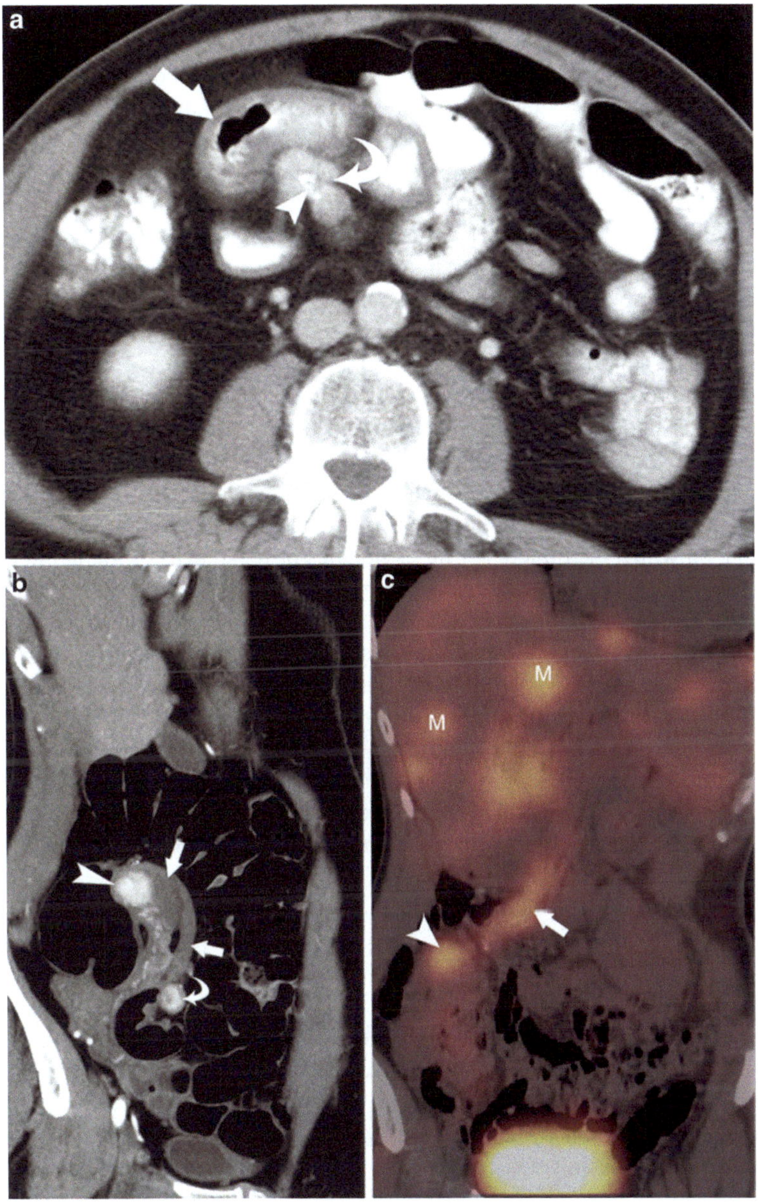

Fig. 5.2 (**a**) Axial CT image demonstrates a thickened segment of ileum (*arrow*) with a fibrotic mass (*curve arrow*) in the mesentery and small calcification (*arrowhead*) due to a carcinoid tumor. (**b**) CT image in an oblique coronal plain defines a hyperdense enhancing nodule (*arrowhead*) in the wall of the terminal ileum (*arrows*) due to a carcinoid tumor. Note is a metastatic node (*curve arrow*) in the mesentery. (**c**) Coronal SPECT image obtained with ^{111}In-octreotide fused with coronal CT (SPECT/CT) demonstrates radiotracer uptake at the ileal carcinoid (*arrowhead*), tumor in the ileocolic vein, and multiple liver metastases (M). The diagnosis was confirmed by surgical resection

radiating dense soft-tissue strands caused by thickened neurovascular bundles (Fig. 5.2a) [15]. A calcified mesenteric mass can be seen (Fig. 5.2a) [15, 16]. The mesenteric vessels may be involved, either directly (as a result of tumor perivascular encasement and venous extension) or indirectly (as a result of the secretion of serotonin that causes fat necrosis and mesenteric fibrosis) [15, 16]. Bowel ischemia may be observed as thickening of the mucosal folds, valvulae conniventes, and small-bowel wall (Fig. 5.2a). Three-dimensional CT angiography using volume rendering is especially useful in these patients with small-bowel carcinoids because of its ability to demonstrate the relationship between tumor and adjacent vascular structures – information that is important for surgical planning [2]. This pattern of small bowel and mesenteric involvement can also be observed in retractile mesenteritis, treated lymphoma, Crohn's disease, and tuberculosis [14].

Similar to CT, MRI may have difficulty visualizing small primary carcinoid tumors of the small bowel .When identified, the tumors may appear as focal, asymmetric bowel-wall thickening with an isointense signal on T1-weighted images and an isointense or mild hyperintense signal on T2-weighted images [7]. The tumors are best visualized on gadolinium-enhanced T1-weighted images obtained with fat suppression, on which the tumors appear as nodules or focal areas of mural thickening with moderately intense gadolinium enhancement [17]. Mesenteric masses range between 2 and 4 cm and are typically isointense to muscle on T1- and T2-weighted images [15]. Desmoplastic stranding manifests as hypointense strands on both T1- and T2-weighted images [18]. Intense enhancement is noted in most patients [15]. Calcification, which is commonly visible on CT, cannot be seen on MRI.

Angiography has a limited role in the diagnosis and localization of carcinoid tumors, as cross-sectional imaging and nuclear scintigraphy have become widely available. Vascular anatomy and the relationship between the tumor and the adjacent major vascular structures can be illustrated by CT or MR angiography.

Appendiceal Carcinoids

The appendix once was the most common site of carcinoid tumors within the GI tract; however, study results have suggested that the incidence of primary appendiceal carcinoid is declining, while the incidence of gastric and rectal carcinoid disease is increasing [11, 19]. This evolution is presumably due to more widespread screening and improvements in diagnostic technology over the last several decades. Carcinoids of the appendix commonly are found incidentally in the pathologic specimen of an appendectomy [20]. These tumors tend to cause symptoms early because of appendiceal luminal obstruction followed by acute appendicitis [15]. Tumor size is the best predictor of prognosis. Typically, most of the tumors are small (<2 cm) and metastases are rare [20]. Approximately one-third of patients with tumors >2 cm present with or develop nodal and distant metastases.

On CT, appendiceal carcinoids may appear as a focal soft-tissue mass within the appendix or as diffuse, circumferential mural thickening [21].

Colorectal Carcinoids

Carcinoid tumors of the colon are very rare, occur more commonly in the right colon, and tend to be large (mean, approximately 5 cm). At the time of diagnosis, 50–60% of patients with colonic carcinoids have metastases to the liver, lymph nodes, or peritoneum. Rectal carcinoids are much more common than colonic carcinoids and their incidence appears to be on the rise, likely due to increased detection related to the widespread use of endoscopy for cancer screening [22]. Rectal carcinoids are often small (<1 cm) with low risk of metastases.

On imaging studies, colorectal carcinoids appears as mural or intraluminal polypoid masses that are indistinguishable from polypoid adenomas or adenocarcinomas [9]. MRI is superior to CT for lesion characterization and, with endoluminal coil, provides high-resolution assessment of the rectal wall layers. Rectal carcinoid is isointense to muscle on T1-weighted images, is isointense to hyperintense on T2-weighted images, and shows homogeneous contrast enhancement [23].

EUS is useful in preoperatively assessing tumor invasion, with a reported accuracy of 90% for localization and staging of colorectal carcinoids [24]. CT, MRI, and somatostatin receptor scintigraphy (SRS) can be helpful for tumor staging, particularly in the larger tumors, which carry a high risk of nodal and distant metastases. The multiplanar and three-dimensional capabilities of CT and MR allow preoperative assessment of the tumor's relationship to adjacent pelvic structures [23].

Hepatic Metastases from Gastrointestinal Carcinoid Tumors

Liver metastases are common, and patients may present with carcinoid syndrome, including flushing, diarrhea, bronchoconstriction, and right-sided heart valve disease [25]. Like the primary tumor, liver metastases are usually hypervascular and are typically well visualized as avidly enhanced masses during the early arterial phase [14]. Multiphasic CT plays an important role in detection of liver metastases. Lesions may be missed if the images are acquired only at the portal venous phase, which is routine for general-purpose scanning, as the tumor become isodense to normal liver parenchyma. In this circumstance, precontrast CT and delayed post contrast images may help demonstrate lesions that show low attenuation in relation to the surrounding liver parenchyma. The appearance of liver metastases on CT can vary. From our experience reviewing CT images, the liver metastases from NETs can appear cystic, which may make it difficult to differentiate the metastases from primary cystic liver tumors, such as biliary cystadenoma or cystadenocarcinoma, or cystic liver metastases from other primary tumor types.

MRI is superior to contrast-enhanced CT in detecting and evaluating liver metastases. Liver metastases have variable appearances on noncontrast MRI, showing hypointensity or isointensity relative to normal liver parenchyma on T1-weighted images and hyperintensity or isointensity on T2-weighted images [17]. The majority of these tumors show moderately intense enhancement during the arterial phase. Larger metastases may become heterogeneously enhanced because of central necrosis, hemorrhage, and degeneration.

Approximately 5% of patients with midgut carcinoids exhibit peritoneal metastases, which may present as miliary peritoneal implants, large masses, or omental cake [26]. Contrast-enhanced CT is superior to MRI for evaluating peritoneal metastases. On MRI, peritoneal metastases are best seen using late postgadolinium fat-suppressed images [17].

Pancreatic Islet-Cell Tumors

Islet-cell tumors are rare neoplasms of the pancreas accounting for approximately 1% of pancreatic cancers by incidence and 10% of pancreatic cancers by prevalence [27]. Islet-cell tumors arise from pancreatic endocrine cells (islets of Langerhans) and can be clinically classified into functioning and nonfunctioning tumors. Functioning islet-cell tumors are usually detected early when they are small because of early clinical manifestation of hormonal overproduction, whereas nonfunctioning tumors are often already large when they are detected.

Insulinoma is the most common functioning endocrine tumor of the pancreas, accounting for approximately 60% of all pancreatic islet-cell tumors, 90% of which are benign [28]. Gastrinoma is the second-most common type of functioning endocrine tumor, accounting for 20–30% of islet-cell tumors, and the majority of these tumors (60%) are malignant. Up to 10% of gastrinomas are extrapancreatic but confined within an anatomic triangle defined superiorly by the common bile duct and cystic duct, inferiorly by the third portion of the duodenum and medially by the pancreatic neck and body. However, gastrinomas in ectopic locations (such as the stomach, mesentery, spleen, and ovaries) have been reported [29, 30]. Associated gastric-wall thickening, indicating peptic ulcer disease and gastric hyperplasia due to effects of gastrin, can bè helpful in diagnosing gastrinoma [28]. The remaining rare functioning islet-cell tumors include glucagonoma, VIPoma, somatostatinoma, and pancreatic polypeptidoma. Islet-cell tumors can occur sporadically or can be associated with some multiple-endocrine organ syndromes such as MEN-1, tuberous sclerosis, von Recklinghausen disease, and von Hippel-Lindau disease.

Imaging of Pancreatic Islet-Cell Tumors

Computed tomography. Generally, a multidetector CT scanner and multiphasic contrast enhancement are required to best evaluate primary tumors and their metastases [14, 31, 32]. Multiphasic contrast enhancement with a dual-phase (arterial and portal venous), triple-phase (early arterial, late arterial, and portal venous), or pancreatic (pancreatic and portal venous) protocol are also recommended for detecting

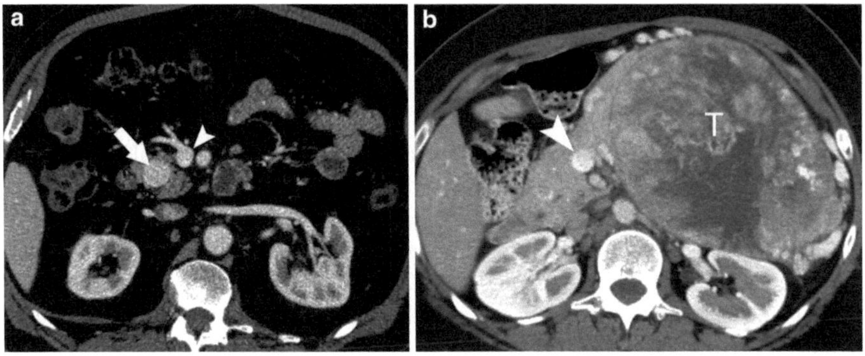

Fig. 5.3 (**a**) Functioning islet cell tumor (insulinoma) in a 65-year-old-man who presented with intermittent profound hypoglycemia. An axial CT image shows a well-defined, hyperdense enhancing tumor (*arrow*) in the head of the pancreas in a patient with an insulinoma. The tumor is clearly separable from the superior mesenteric vein (*arrowhead*). (**b**) Nonfunctioning islet cell tumor in a 38-year-old-woman who presented with palpable mass at left-sided abdomen. Axial CT demonstrates a large, nonfunctioning islet cell tumor (T) in the tail of the pancreas. Note the mixed areas of tumor necrosis and solid-enhancing nodules. The tumor grows into the splenic vein (not shown), but the superior mesenteric vein is patent (*arrowhead*)

the characteristic early arterial enhancement of islet-cell tumors. Maximizing the contrast between the tumor and the adjacent normal parenchyma is particularly important when trying to localize small islet-cell tumors (Fig. 5.3a). A negative oral contrast agent such as water allows optimum visualization of the duodenum, improving the detection of duodenal gastrinomas [33].

Functioning islet-cell tumors, insulinomas, and gastrinomas are usually small (with an average size of <2 cm for insulinomas and 4 cm for gastrinomas) and can occur in multiples. The characteristic appearance of small functioning islet-cell tumors is of a homogeneous-enhancing mass during the arterial and pancreatic or portal venous phases of imaging (Fig. 5.3a). Islet-cell tumors can have a cystic appearance, which sometimes may be difficult to differentiate from cystic lesions such as pseudocysts, mucinous cystadenomas, or serous cystadenomas [34, 35]. The larger functioning tumors may exhibit more postcontrast heterogeneity than smaller tumors, with central necrosis and ring-like enhancement [32]. The other rare functioning tumors, such as glucagonomas and somatostatinomas, are typically larger and have features that mimic nonfunctioning tumors.

Nonfunctioning islet-cell tumors tend to be large (4–24 cm) and heterogeneous, and they may contain cystic areas of degeneration and necrosis (Fig. 5.3b) [34, 36, 37]. Nonfunctioning tumors are detected more easily by mass effect than are functioning tumors, and they may cause pancreatic or bile duct obstruction. In our experience, we have seen tumor extension into the pancreatic duct. Enhancing tumor thrombus has been reported and is more suggestive of an islet-cell tumor than of a pancreatic ductal carcinoma. Approximately 20% of islet-cell tumors demonstrate calcification on imaging [29]. Nodal and liver metastases are commonly present [36, 37]. Peritoneal carcinomatosis is relatively rare.

The overall sensitivity of multidetector CT for the detection of functioning islet-cell tumors ranges from 64 to 82% [31–33]. False-negatives can occur when tumors are very small, adjacent to vessels, pedunculated in their morphology, and nonenhancing [31].

Magnetic resonance imaging. MRI offers the advantage of greater soft-tissue contrast than CT and increasingly has been used in pancreatic imaging. Generally, islet-cell tumors show low signal intensity on T1-weighted images and high signal intensity on T2-weighted images [38]. Islet-cell tumors are well visualized on T1- and T2-weighted images with fat suppression [28]. Small functioning islet-cell tumors typically enhance homogeneously on immediate postgadolinium images [29]. Large tumors (>2 cm) often enhance heterogeneously or show ring enhancement [31].

Liver metastases typically show low signal intensity on T1-weighted images, moderately high signal intensity on T2-weighted images with fat suppression, and moderately intense enhancement during the hepatic arterial phase. Precontrast T1- and T2-weighted images do not have the problem of variations in the timing of phases of contrast enhancement and therefore provide another useful technique for measuring lesions to assess treatment response.

Paraganglioma and Pheochromocytoma

Paragangliomas are rare NETs that arise from paraganglionic tissue derived from neural crest and chromaffin cells of the APUD system. Paraganglionic tissues are distributed from the base of the skull to the pelvic floor. These tissues are found in the adrenal medulla, sympathetic and parasympathetic ganglia along the prevertebral and paravertebral sympathetic chains, and connective tissue in or near the wall of the pelvic organs. In 2004, the WHO classification of endocrine tumors defined a pheochromocytoma as an intra-adrenal paraganglioma, whereas tumors of extra-adrenal sympathetic or parasympathetic paraganglia were classified as extra-adrenal paragangliomas [39].

Extra-adrenal paragangliomas account for approximately 10–20% of catecholamine-producing paragangliomas, up to 80% of which are in the abdomen and the remainder of which are in the chest or neck. Common locations include the organ of Zuckerkandl, bladder wall, retroperitoneum, paracardiac region, and carotid and glomus jugulare bodies.

Paragangliomas are associated with several familial syndromes, including MEN-2A, MEN-2B, neurofibromatosis type 1, von Hippel-Lindau (VHL) disease, Carney's triad, and familial paragangliomas [40]. Pheochromocytomas are frequently functioning, whereas extra-adrenal paraganglioma may be functioning (producing catecholamines) or nonfunctioning. Malignant pheochromocytomas and paragangliomas are uncommon, and their metastases typically affect the bones, liver, lungs, and lymph nodes [41].

The diagnosis of pheochromocytoma is based on the elevation of catecholamines and metabolites in plasma or a 24-h urine specimen. After confirming the clinical diagnosis of pheochromocytoma, imaging studies are an important part of localizing the tumor and determining its extent for effective treatment planning.

Adrenal Pheochromocytoma

MRI has been used increasingly because of its multiplanar capability, high sensitivity for contrast enhancement, and lack of ionizing radiation [42]. MRI protocol should consist of a coronal localizer pulse sequence followed by axial spin-echo T1-weighted and axial fast spin-echo T2-weighted scans. Imaging in the coronal and sagittal planes helps to show invasion by large lesions into adjacent structures. Paramagnetic contrast media are commonly used because most pheochromytomas are hypervascular and are brightly enhanced during the early phase of contrast enhancement.

On MRI, pheochromocytomas typically exhibit high signal intensity on T2-weighted imaging, best appreciated with the use of fat suppression [43]. These pheochromocytomas can be heterogeneous and may demonstrate areas of cystic, necrotic, hemorrhagic, or calcific degeneration. Although the classic T2-weighted appearance of these tumors has been described as a light bulb-bright signal, this sign is neither specific nor sensitive and the use of this sign alone thus may lead to the misdiagnosis of pheochromocytoma in up to 35% of cases [44]. Pheochromocytomas usually enhance minimally on immediate postgadolinium images and demonstrate progressive enhancement on later interstitial-phase images, although relatively intense early enhancement may be observed.

On CT, pheochromocytomas are seen as rounded or oval masses of density similar to that of the surrounding soft-tissue structures on noncontrast scans. Scattered parenchymal calcification can be observed in about 10% of the tumors. The tumor tends to be large (mean, 5 cm) and then often shows central necrosis and cystic appearance [45, 46]. Most tumors enhance markedly after administration of IV contrast material (Fig. 5.4). Multiphasic CT also has the potential to demonstrate arterial supply and venous drainage of the pheochromocytoma for proper preoperative planning. When ionic contrast media are used, alpha-adrenergic blockade is necessary to prevent a hypertensive crisis. No blockade is necessary with nonionic contrast media.

Extra-Adrenal Paragangliomas

On contrast-enhanced CT scans, extra-adrenal paragangliomas appear as paraaortic hypervascular soft-tissue masses that are either homogeneous (Fig. 5.5) or have central areas of low attenuation [47, 48]. Smaller tumors are more likely to be homogeneous in attenuation and sharply marginated than are larger tumors. Punctate calcification or focal areas of high attenuation caused by acute hemorrhage may be seen in some tumors.

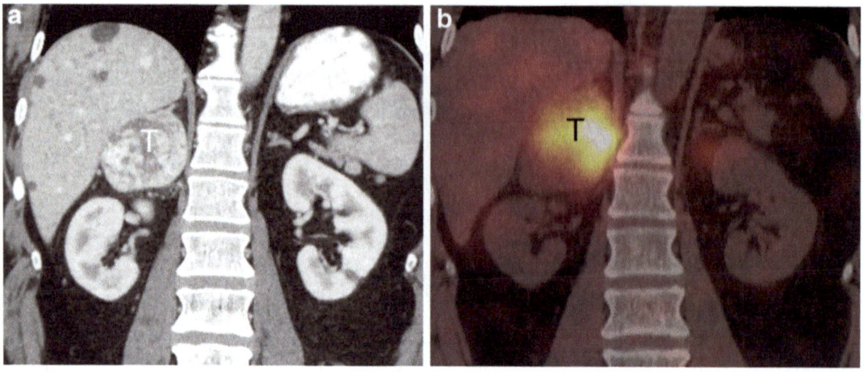

Fig. 5.4 (**a**) Adrenal pheochromocytoma in a 53-year-old-man who underwent CT staging for prostate cancer and was found to have right adrenal mass. A coronal view of CT after intravenous contrast enhancement shows a hyperdense-enhancing tumor (T) in the right adrenal gland. Multiple cysts were noted in the liver. (**b**) Coronal SPECT image obtained with ^{123}I-MIBG fused with coronal CT demonstrates radiotracer uptake at the right adrenal mass (T), compatible with a pheochromocytoma. Note normal left adrenal gland. The diagnosis was confirmed by biochemical profile and surgical resection

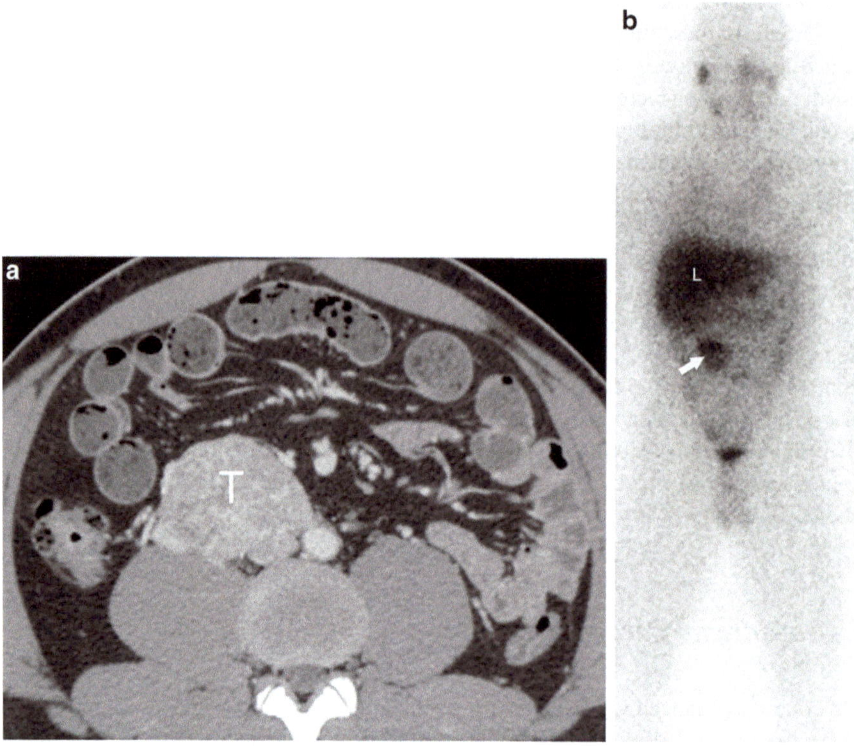

Fig. 5.5 (**a**) Paraganglioma in a 26-year-old-man who had hypertension and presented with ischemic cerebrovascular accident. Axial CT image after intravenous contrast administration shows a hyperdense enhancing tumor (T) in the retroperitoneum anterior to the inferior vena cava. (**b**) Anterior whole-body image obtained with ^{123}I-MIBG shows radiotracer uptake at the right retroperitoneal mass (*arrows*), compatible with extraadrenal paraganglioma. The diagnosis was confirmed by biochemical profile and surgical resection. L = liver

Extra-adrenal paragangliomas are usually hypointense or isointense to the liver parenchyma on T1-weighted MR images and are markedly hyperintense on T2-weighted MR images [49]. Similar to tumors of adrenal origin, extra-adrenal paragangliomas show marked enhancement, which may be either homogeneous or heterogeneous enhancement depending on whether the tumor contains cystic or necrotic areas.

Radionuclide Imaging

Radionuclide imaging provides functional information about the tumors, which is often complementary to anatomical information obtained from conventional diagnostic imaging. These functional images are useful not only in localization of primary tumors and their metastases but also in evaluation of prognosis and response to therapy. The three most commonly used radionuclide imaging techniques for NETs are SRS, positron-emission tomography (PET), and radiolabeled metaiodobenzylguanidine (^{123}I-MIBG) scintigraphy.

Somatostatin Receptor Scintigraphy (SRS)

Somatostatin is a peptide hormone that inhibits hormone synthesis of neuroendocrine cells [50]. Somatostatin binds to the somatostatin receptors, which are structurally related membrane glycoproteins that are highly expressed in NETs [51–53]. Theoretically, radionuclide-labeled somatostatin could bind to NETs and thereby facilitate the identification and imaging of the tumors and their metastases [53]. However, because of the instability and short biological half-life of the radiolabeled somatostatin in the circulation, the long-acting somatostatin analog (octreotide) was developed [53]. Of the five subtypes of somatostatin receptors, octreotide binds with high affinity to receptor subtypes 2 and 5, which are present on the majority (>80%) of NETs [54].

SRS has been used widely to manage carcinoid tumors, and ^{111}Indium (In) pentetreotide is the most commonly used radioactively labeled octreotide [55]. SRS has been used for diagnosis, localization, and staging of primary or recurrent carcinoid tumors, prediction of tumor response to octreotide analog therapy, and as a therapeutic guide for Y-90 octreotide or analogs. The sensitivity of SRS has been estimated to be in the range of 80–90% in patients with asymptomatic GI NETs and more than 90% in patients with symptoms of carcinoid syndrome [55–57].

SRS can also detect islet-cell tumors with the sensitivity of approximately 50% for insulinomas and 80–90% for other tumors. Failure to visualize some insulinomas may be related to higher affinity binding for somatostatin receptor type 3 than for types 2 or 5. Pancreatic adenocarcinomas typically are not detected on SRS.

The sensitivity of SRS can be affected by the administered peptide dose, the duration of image acquisition, and the use of single photon emission computed tomography (SPECT) [52]. Since the resolution of scintigraphy is poor, the use of SPECT or SPECT-CT fusion have been shown to improve sensitivity of SRS [52].

Poorly differentiated NETs usually do not have somatostatin receptors, so they cannot be reliably imaged with SRS [58]. However, their poor differentiation and high proliferative rate are associated with increased use of glucose, which makes F-labeled fluorodeoxyglucose positron emission tomography (FDG-PET), a highly accurate imaging method for localizing and detecting metastases [59, 60].

NETs may remain visible during treatment with octreotide, although the tumor uptake may be up to 50% less than tumor uptake without octreotide treatment. Octreotide therapy must be discontinued 72 h before injection of ^{111}In pentetreotide because octreotide and ^{111}In pentetreotide competitively bind to somatostatin receptors, thereby decreasing the sensitivity of imaging with ^{111}In pentetreotide [53].

Metaiodobenzylguanidine Scintigraphy

Metaiodobenzylguanidine (MIBG) is a norepinephrine analog, and ^{131}I- and ^{123}I-MIBG have been used widely for the diagnosis of pheochromocytoma and paraganglioma (Figs. 5.4 and 5.5). ^{123}I-MIBG achieves better image quality, greater sensitivity, and reduced radiation exposure because of higher photon flow and shorter half-life. However, ^{131}I-MIBG is still commonly used because of lower cost and possibility of obtaining delayed scans. MIBG has high specificity and ability to detect both primary tumors and metastatic lesions when compared with morphologic imaging methods such as CT and MRI [61]. The overall sensitivity of MIBG for the detection of pheochromocytoma ranges from 90 to 95% with a specificity up to 99%.

F-Labeled Fluorodeoxyglucose Positron Emission Tomography (FDG-PET)

FDG-PET imaging is not useful in low-grade NETs because the tumors are well-differentiated, slow growing, and have a low metabolic rate [58]. Recent advances in developing PET radiotracers, such as carbon 11-5-hydroxyl tryptophan, copper 64-tetraazocyclotetradecane octreotide, fluorodopa F 18 (18 F-DOPA) [62], and gallium 68-tetraazocyclododecane tetraacetic acid octreotide (^{68}GA-DOTATOC) [63], have shown potential for evaluating NETs with better result than with SRS. However, these radiotracers are available only in a few highly specialized centers.

Imaging Evaluation of Patients with Metastatic Neuroendocrine Tumors of Unknown Primary

Patients with NETs may present with metastatic disease such as hepatic metastases, lymph node metastases, or pulmonary metastases. Tissue diagnosis from the metastatic site and biochemical markers may be confirmed as a NET, but the primary site of tumors may not be apparent at presentation. In such circumstances, we recommend mutiphasic, thin-section (3 mm or less), multidetector helical CT with pancreatic protocol using water as oral contrast to search for a primary in the pancreas. We also use multiphasic, helical CT with water or Volumen® (E-Z-Em, Inc., Westbury, N.Y.) as a negative enteric contrast agent for the small bowel, and chest CT to detect small carcinoid tumors in those patients with carcinoid syndrome. Somatostatin receptor SPECT-CT (Octreoscan) may also be used to localize the primary tumor.

Summary

Imaging plays an important role in preoperative localization of primary NETs and detection of their metastases. The majority of the primary tumors and metastases are hypervascular and some can be small, which requires careful attention to imaging technique. At this time, no single imaging modality exists that is 100% effective. The contribution of each imaging technique varies according to the primary tumor site. Moreover, the cost, availability, and local expertise should be considered when choosing an imaging method.

References

1. National Comprehensive Cancer Network. Clinical Practice Guidelines in Oncology: Neuroendocrine Tumors V.2.2009.
2. Horton KM, Kamel I, Hofmann L, Fishman EK. Carcinoid tumors of the small bowel: a multitechnique imaging approach. AJR Am J Roentgenol. 2004;182:559–67.
3. Williams ED, Sandler M. The classification of carcinoid tum ours. Lancet. 1963;1(7275):238–9.
4. Oberg K, Astrup L, Eriksson B, et al. Guidelines for the management of gastroenteropancreatic neuroendocrine tumours (including bronchopulmonary and thymic neoplasms). Part II-specific NE tumour types. Acta Oncol. 2004;43:626–36.
5. Borch K, Ahren B, Ahlman H, Falkmer S, Granerus G, Grimelius L. Gastric carcinoids: biologic behavior and prognosis after differentiated treatment in relation to type. Ann Surg. 2005;242:64–73.
6. Delle Fave G, Capurso G, Annibale B, Panzuto F. Gastric neuroendocrine tumors. Neuroendocrinology 2004;80 Suppl 1:16–19.
7. Gore RM, Berlin JW, Mehta UK, Newmark GM, Yaghmai V. GI carcinoid tumours: appearance of the primary and detecting metastases. Best Pract Res Clin Endocrinol Metab. 2005;19:245–63.
8. Gourtsoyiannis N, Grammatikakis J, Prassopoulos P. Role of conventional radiology in the diagnosis and staging of gastrointestinal tract neoplasms. Semin Surg Oncol. 2001;20:91–108.

9. Levy AD, Sobin LH. From the archives of the AFIP: Gastrointestinal carcinoids: imaging features with clinicopathologic comparison. Radiographics. 2007;27:237–57.
10. Kulke MH, Mayer RJ. Carcinoid tumors. N Engl J Med. 1999;340:858–68.
11. Modlin IM, Lye KD, Kidd M. A 5-decade analysis of 13,715 carcinoid tumors. Cancer. 2003;97:934–59.
12. Moertel CG, Sauer WG, Dockerty MB, Baggenstoss AH. Life history of the carcinoid tumor of the small intestine. Cancer. 1961;14:901–12.
13. Sippel RS, Chen H. Carcinoid tumors. Surg Oncol Clin N Am. 2006;15:463–78.
14. Tamm EP, Kim EE, Ng CS. Imaging of neuroendocrine tumors. Hematol Oncol Clin North Am. 2007;21:409–32.
15. Chang S, Choi D, Lee SJ, et al. Neuroendocrine neoplasms of the gastrointestinal tract: classification, pathologic basis, and imaging features. Radiographics. 2007;27:1667–79.
16. Pantongrag-Brown L, Buetow PC, Carr NJ, Lichtenstein JE, Buck JL. Calcification and fibrosis in mesenteric carcinoid tumor: CT findings and pathologic correlation. AJR Am J Roentgenol. 1995;164:387–91.
17. Bader TR, Semelka RC, Chiu VC, Armao DM, Woosley JT. MRI of carcinoid tumors: spectrum of appearances in the gastrointestinal tract and liver. J Magn Reson Imaging. 2001;14:261–9.
18. Kim KW, Ha HK. MRI for small bowel diseases. Semin Ultrasound CT MR. 2003;24:387–402.
19. Modlin IM, Lye KD, Kidd M. A 50-year analysis of 562 gastric carcinoids: small tumor or larger problem? Am J Gastroenterol. 2004;99:23–32.
20. Kvols L. Carcinoids of the appendix. Neuroendocrinology. 2004;80 Suppl 1:33–4.
21. Pickhardt PJ, Levy AD, Rohrmann Jr CA, Kende AI. Primary neoplasms of the appendix: radiologic spectrum of disease with pathologic correlation. Radiographics. 2003;23:645–62.
22. Yao JC, Hassan M, Phan A, et al. One hundred years after "carcinoid": epidemiology of and prognostic factors for neuroendocrine tumors in 35,825 cases in the United States. J Clin Oncol. 2008;26:3063–72.
23. Rouse HC, Godoy MC, Lee WK, Phang PT, Brown CJ, Brown JA. Imaging findings of unusual anorectal and perirectal pathology: a multi-modality approach. Clin Radiol. 2008;63:1350–60.
24. Yoshida M, Tsukamoto Y, Niwa Y, et al. Endoscopic assessment of invasion of colorectal tumors with a new high-frequency ultrasound probe. Gastrointest Endosc. 1995;41:587–92.
25. Robiolio PA, Rigolin VH, Wilson JS, et al. Carcinoid heart disease. Correlation of high serotonin levels with valvular abnormalities detected by cardiac catheterization and echocardiography. Circulation. 1995;92:790–5.
26. Modlin IM, Kidd M, Latich I, Zikusoka MN, Shapiro MD. Current status of gastrointestinal carcinoids. Gastroenterology. 2005;128:1717–51.
27. Yao JC, Eisner MP, Leary C, et al. Population-based study of islet cell carcinoma. Ann Surg Oncol. 2007;14:3492–500.
28. Rha SE, Jung SE, Lee KH, Ku YM, Byun JY, Lee JM. CT and MR imaging findings of endocrine tumor of the pancreas according to WHO classification. Eur J Radiol. 2007;62:371–7.
29. Noone TC, Hosey J, Firat Z, Semelka RC. Imaging and localization of islet-cell tumours of the pancreas on CT and MRI. Best Pract Res Clin Endocrinol Metab. 2005;19:195–211.
30. Norton JA, Alexander HR, Fraker DL, Venzon DJ, Gibril F, Jensen RT. Possible primary lymph node gastrinoma: occurrence, natural history, and predictive factors: a prospective study. Ann Surg. 2003;237:650–7. discussion 657–659.
31. Fidler JL, Fletcher JG, Reading CC, et al. Preoperative detection of pancreatic insulinomas on multiphasic helical CT. AJR Am J Roentgenol. 2003;181:775–80.
32. Sheth S, Hruban RK, Fishman EK. Helical CT of islet cell tumors of the pancreas: typical and atypical manifestations. AJR Am J Roentgenol. 2002;179:725–30.
33. Van Hoe L, Gryspeerdt S, Marchal G, Baert AL, Mertens L. Helical CT for the preoperative localization of islet cell tumors of the pancreas: value of arterial and parenchymal phase images. AJR Am J Roentgenol. 1995;165:1437–9.
34. Buetow PC, Parrino TV, Buck JL, et al. Islet cell tumors of the pancreas: pathologic-imaging correlation among size, necrosis and cysts, calcification, malignant behavior, and functional status. AJR Am J Roentgenol. 1995;165:1175–9.

35. Ahrendt SA, Komorowski RA, Demeure MJ, Wilson SD, Pitt HA. Cystic pancreatic neuroendocrine tumors: is preoperative diagnosis possible? J Gastrointest Surg. 2002;6:66–74.
36. Eelkema EA, Stephens DH, Ward EM, Sheedy 2nd PF. CT features of nonfunctioning islet cell carcinoma. AJR Am J Roentgenol. 1984;143:943–8.
37. Stafford-Johnson DB, Francis IR, Eckhauser FE, Knol JA, Chang AE. Dual-phase helical CT of nonfunctioning islet cell tumors. J Comput Assist Tomogr. 1998;22:335–9.
38. Kraus BB, Ros PR. Insulinoma: diagnosis with fat-suppressed MR imaging. AJR Am J Roentgenol. 1994;162:69–70.
39. Havekes B, van der Klaauw AA, Weiss MM, et al. Pheochromocytomas and extra-adrenal paragangliomas detected by screening in patients with SDHD-associated head-and-neck paragangliomas. Endocr Relat Cancer. 2009;16:527–36.
40. Sahdev A, Sohaib A, Monson JP, Grossman AB, Chew SL, Reznek RH. CT and MR imaging of unusual locations of extra-adrenal paragangliomas (pheochromocytomas). Eur Radiol. 2005;15:85–92.
41. Takano A, Oriuchi N, Tsushima Y, et al. Detection of metastatic lesions from malignant pheochromocytoma and paraganglioma with diffusion-weighted magnetic resonance imaging: comparison with 18 F-FDG positron emission tomography and 123I-MIBG scintigraphy. Ann Nucl Med. 2008;22:395–401.
42. Elsayes KM, Narra VR, Leyendecker JR, Francis IR, Lewis Jr JS, Brown JJ. MRI of adrenal and extraadrenal pheochromocytoma. AJR Am J Roentgenol. 2005;184:860–7.
43. Blake MA, Kalra MK, Maher MM, et al. Pheochromocytoma: an imaging chameleon. Radiographics. 2004;24 Suppl 1:S87–99.
44. Varghese JC, Hahn PF, Papanicolaou N, Mayo-Smith WW, Gaa JA, Lee MJ. MR differentiation of phaeochromocytoma from other adrenal lesions based on qualitative analysis of T2 relaxation times. Clin Radiol. 1997;52:603–6.
45. Welch TJ, Sheedy 2nd PF, van Heerden JA, Sheps SG, Hattery RR, Stephens DH. Pheochromocytoma: value of computed tomography. Radiology. 1983;148:501–3.
46. Mukherjee JJ, Peppercorn PD, Reznek RH, et al. Pheochromocytoma: effect of nonionic contrast medium in CT on circulating catecholamine levels. Radiology. 1997;202:227–31.
47. Lee KY, Oh YW, Noh HJ, et al. Extraadrenal paragangliomas of the body: imaging features. AJR Am J Roentgenol. 2006;187:492–504.
48. Hayes WS, Davidson AJ, Grimley PM, Hartman DS. Extraadrenal retroperitoneal paraganglioma: clinical, pathologic, and CT findings. AJR Am J Roentgenol. 1990;155:1247–50.
49. van Gils AP, Falke TH, van Erkel AR, et al. MR imaging and MIBG scintigraphy of pheochromocytomas and extraadrenal functioning paragangliomas. Radiographics. 1991;11:37–57.
50. Kvols LK. Somatostatin-receptor imaging of human malignancies: a new era in the localization, staging, and treatment of tumors. Gastroenterology. 1993;105:1909–11.
51. Gibril F, Reynolds JC, Doppman JL, et al. Somatostatin receptor scintigraphy: its sensitivity compared with that of other imaging methods in detecting primary and metastatic gastrinomas. A prospective study. Ann Intern Med. 1996;125:26–34.
52. Lamberts SW, Bakker WH, Reubi JC, Krenning EP. Somatostatin-receptor imaging in the localization of endocrine tumors. N Engl J Med. 1990;323:1246–9.
53. Intenzo CM, Jabbour S, Lin HC, et al. Scintigraphic imaging of body neuroendocrine tumors. Radiographics. 2007;27:1355–69.
54. de Herder WW, Hofland LJ, van der Lely AJ, Lamberts SW. Somatostatin receptors in gastroentero-pancreatic neuroendocrine tumours. Endocr Relat Cancer. 2003;10:451–8.
55. Oberg K, Kvols L, Caplin M, et al. Consensus report on the use of somatostatin analogs for the management of neuroendocrine tumors of the gastroenteropancreatic system. Ann Oncol. 2004;15:966–73.
56. Kwekkeboom DJ, Krenning EP. Somatostatin receptor imaging. Semin Nucl Med. 2002;32:84–91.
57. Ramage JK, Davies AH, Ardill J, et al. Guidelines for the management of gastroenteropancreatic neuroendocrine (including carcinoid) tumours. Gut. 2005;54 Suppl 4:1–16.

58. Ezziddin S, Logvinski T, Yong-Hing C, et al. Factors predicting tracer uptake in somatostatin receptor and MIBG scintigraphy of metastatic gastroenteropancreatic neuroendocrine tumors. J Nucl Med. 2006;47:223–33.
59. Pasquali C, Rubello D, Sperti C, et al. Neuroendocrine tumor imaging: can 18 F-fluorodeoxyglucose positron emission tomography detect tumors with poor prognosis and aggressive behavior? World J Surg. 1998;22:588–92.
60. Rambaldi PF, Cuccurullo V, Briganti V, Mansi L. The present and future role of (111)In pentetreotide in the PET era. Q J Nucl Med Mol Imaging. 2005;49:225–35.
61. van der Harst E, de Herder WW, Bruining HA, et al. [(123)I]metaiodobenzylguanidine and [(111)In]octreotide uptake in begnign and malignant pheochromocytomas. J Clin Endocrinol Metab. 2001;86:685–93.
62. Hoegerle S, Altehoefer C, Ghanem N, et al. Whole-body 18 F dopa PET for detection of gastrointestinal carcinoid tumors. Radiology. 2001;220:373–80.
63. Bohuslavizki KH. Somatostatin receptor imaging: current status and future perspectives. J Nucl Med. 2001;42:1057–8.

Chapter 6
Surgical Management of Sporadic Gastrointestinal Neuroendocrine Tumors

Glenda G. Callender and Jason B. Fleming

Abstract Sporadic neuroendocrine tumors of the gut and pancreas are relatively uncommon, and are generally considered to be slow-growing and indolent. However, these tumors can result in significant morbidity related to hormone overproduction, and are sometimes aggressive and treatment-resistant. Surgical therapy forms a critical component of the multidisciplinary treatment of patients with primary neuroendocrine tumors, and can often play a role in the management of metastatic disease. The purpose of this chapter is to discuss the surgical management of carcinoid tumors and pancreatic islet cell carcinomas that occur in the absence of an inherited syndrome.

Keywords Hormone overproduction • Surgical therapy • Metastatic disease • Carcinoid tumors • Pancreatic islet cell tumors

Introduction

Sporadic neuroendocrine tumors of the gut and pancreas are relatively uncommon, and are generally considered to be slow-growing and indolent. However, these tumors can result in significant morbidity related to hormone overproduction, and are sometimes aggressive and treatment-resistant. Surgical therapy forms a critical component of the multidisciplinary treatment of patients with primary neuroendocrine tumors, and can often play a role in the management of metastatic disease. The purpose of this chapter is to discuss the surgical management of carcinoid tumors and pancreatic islet cell carcinomas that occur in the absence of an inherited syndrome.

J.B. Fleming (✉)
Department of Surgical Oncology, The University of Texas
M.D. Anderson Cancer Center, Houston, TX 77030, USA
e-mail: jbflemin@mdanderson.org

J.C. Yao et al. (eds.), *Neuroendocrine Tumors*, Current Clinical Oncology,
DOI 10.1007/978-1-60327-997-0_6,

Carcinoid Tumors

The term "Karzinoide" (carcinoma-like) was first used by Oberndorfer in 1907 to describe tumors of the gastrointestinal tract that were more indolent than adenocarcinomas [1]. Today, the term "carcinoid" simply cannot convey the diverse range of tumor types and secreted hormones that can originate from neuroendocrine cells throughout the gut. The WHO classification utilizes the term *neuroendocrine tumor* to describe tumors of benign behavior or uncertain malignant potential, and distinguishes this from *neuroendocrine carcinoma* which can be well-differentiated (low-grade malignancy) or poorly differentiated (high-grade malignancy). Essentially, *carcinoid* is synonymous with *neuroendocrine tumor*, and *malignant carcinoid* is synonymous with *neuroendocrine carcinoma* [2].

Carcinoid tumors are commonly classified based upon their site of origin in the embryonic gut. Foregut tumors include bronchial and gastric carcinoid tumors; midgut tumors include carcinoid tumors of the small intestine and appendix; and hindgut tumors include colon and rectal carcinoid tumors. A recent analysis of 10,878 carcinoid tumors from the Surveillance, Epidemiology, and End Result Program (SEER) demonstrated that 28% of carcinoid tumors originate in the lungs or bronchi, and 64% originate within the gastrointestinal tract (Table 6.1) [3]. The American Joint Committee on Cancer (AJCC) Tumor, Node, Metastasis (TNM) staging system for carcinoid tumors was recently updated and is outlined in Table 6.2. Table 6.3 contains the AJCC stage grouping and survival for carcinoid tumors. The remainder of this section will discuss the surgical management of gastrointestinal carcinoid tumors.

Gastric Carcinoid Tumors

Gastric carcinoid tumors account for less than 1% of gastric tumors, and 5–7% of all carcinoids [3, 4]. There are three distinct types: type I tumors are associated with chronic atrophic gastritis; type II tumors are associated with MEN1-related Zollinger-Ellison syndrome; type III tumors are sporadic [5]. They may present with bleeding or ulcer symptoms, but are often diagnosed on routine endoscopy.

Type I and II gastric carcinoids are generally indolent and metastasize in only 8–12% of patients [6]. These can be managed by endoscopic resection if lesions are less than 1 cm in diameter and less than five in number. For larger lesions and lesions that recur after polypectomy, operative local excision is indicated. At the time of surgery, some authors advocate performing antrectomy if the patient has type I gastric carcinoid to remove the gastrin stimulus, as this has been shown to result in disease regression [7, 8]. However, some tumors can become gastrin-independent,

Table 6.1 Distribution of carcinoid tumors, stage, and overall 5-year survival rates

Carcinoid site	% of all carcinoids*	% Localized	5-Year survival (localized)	% Regional	5-Year survival (regional)	% Distant	5-Year survival (distant)	Overall 5-year survival
Lung	27.9	65.4	81.1	5.2	76.7	0.5	25.6	73.5
Stomach	4.6	67.5	69.1	3.1	n/a	6.5	21.2	63
Small intestine	28.5	35.9	59.9	35.9	72.8	22.4	50	60.5
Appendix	4.8	55.4	80.8	28.9	88.1	9.9	9.6	71
Colon	10.2	33.4	76	25.8	71.6	29.5	30	61.8
Rectum	13.6	81.7	90.8	2.2	48.9	1.7	32.3	88.3

*Data from SEER 1973 to 1999; remainder of data from SEER 1992 to 1999 [3]

Table 6.2 AJCC TNM staging for neuroendocrine (carcinoid) tumors [68]

Disease site	Definition of TNM stage		
Stomach	T	TX	Primary tumor cannot be assessed
		T0	No evidence of primary tumor
		Tis	Carcinoma in situ/dysplasia (tumor size <0.5 mm), confined to mucosa
		T1	Tumor invades lamina propria or submucosa and ≤ 1cm in size
		T2	Tumor invades muscularis propria or >1 cm in size
		T3	Tumor penetrates subserosa
		T4	Tumor invades visceral peritoneum (serosa) or other organs or adjacent structures
	N	NX	Regional lymph nodes cannot be assessed
		N0	No regional lymph node metastasis
		N1	Regional lymph node metastasis
	M	M0	No distant metastasis
		M1	Distant metastasis
Duodenum, ampulla, jejunum, ileum	T	TX	Primary tumor cannot be assessed
		T0	No evidence of primary tumor
		T1	Tumor invades lamina propria or submucosa and size ≤ 1 cm (small intestinal tumors); tumor ≤ 1 cm (ampullary tumors)
		T2	Tumor invades muscularis propria or size >1 cm (small intestinal tumors); tumor >1 cm (ampullary tumors)
		T3	Tumor invades through the muscularis propria into subserosal tissue without penetration of overlying serosa (jejunal or ileal tumors) or invades pancreas or retroperitoneum (ampullary or duodenal tumors) or into nonperitonealized tissues
		T4	Tumor invades visceral peritoneum (serosa) or invades other organs
	N	NX	Regional lymph nodes cannot be assessed
		N0	No regional lymph node metastasis
		N1	Regional lymph node metastasis
	M	M0	No distant metastasis
		M1	Distant metastasis

(continued)

Table 6.2 (continued)

Disease site	Definition of TNM stage		
Colon, rectum	T	TX	Primary tumor cannot be assessed
		T0	No evidence of primary tumor
		T1	Tumor invades lamina propria or submucosa and size ≤ 2 cm
		T1a	Tumor size <1 cm in greatest dimension
		T1b	Tumor size 1–2 cm in greatest dimension
		T2	Tumor invades muscularis propria or size >2 cm with invasion of lamina propria or submucosa
		T3	Tumor invades through the muscularis propria into the subserosa, or into nonperitonealized pericolic or perirectal tissues
		T4	Tumor invades peritoneum or other organs
	N	NX	Regional lymph nodes cannot be assessed
		N0	No regional lymph node metastasis
		N1	Regional lymph node metastasis
	M	M0	No distant metastasis
		M1	Distant metastasis
Appendix	T	TX	Primary tumor cannot be assessed
		T0	No evidence of primary tumor
		T1	Tumor 2 cm or less in greatest dimension
		T1a	Tumor 1 cm or less in greatest dimension
		T1b	Tumor more than 1 cm but not more than 2 cm
		T2	Tumor more than 2 cm but not more than 4 cm or with extension to the cecum
		T3	Tumor more than 4 cm or with extension to the ileum
		T4	Tumor directly invades other adjacent organs or structures, e.g., abdominal wall and skeletal muscle
	N	NX	Regional lymph nodes cannot be assessed
		N0	No regional lymph node metastasis
		N1	Regional lymph node metastasis
	M	M0	No distant metastasis
		M1	Distant metastasis

Used with the permission of the American Joint Committee on Cancer (AJCC), Chicago, Illinois. The original source for this material is the AJCC Cancer Staging Manual, Seventh Edition (2010) published by Springer Science and Business Media LLC, www.springer.com

and therefore patients still require lifelong endoscopic surveillance. Medical management with somatostatin analogs has been shown to result in tumor regression in type II gastric carcinoids [9].

Type III gastric carcinoids account for 21% of gastric carcinoids and are significantly more aggressive than type I or type II tumors, with metastasis in 25–55% of cases [5]. These tumors should be treated like gastric adenocarcinoma, and require gastrectomy (total or partial, depending upon the location of the tumor) with regional lymph node dissection.

Table 6.3 AJCC stage grouping and survival for neuroendocrine (carcinoid) tumors [68]

Stage group	T stage	N stage	M stage	5-Year survival
Stomach, duodenum, ampulla, jejunum, ileum, colon and rectum				
0	Tis	N0	M0	N/A
I	T1	N0	M0	86%
IIA	T2	N0	M0	75%
IIB	T3	N0	M0	72%
IIIA	T4	N0	M0	59%
IIIB	Any T	N1	M0	70%
IV	Any T	Any N	M1	40%
Appendix				
I	T1	N0	M0	Prognostic significance of staging is controversial
II	T2-3	N0	M0	
III	T4	N0	M0	
	Any T	N1	M0	
IV	Any T	Any N	M1	

Used with the permission of the American Joint Committee on Cancer (AJCC), Chicago, Illinois. The original source for this material is the AJCC Cancer Staging Manual, Seventh Edition (2010) published by Springer Science and Business Media LLC, www.springer.com

Midgut Carcinoid Tumors

The jejunum and ileum are the most common locations for carcinoid tumors (28%), with the incidence rising with proximity to the ileocecal valve [3]. Carcinoids are also the most common tumor of the small intestine [10]. Patients usually present with symptoms of intestinal obstruction, bleeding, or ischemia; a small percentage of patients present with symptoms of carcinoid syndrome and almost all such patients are discovered to have liver metastases. Over 60% of jejunoileal carcinoids are metastatic to lymph nodes or liver at the time of diagnosis [3, 11]; this is possibly because most are not discovered on screening endoscopy, and instead are discovered when symptomatic and already advanced.

The risk of lymph node metastasis has previously been considered to be small in tumors that are less than 2 cm or have a depth of invasion that does not extend beyond the submucosa [12]. However, recent studies have demonstrated a significant risk of lymph node metastasis even these patients [13, 14]. The risk of lymph node metastasis in tumors limited to the submucosa is as high as 16%; in tumors ranging from 5 to 10 mm in size, the risk is 13%; and even in tumors less than or equal to 5 mm in size, the risk is 6% [14]. This underscores the need for adequate lymph node dissection even in carcinoids considered to be of low risk.

The primary treatment for localized midgut carcinoid is surgical resection with regional lymph node dissection. The extent of lymphadenectomy required is unclear. Analysis of the SEER data from 1973 to 2004 revealed that the median survival for

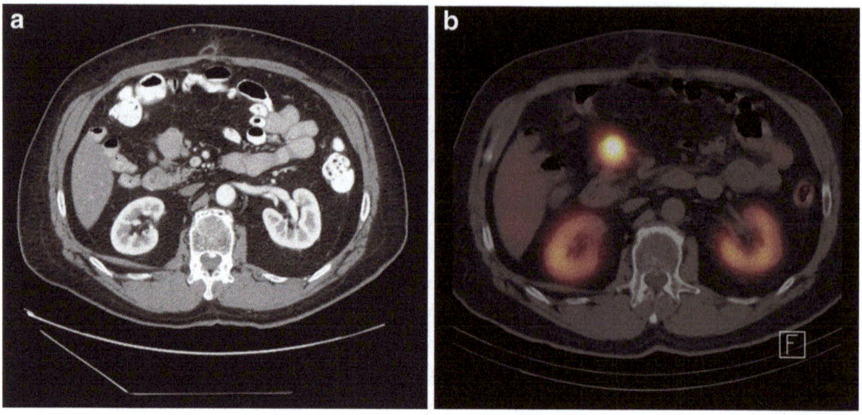

Fig. 6.1 A 63-year-old man underwent routine screening colonoscopy and was found to have an ulcerated mass at the ileocecal valve, with biopsy revealing well-differentiated neuroendocrine carcinoma. Right hemicolectomy was performed. Postoperative imaging demonstrated a large mesenteric lymph node metastasis seen on (**a**) CT scan and (**b**) octreotide single positron emission CT (SPECT) scan

patients with localized duodenal or small bowel carcinoids is not substantially different from the median survival for patients with regional duodenal or small bowel carcinoids (duodenal: 107 vs. 101 months, respectively; small bowel: 111 vs. 105 months, respectively), whereas the median survival for patients with regional disease was significantly lower than the median survival for patients with localized disease for all other carcinoid locations [11]. This data suggest that in fact many of the patients in the category of "localized disease" were simply understaged because an inadequate or no lymph node dissection was performed. Therefore, it appears that current surgical practice is achieving inadequate lymphadenectomy for this disease location, and complete resection of the associated mesentery should be performed (Fig. 6.1).

Patients with midgut carcinoid often present with an unclear primary and bulky mesenteric disease causing symptoms of intestinal obstruction or ischemia. Surgical resection of the mesenteric disease (and any identified primary tumor) is indicated in these patients for symptom palliation. However, even in asymptomatic patients, resection of mesenteric disease may confer a survival benefit. A recent study examined the median survival of patients who underwent resection or no resection of mesenteric disease either in the setting of no distant disease or in the setting of liver metastases. In both cases, patients had increased survival after resection of mesenteric disease (12.4 vs. 7.4 years in patients with no distant disease; 7.8 vs. 3.8 years in the setting of liver metastasis) [15].

Management of an asymptomatic primary midgut carcinoid in the setting of liver metastasis is controversial. Because the life expectancy of patients with liver metastasis is likely to be at least several years, many authors advocate surgical resection to avoid the potential long-term complications of a primary tumor (intestinal obstruction, bleeding, ischemia). The primary tumor is often not able to be identified on preoperative imaging studies, but careful exploration will reveal the primary tumor in up to 80% of cases [16].

A recent study has proposed resection of an asymptomatic primary tumor in the setting of metastatic disease for survival benefit. In 84 patients with midgut carcinoid and liver metastasis, a greater median progression-free and overall survival was seen in patients whose primary tumor was resected vs. patients whose primary tumor was not resected (56 vs. 25 months, and 159 vs. 47 months, respectively), even when controlling for the amount of liver involved with tumor [17]. It is difficult to explain a physiologic reason for these findings, and further investigation is clearly warranted.

Appendiceal Carcinoid Tumors

The appendix has historically been the most common location for carcinoid tumors and was thought to account for 35–45% of all carcinoids [3]. However, the vast majority of these tumors were discovered as incidental findings after appendectomy performed for other reasons.

The predicted clinical behavior and ensuing recommendations for surgical management of appendiceal carcinoid tumors is related to the size of the tumor. Because so many of these tumors are incidental findings, more than 95% of appendiceal carcinoids measure less than 2 cm in diameter at the time of diagnosis [3]. The incidence of metastatic disease in such cases is approximately 3%. However, the incidence of metastasis (usually to lymph nodes or the liver) is 30–60% in patients with tumors measuring more than 2 cm in diameter [18]. Therefore, simple appendectomy is sufficient treatment for appendiceal carcinoids measuring less than 2 cm, but tumors larger than 2 cm in diameter should be managed by formal right hemicolectomy in order to perform an adequate lymph node dissection.

Colon Carcinoid Tumors

Carcinoid tumors of the colon account for approximately 8% of all carcinoid tumors, and occur most frequently in the cecum (40–50%) [3, 19]. Most present with similar symptoms as colon adenocarcinoma. As with appendiceal carcinoid tumors, metastasis is rare if tumors are less than 2 cm in diameter and demonstrate minimal invasion through the colon wall (i.e., invasion limited to the submucosa); such tumors can theoretically be managed with local excision or limited resection. In reality, however, the majority of colon carcinoids are larger than 2 cm and involve at least the muscularis propria at the time of presentation [19]. Metastasis is present in more than two-thirds of such patients, and therefore they should be managed as colon adenocarcinomas, with formal colon resection and adequate lymph node dissection.

Rectal Carcinoid Tumors

Rectal carcinoid tumors account for approximately 14% of all carcinoid tumors. More than half are asymptomatic and are discovered incidentally during routine endoscopy [3]. Over 80% of rectal carcinoids are less than 1 cm in diameter at diagnosis, and metastases are present in only 5% of these [20, 21]. Therefore, such lesions can safely be managed with local excision (transanal or endoscopic). The management of larger lesions is controversial. Tumors between 1 and 2 cm in diameter have a 30% incidence of regional metastasis [20], and should be evaluated with endorectal ultrasound. If there is no evidence of muscular invasion, no ulceration, and lymph nodes are negative, local excision may be adequate; otherwise, consideration should be given to proctectomy with total mesorectal excision. Tumors greater than 2 cm in diameter have a 60–80% incidence of regional metastases [20], and traditional teaching has been that these lesions should be managed with proctectomy and total mesorectal excision (low anterior resection or abdominoperineal resection). However, this approach has been questioned in light of the significant morbidity and lifestyle concerns associated with radical rectal surgery (wound complications, sexual and bladder dysfunction, anal sphincter incompetence) balanced against the relatively indolent nature of carcinoid tumors [22, 23]. Thus, in the case of rectal carcinoids, an individualized approach to therapy that takes into consideration patient age, comorbidities, and preferences is more appropriate.

Pancreatic Islet Cell Carcinomas

Islet cell tumors are neuroendocrine tumors of the pancreas and periampullary region of the small intestine. As with carcinoid, they are classified into three general categories: *well-differentiated neuroendocrine tumors* (benign tumors or tumors of uncertain malignant potential), *well-differentiated neuroendocrine carcinomas* (low- to intermediate-grade malignancy) or *poorly differentiated neuroendocrine carcinomas* (high-grade malignancy). The only reliable criteria for determining malignancy include locoregional invasion (e.g., of other organs), the presence of tumor cells in lymph nodes, or distant metastases [2].

Islet cell tumors are also subdivided into functioning and nonfunctioning tumors. Functioning tumors result in very characteristic and well-defined clinical syndromes as a result of overproduction of a specific hormone or hormones. Nonfunctioning tumors do not produce symptoms of hormone overproduction, although excess hormone levels can often be detected biochemically.

Islet cell tumors are rare, and account for only about 2% of all pancreatic neoplasms [24]. They are usually sporadic, but may also be seen in the context of several genetic syndromes, including MEN1, VHL, and NF1. The AJCC TNM staging system for pancreatic neuroendocrine (islet cell) tumors was recently updated and is outlined in Table 6.4. Table 6.5 contains the AJCC stage grouping and survival for pancreatic neuroendocrine (islet cell) tumors. The remainder of this section will describe the surgical management of pancreatic islet cell carcinomas. Table 6.6 contains a brief summary of the clinical syndrome of each tumor, with key elements for diagnosis and surgical planning.

Table 6.4 AJCC TNM staging for pancreatic neuroendocrine (islet cell) tumors [68]

T	TX	Primary tumor cannot be assessed
	T0	No evidence of primary tumor
	Tis	Carcinoma in situ
	T1	Tumor limited to the pancreas, 2 cm or less in greatest dimension
	T2	Tumor limited to the pancreas, more than 2 cm in greatest dimension
	T3	Tumor extends beyond the pancreas but without involvement of the celiac axis or the superior mesenteric artery
	T4	Tumor involves the celiac axis or the superior mesenteric artery (unresectable primary tumor)
N	NX	Regional lymph nodes cannot be assessed
	N0	No regional lymph node metastasis
	N1	Regional lymph node metastasis
M	M0	No distant metastasis
	M1	Distant metastasis

Table 6.5 AJCC stage grouping and survival for pancreatic neuroendocrine (islet cell) tumors [68, 69]

Stage group	T stage	N stage	M stage	5-Year survival
0	Tis	N0	M0	N/A
IA	T1	N0	M0	61%
IB	T2	N0	M0	
IIA	T3	N0	M0	52%
IIB	T1-3	N1	M0	
III	T4	Any N	M0	41%
IV	Any T	Any N	M1	16%

Table 6.6 Diagnosis and management of islet cell tumors

Tumor	Hormone	Syndrome	% MEN1	Diagnosis	Site of origin	% Malignant	Operation
Gastrinoma	Gastrin	Peptic ulcer disease, abdominal pain, esophagitis, diarrhea	20%	Gastrin level with gastric pH	75% gastrinoma triangle 75% duodenal	>50%	Resection with regional lymph node dissection; include duodenotomy with careful search for additional tumors
Insulinoma	Insulin	Hypoglycemia, weight gain	<10%	Witnessed fast	Anywhere throughout pancreas	<10%	Enucleation or resection; usually no regional lymph node dissection
Glucagonoma	Glucagon	Diabetes, weight loss, anemia, necrolytic migratory erythema	Rare	Glucagon level	Pancreas; 90% in body and tail	>70%	Distal pancreatectomy, splenectomy, regional lymph node dissection
VIPoma	Vasoactive intestinal peptide	Watery diarrhea, hypokalemia, achlorhydria	Rare	VIP level	75% pancreas 20% neurogenic 5% duodenum (if in pancreas: 75% body/tail)	>50%	Resection with regional lymph node dissection (usually distal pancreatectomy and splenectomy)
Somatostatinoma	Somatostatin	Steatorrhea, diabetes, cholelithiasis, hypochlorhydria	Rare	Somato-statin level	66% pancreas 33% duodenal (if in pancreas: 66% head)	>70%	Resection with regional lymph node dissection (usually pancreatico-duodenectomy)
Nonfunctioning PET	Pancreatic polypeptide; other; none	None	>15%	Imaging PP level	60% pancreatic head	>60%	Resection with regional lymph node dissection; no role for incomplete debulking

Gastrinoma

Gastrinoma, also known as the Zollinger-Ellison syndrome [25], is a tumor that secretes the gastrointestinal hormone gastrin. It is sporadic in 70–80% of cases and is associated with MEN1 in 20–30% of cases [26]. The management of sporadic gastrinoma differs considerably from the management of MEN1-associated gastrinoma because patients with sporadic gastrinomas are more likely to have the more aggressive form of the disease [27, 28]; in addition, patients with MEN1-associated gastrinoma typically have multiple small tumors and usually cannot be cured with surgery [29].

Gastrinoma often presents as refractory peptic ulcer disease, with abdominal pain, esophagitis, and/or diarrhea. The diagnosis is made by measuring a serum gastrin level drawn when the patient has discontinued proton-pump inhibitors for at least 2 weeks. The gastrin level is usually greater than 1,000 pg/ml in a patient with gastrinoma. A simultaneous gastric pH of less than 2.5 is diagnostic of gastrinoma. However, if the gastrin level is equivocal, a secretin stimulation test can be performed; if the gastrin level increases by 200 pg/ml or more, the diagnosis is confirmed.

More than 75% of gastrinomas occur within the gastrinoma triangle (the area between the confluence of the cystic and common bile duct, the junction of the second and third portions of the duodenum, and the junction of the neck and body of the pancreas) [30]. The remainder is located in the body of the pancreas and the distal duodenum. Overall, duodenal tumors are 3–10 times more common than pancreatic tumors, and patients with duodenal tumors have a better prognosis, although tumors at both locations carry similar rates of malignancy. Lymph node metastases are found in 40–70% of patients at the time of diagnosis; liver metastasis occurs in approximately 5% [29]. Tumor localization is best accomplished by a combination of octreotide scan, CT or MRI, and endoscopic ultrasonography (EUS).

There is evidence to support routine surgical management of gastrinoma in sporadic cases; surgery is associated with little morbidity, and can provide a postoperative cure rate of 60%, with a third of patients achieving long-term cure (10 years) [31, 32]. The goal of surgery is to perform a complete resection of disease and preserve the maximal amount of pancreas. Tumors in the tail of the pancreas can be managed by distal pancreatectomy. Tumors in the head of the pancreas can often be managed by enucleation. Duodenal tumors can be managed by full-thickness excision. Duodenotomy with careful palpation of the duodenum or endoscopic transillumination should be performed routinely, even for patients who do not have a diagnosed duodenal primary, as duodenal tumors in patients with gastrinoma are extremely common, and can be multiple and very small. Routine peripancreatic lymph node dissection should also be performed because of the high incidence of lymph node metastasis at the time of diagnosis. There is growing evidence to support more extensive surgery (pancreaticoduodenectomy) in certain cases: the presence of a large duodenal or pancreatic head tumor that is not amenable to enucleation; the presence of multiple duodenal tumors or multiple enlarged lymph nodes; and failure of cure after routine surgical management [29]. Minimally invasive options, such as endoscopic resection of duodenal tumors, or laparoscopic pancreatic procedures can also play a role in selected cases.

Insulinoma

Insulinoma is a tumor that secretes insulin. It is usually sporadic, but may occur in association with MEN1 in 4–10% of cases [33]. Sporadic insulinomas are almost always solitary tumors; in fact, the presence of multiple insulinomas in a single patient should suggest the diagnosis of MEN1. Unlike other pancreatic islet cell carcinomas, insulinomas are almost always benign.

Insulinoma classically presents as "Whipple's triad" [34] of fasting or exercise-induced hypoglycemia, plasma glucose level less than 50 mg/dl, and reversal of symptoms with administration of glucose. The diagnosis is confirmed with a monitored 72-h fast in which plasma glucose and insulin levels are measured every 4–6 h. An inappropriately high insulin level in the presence of a low glucose level (insulin to glucose ratio greater than 0.4) is indicative of insulinoma. A serum C-peptide level and sulfonylurea screen should be obtained to exclude the possibility of surreptitious use if antihyperglycemic agents.

Insulinomas may be located anywhere throughout the pancreas, and therefore, preoperative localization studies are essential. CT and EUS (as well as intraoperative US) are the best tests for localization. Octreotide scanning is of limited value, as insulinomas express few somatostatin receptors.

The management of insulinomas is surgical. Although nearly all sporadic insulinomas are solitary, careful exploration at the time of surgery is essential in order to identify the presence of multiple tumors; intraoperative US is often a valuable tool. Ideal management of insulinomas involves enucleation of the tumor. However, tumors that lie close to the main pancreatic duct may be more safely managed by formal pancreatic resection (pancreaticoduodenectomy for pancreatic head tumors or distal pancreatectomy for tumors in the pancreatic tail). If enucleation is performed and a pancreatic duct leak is identified intraoperatively, a formal resection can then be performed, or alternatively, a roux limb of jejunum can be anastomosed to the pancreatic defect. Distal pancreatectomy can almost always be spleen-sparing, as there is little need to remove lymph nodes in this disease that is almost always benign. Laparoscopic operations for insulinoma are often appropriate and are becoming routine [35].

Other Functioning Pancreatic Islet Cell Carcinomas

Glucagonomas, VIPomas, and somatostatinomas are other functioning pancreatic islet cell carcinomas that secrete glucagon, vasoactive intestinal peptide (VIP), and somatostatin, respectively. They are extremely rare and account for approximately 7% of pancreatic islet cell carcinomas [36]. They are almost always solitary, sporadic tumors, and only rarely are associated with MEN1.

Glucagonomas present with the syndrome of diabetes, weight loss, anemia, and necrolytic migratory erythema. A serum glucagon level greater than 1,000 pg/ml confirms the diagnosis, although a secretin stimulation test or skin biopsy may also be useful in equivocal situations. More than 80% of glucagonomas ultimately display malignant behavior; over 50% of patients have regional or distant metastatic disease at the time of diagnosis [37]. Glucagonomas are always located in the pancreas, and 90% are located in the body and tail. They are often very large tumors that are best managed by distal pancreatectomy and splenectomy, with regional lymph node dissection.

VIPomas present with the syndrome of severe intermittent watery diarrhea, hypokalemia, and achlorhydria (Verner-Morrison [38] or WDHA syndrome). The diagnosis is made by a fasting serum VIP level greater than 200 pg/ml, although most patients will have levels of greater than 1,000 pg/ml [37]. VIPomas are usually located in the pancreas [39], but up to 20% are neurogenic (arising from the splanchnic nervous system), and 5% are located within the duodenum and jejunum [40]. Approximately half of pancreatic VIPomas are malignant, with metastases most commonly to regional lymph nodes and the liver. Neurogenic VIPomas are nearly always benign. Pancreatic VIPomas are located in the body and tail of the pancreas 75% of the time, and formal resection (usually distal pancreatectomy and splenectomy) with regional lymph node dissection is the ideal management.

Somatostatinomas present with steatorrhea, diabetes, cholelithiasis, and hypochlorhydria. The diagnosis is confirmed by a fasting serum somatostatin level greater than 100 pg/ml. Approximately two-thirds of somatostatinomas are located in the pancreas, and the rest are periampullary, duodenal, or small bowel in origin. About half of somatostatinomas are malignant, regardless of their location. Duodenal somatostatinomas have an association with neurofibromatosis type 1; therefore, pheochromocytoma should be ruled out preoperatively in these patients [41]. Management is surgical resection, with regional lymph node dissection, and because two-thirds of pancreatic somatostatinomas are located in the head of the pancreas, resection involves pancreaticoduodenectomy.

Nonfunctioning Pancreatic Islet Cell Carcinomas

Nonfunctioning pancreatic endocrine tumors (PETs) account for the largest subgroup of islet cell carcinomas (15–30%) [24]. Pancreatic polypeptidoma (PPoma) is considered together with nonfunctioning PETs because oversecretion of pancreatic polypeptide does not produce a clinical syndrome. Although some amount of hormone can often be detected biochemically, nonfunctioning PETs are usually diagnosed because of the mechanical effects from local growth or metastatic disease (e.g., pain, jaundice). Thus, most nonfunctioning PETs are diagnosed when the primary tumor is large or has already metastasized; only 25% of patients are candidates for a potentially curative resection at the time of diagnosis [42]. These tumors are malignant in more than 60% of cases, with metastasis most commonly to lymph nodes and liver.

Approximately 60% of nonfunctioning PETs are located in the pancreatic head [43]. Surgical resection (pancreaticoduodenectomy or distal pancreatectomy) with lymph node dissection is indicated for localized resectable tumors (Fig. 6.2). However, only approximately 50% of those patients experience long-term cure [42]. There is no survival benefit to incomplete resection of a primary tumor (cytoreduction or debulking), and patients experience considerable morbidity and mortality [44].

The surgical management of patients who present with a localized but unresectable tumor is controversial. Because the majority of nonfunctioning PETs are located in the pancreatic head, local growth will eventually result in bile duct and duodenal

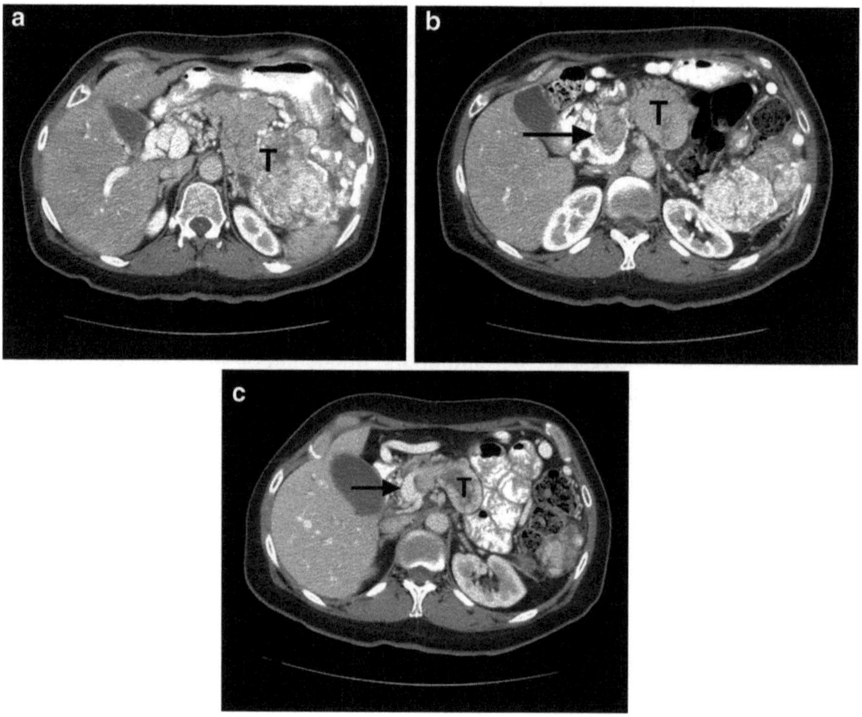

Fig. 6.2 A 54-year-old woman experienced decreased appetite and weight loss. Workup ultimately revealed a large nonfunctioning pancreatic neuroendocrine tumor. On CT scan, the tumor was found to (**a**) completely replace the body and tail of the pancreas, with (**b**) a large tumor thrombus expanding and completely occluding the splenoportal confluence. After nine cycles of chemotherapy with 5-fluorouracil, adriamycin, and streptozocin, the tumor and tumor thrombus decreased dramatically in size (**c**). The patient underwent distal pancreatectomy and splenectomy, with removal of tumor thrombus and primary repair of the portal vein (*T* tumor; *arrow* points to splenoportal confluence with tumor thrombus)

obstruction. Although endoscopic stents can be used to manage these situations in patients with localized but unresectable tumors, we prefer surgical biliary and gastric bypass. Such patients typically have a median survival of 5 years [42], and surgical bypass provides a much more durable response than endoscopic stenting.

The management of an intact primary tumor in the setting of metastatic disease is also controversial. A small number of patients (less than 5%) will be candidates for complete resection of the primary tumor and all metastatic disease, and may experience a survival benefit [42]. There is no evidence that surgical resection of the primary tumor without complete resection of all metastatic disease results in increased survival [42, 43]. The only indication for surgery in this subpopulation of patients is symptom palliation. In the case of tumors in the body and tail of the pancreas, symptoms are unusual, even with tumors that become very large. However, surgical resection may be considered for symptom palliation of tumors in the pancreatic head, especially in the setting of low-volume metastatic disease and a low-risk patient. In such a situation, biliary and duodenal obstruction or gastrointestinal hemorrhage from erosion into the duodenum may be managed better by pancreaticoduodenectomy than by palliative bypass alone.

Neuroendocrine Carcinomas Metastatic to the Liver

A recent analysis of the SEER Program registries revealed that metastatic disease is present at the time of diagnosis in 21% of patients with well-differentiated neuroendocrine tumors, 30% of patients with moderately differentiated neuroendocrine tumors, and 50% of patients with poorly differentiated or undifferentiated neuroendocrine tumors [11]. The liver is the most common site of metastatic disease, and eventually, up to 75% of patients will develop liver metastases [45]. Primary neuroendocrine tumors can secrete a variety of hormones (e.g., serotonin, bradykinin, and histamine) which are usually cleared by the liver, and therefore patients are usually asymptomatic. However, liver metastases can secrete hormones which are dispersed systemically before first-pass clearance by the liver and are therefore frequently associated with a hormonal syndrome. In patients who present with carcinoid syndrome, which can include debilitating diarrhea, flushing, asthma, and right heart valvular disease, almost all have liver metastases. Surgical or other interventional therapy is often effective in the palliation of symptoms, and can occasionally be performed for cure.

Surgical Resection

The largest early series of patients undergoing hepatic resection for metastatic neuroendocrine carcinoma was published by McEntee and colleagues at the Mayo Clinic and reflected their experience from 1970 to 1989. Hepatic resection was performed in 37 patients, 17 with curative intent, and 20 with palliative intent. At a median follow-up of 19 months, disease-free survival was 75% in the group undergoing resection for curative intent. Of the patients undergoing palliative resection, 60% achieved complete relief from symptoms and an additional 35% experienced partial relief from symptoms. The authors concluded that surgery was effective if all disease could be resected or at least 90% of disease could be debulked [46].

Que et al. reported the largest recent series of patients undergoing hepatic resection for metastatic neuroendocrine carcinoma, which represented the Mayo Clinic experience from 1989 to 1994. In this series, 74 patients with completely resectable disease or disease amenable to at least 90% debulking underwent surgery. Symptom relief was achieved in 90% of patients. There was no statistically significant difference in survival between patients undergoing surgery for curative vs. palliative intent; however, overall survival at 4 years was 73%, which compared very favorably to historical controls with overall survival rates of 30–40% [47].

Several recent studies have reported that surgical resection of hepatic metastases from neuroendocrine tumors improves survival compared with nonsurgical treatment [48–51]. However, these studies must be interpreted in light of the considerable bias that exists when patients are selected for surgical vs. nonsurgical management. Only 10% of patients with liver metastases are candidates for surgical resection with curative intent, and in these, R0 resection is only possible in approximately 50% because of more extensive liver disease than anticipated or extra-hepatic disease undiagnosed on preoperative imaging [48]. Even in patients who undergo R0 resection, early disease recurrence is common, and only approximately 25% of patients remain disease-free at 2 years [48]. On the other hand, 80–95% of patients experience a significantly higher quality of life after surgery [52], even in situations in which less than 90% of their tumor burden was able to be debulked; [45] therefore, low-volume residual disease may not be of significant consequence.

We currently advocate surgical intervention for liver metastasis in the setting of neuroendocrine tumors in patients with solitary metastasis, or disease that is completely treatable by surgery or a combination of surgery and other ablative techniques. Histology is also important; liver resection should only be considered for low-grade tumors. A period of maximal medical management (octreotide for carcinoid; systemic chemotherapy for islet cell tumors) and/or hepatic artery chemoembolization can be useful in distinguishing patients whose disease is likely to be indolent and less aggressive over time, and therefore may achieve maximal benefit from surgery.

Liver transplantation has been explored as a treatment option for patients with otherwise unresectable hepatic disease. However, no randomized data are available, and the number of patients treated is small. A multicenter study from Europe reported a 5-year overall survival rate of 36% in 31 patients who underwent liver transplantation for neuroendocrine tumor metastases. Three-year survival was greater for patients with metastases from carcinoid tumors compared with islet cell tumors (69 vs. 15%) [53]. In a generally indolent disease process such as carcinoid, it is difficult to ascertain the potential benefit of a treatment with the substantial morbidity and mortality of liver transplantation.

Hepatic Artery Embolization and Chemoembolization

The peculiarities of the dual blood supply to the liver contribute to the effectiveness of hepatic arterial embolization techniques in the treatment of liver metastases. Normal liver derives only 25% of its blood supply from the hepatic artery; the remainder is from the portal vein. However, liver metastases derive 95% of their blood supply from the hepatic artery. Thus, interruption of hepatic artery blood supply results in ischemic necrosis of the metastases, but spares normal liver. Hepatic arterial occlusion techniques have been evaluated in the treatment of liver metastases since the 1980s. Initially, these involved laparotomy and ligation of the common hepatic artery, but percutaneous techniques have permitted a much more selective approach. Trials of hepatic artery ligation or embolization in neuroendocrine metastasis have demonstrated a 30–40% tumor response [54–56].

Liver-directed chemotherapy provides high concentrations of drug in the liver, yet spares the systemic circulation and thus limits toxicity [57]. Not surprisingly, liver-directed chemotherapy given via the hepatic artery results in a tenfold higher intratumoral drug concentration than chemotherapy given via the portal vein [58]. The combination of intra-arterial chemotherapy followed by embolization (chemoembolization) has led to tumor response rates up to 60% [59–61].

The experience in our institution was recently reported [59]. A total of 123 patients (69 carcinoid; 54 pancreatic islet cell tumors) underwent hepatic arterial embolization (HAE) or chemoembolization (HACE). Patients with carcinoid tumors had a higher overall response rate (66 vs. 35%), progression-free survival (23 vs. 16 months), and overall survival (33.8 vs. 23.2 months) than patients with pancreatic islet cell tumors, a finding which has also been reported by others [56, 62–64]. The addition of chemotherapy to hepatic arterial embolization appeared to have a somewhat deleterious effect on patients with carcinoid metastases; those treated with HAE had a higher response rate than those treated with HACE (81 vs. 44%). However, there was a trend toward significant improvement outcome for patients with pancreatic islet cell metastases treated with HACE vs. HAE (50 vs. 25%; $p = 0.06$), which likely reflects the overall greater sensitivity of pancreatic islet cell tumors to chemotherapy compared with carcinoid tumors [59].

Radiofrequency Ablation

Radiofrequency ablation (RFA) is a technique that utilizes high-frequency radio waves to generate thermal energy for tumor destruction. The electrode can be inserted percutaneously under imaging guidance, or can be used at laparoscopy or laparotomy using intraoperative ultrasound. RFA has been used successfully in the treatment of hepatocellular carcinoma and liver metastases from colorectal cancer and has recently been explored in the setting of liver metastases from neuroendocrine tumors with encouraging initial results. When used alone, RFA can provide symptomatic relief in 70–80% of patients, with recurrence rates of 15–30% and minimal morbidity [65–67]. Often, however, RFA is used as an adjunct to surgery or hepatic artery chemoembolization.

Other Therapies

Other less-explored options for the treatment of metastatic neuroendocrine tumors include cryotherapy, percutaneous ethanol injection, stereotactic radiosurgery, and intra-arterial radiation radiation therapy (e.g., with yttrium-90 microspheres or iodine-131 lipiodol). Extremely limited data exist with regards to any of these therapies, but it is possible that they may play a role in the highly individualized multidisciplinary management of patients with neuroendocrine tumor liver metastasis.

Summary

Carcinoid and islet cell tumors are rare neuroendocrine tumors of the gut and pancreas. They are often indolent, but can result in significant morbidity from hormone overproduction, and can sometimes be aggressive and resistant to treatment. Surgical resection is the main treatment for primary tumors and regional disease. In the setting of metastatic disease, it is often not possible to offer patients long-term cure with surgery; however, surgical resection and other interventional techniques can play a significant role in symptom palliation and multidisciplinary management of these patients.

References

1. Oberndorfer S. Karzinoide Tumoren des Dunndarms. Frankfurter Zeitschrift fur Pathologie. 1907;1:425–9.
2. Solcia E, Kloppel G, Sobin L. Histological typing of endocrine tumors. WHO international classification of tumours. 2nd ed. Berlin: Springer; 2000.
3. Modlin IM, Lye KD, Kidd M. A 5-decade analysis of 13,715 carcinoid tumors. Cancer. 2003;97(4):934–59.
4. Modlin IM, Gilligan CJ, Lawton GP, Tang LH, West AB, Darr U. Gastric carcinoids. The Yale experience. Arch Surg Mar. 1995;130(3):250–5. discussion 255-256.
5. Rindi G, Luinetti O, Cornaggia M, Capella C, Solcia E. Three subtypes of gastric argyrophil carcinoid and the gastric neuroendocrine carcinoma: a clinicopathologic study. Gastroenterology. 1993;104(4):994–1006.
6. Modlin IM, Lye KD, Kidd M. A 50-year analysis of 562 gastric carcinoids: small tumor or larger problem? Am J Gastroenterol. 2004;99(1):23–32.
7. Eckhauser FE, Lloyd RV, Thompson NW, Raper SE, Vinik AI. Antrectomy for multicentric, argyrophil gastric carcinoids: a preliminary report. Surgery. 1988;104(6):1046–53.

8. Hirschowitz BI, Griffith J, Pellegrin D, Cummings OW. Rapid regression of enterochromaffinlike cell gastric carcinoids in pernicious anemia after antrectomy. Gastroenterology. 1992;102 (4 Pt 1):1409–18.
9. Tomassetti P, Migliori M, Caletti GC, Fusaroli P, Corinaldesi R, Gullo L. Treatment of type II gastric carcinoid tumors with somatostatin analogues. N Engl J Med. 2000;343(8):551–4.
10. Barclay TH, Schapira DV. Malignant tumors of the small intestine. Cancer. 1983;51(5):878–81.
11. Yao JC, Hassan M, Phan A, et al. One hundred years after "carcinoid": epidemiology of and prognostic factors for neuroendocrine tumors in 35,825 cases in the United States. J Clin Oncol. 2008;26(18):3063–72.
12. Burke AP, Thomas RM, Elsayed AM, Sobin LH. Carcinoids of the jejunum and ileum: an immunohistochemical and clinicopathologic study of 167 cases. Cancer. 1997;79(6):1086–93.
13. Mullen JT, Wang H, Yao JC, et al. Carcinoid tumors of the duodenum. Surgery. 2005;138(6):971–7. discussion 977-978.
14. Soga J. Early-stage carcinoids of the gastrointestinal tract: an analysis of 1914 reported cases. Cancer. 2005;103(8):1587–95.
15. Hellman P, Lundstrom T, Ohrvall U, et al. Effect of surgery on the outcome of midgut carcinoid disease with lymph node and liver metastases. World J Surg. 2002;26(8):991–7.
16. Boudreaux JP, Putty B, Frey DJ, et al. Surgical treatment of advanced-stage carcinoid tumors: lessons learned. Ann Surg. 2005;241(6):839–45. discussion 845-836.
17. Givi B, Pommier SJ, Thompson AK, Diggs BS, Pommier RF. Operative resection of primary carcinoid neoplasms in patients with liver metastases yields significantly better survival. Surgery. 2006;140(6):891–7. discussion 897-898.
18. Moertel CG, Weiland LH, Nagorney DM, Dockerty MB. Carcinoid tumor of the appendix: treatment and prognosis. N Engl J Med. 1987;317(27):1699–701.
19. Spread C, Berkel H, Jewell L, Jenkins H, Yakimets W. Colon carcinoid tumors. A population-based study. Dis Colon Rectum May. 1994;37(5):482–91.
20. Soga J. Carcinoids of the rectum: an evaluation of 1271 reported cases. Surg Today. 1997;27(2):112–9.
21. Naunheim KS, Zeitels J, Kaplan EL, et al. Rectal carcinoid tumors–treatment and prognosis. Surgery. 1983;94(4):670–6.
22. Sauven P, Ridge JA, Quan SH, Sigurdson ER. Anorectal carcinoid tumors. Is aggressive surgery warranted? Ann Surg. 1990;211(1):67–71.
23. Koura AN, Giacco GG, Curley SA, Skibber JM, Feig BW, Ellis LM. Carcinoid tumors of the rectum: effect of size, histopathology, and surgical treatment on metastasis free survival. Cancer. 1997;79(7):1294–8.
24. Warner RR. Enteroendocrine tumors other than carcinoid: a review of clinically significant advances. Gastroenterology. 2005;128(6):1668–84.
25. Zollinger RM, Ellison EH. Primary peptic ulcerations of the jejunum associated with islet cell tumors of the pancreas. Ann Surg. 1955;142(4):709–23. discussion, 724-708.
26. Roy PK, Venzon DJ, Shojamanesh H, et al. Zollinger-Ellison syndrome. Clinical presentation in 261 patients. Medicine (Baltimore). 2000;79(6):379–411.
27. Weber HC, Venzon DJ, Lin JT, et al. Determinants of metastatic rate and survival in patients with Zollinger-Ellison syndrome: a prospective long-term study. Gastroenterology. 1995;108(6):1637–49.
28. Yu F, Venzon DJ, Serrano J, et al. Prospective study of the clinical course, prognostic factors, causes of death, and survival in patients with long-standing Zollinger-Ellison syndrome. J Clin Oncol. 1999;17(2):615–30.
29. Norton JA, Jensen RT. Resolved and unresolved controversies in the surgical management of patients with Zollinger-Ellison syndrome. Ann Surg. 2004;240(5):757–73.
30. Stabile BE, Morrow DJ, Passaro Jr E. The gastrinoma triangle: operative implications. Am J Surg. 1984;147(1):25–31.

31. Fraker DL, Norton JA, Alexander HR, Venzon DJ, Jensen RT. Surgery in Zollinger-Ellison syndrome alters the natural history of gastrinoma. Ann Surg. 1994;220(3):320–8. discussion 328-330.
32. Norton JA, Fraker DL, Alexander HR, et al. Surgery to cure the Zollinger-Ellison syndrome. N Engl J Med. 1999;341(9):635–44.
33. Stefanini P, Carboni M, Patrassi N, Basoli A. Beta-islet cell tumors of the pancreas: results of a study on 1,067 cases. Surgery. 1974;75(4):597–609.
34. Whipple AO, Frantz VK. Adenoma of islet cells with hyperinsulinism: a review. Ann Surg. 1935;101(6):1299–335.
35. Fernandez-Cruz L, Saenz A, Astudillo E, et al. Outcome of laparoscopic pancreatic surgery: endocrine and nonendocrine tumors. World J Surg. 2002;26(8):1057–65.
36. van Heerden JA, Thompson GB. Islet call tumours of the pancreas. In: Trede M, Carter DC, editors. Surgery of the pancreas. Edinburgh: Churchill Livingstone; 1993. p. 545–61.
37. Thompson GB. Rare Functioning Tumors: VIPoma, Glucagonoma, Somatostatinoma. In: Von Hoff DD, Evans DB, Hruban RH, editors. Pancreatic Cancer. Sudbury, MA: Jones and Bartlett; 2005. p. 623–30.
38. Verner JV, Morrison AB. Islet cell tumor and a syndrome of refractory watery diarrhea and hypokalemia. Am J Med. 1958;25(3):374–80.
39. Capella C, Polak JM, Buffa R, et al. Morphologic patterns and diagnostic criteria of VIP-producing endocrine tumors. A histologic, histochemical, ultrastructural, and biochemical study of 32 cases. Cancer. 1983;52(10):1860–74.
40. Long RG, Bryant MG, Mitchell SJ, Adrian TE, Polak JM, Bloom SR. Clinicopathological study of pancreatic and ganglioneuroblastoma tumours secreting vasoactive intestinal polypeptide (vipomas). Br Med J (Clin Res Ed). 1981;282(6278):1767–71.
41. Usui M, Matsuda S, Suzuki H, Hirata K, Ogura Y, Shiraishi T. Somatostatinoma of the papilla of Vater with multiple gastrointestinal stromal tumors in a patient with von Recklinghausen's disease. J Gastroenterol. 2002;37(11):947–53.
42. Solorzano CC, Lee JE, Pisters PW, et al. Nonfunctioning islet cell carcinoma of the pancreas: survival results in a contemporary series of 163 patients. Surgery. 2001;130(6):1078–85.
43. Evans DB, Skibber JM, Lee JE, et al. Nonfunctioning islet cell carcinoma of the pancreas. Surgery. 1993;114(6):1175–81. discussion 1181–1172.
44. Bloomston M, Muscarella P, Shah MH, et al. Cytoreduction results in high perioperative mortality and decreased survival in patients undergoing pancreatectomy for neuroendocrine tumors of the pancreas. J Gastrointest Surg. 2006;10(10):1361–70.
45. Knox CD, Feurer ID, Wise PE, et al. Survival and functional quality of life after resection for hepatic carcinoid metastasis. J Gastrointest Surg. 2004;8(6):653–9.
46. McEntee GP, Nagorney DM, Kvols LK, Moertel CG, Grant CS. Cytoreductive hepatic surgery for neuroendocrine tumors. Surgery. 1990;108(6):1091–6.
47. Que FG, Nagorney DM, Batts KP, Linz LJ, Kvols LK. Hepatic resection for metastatic neuroendocrine carcinomas. Am J Surg. 1995;169(1):36–42. discussion 42–33.
48. Chamberlain RS, Canes D, Brown KT, et al. Hepatic neuroendocrine metastases: does intervention alter outcomes? J Am Coll Surg. 2000;190(4):432–45.
49. Touzios JG, Kiely JM, Pitt SC, et al. Neuroendocrine hepatic metastases: does aggressive management improve survival? Ann Surg. 2005;241(5):776–83. discussion 783–775.
50. Musunuru S, Chen H, Rajpal S, et al. Metastatic neuroendocrine hepatic tumors: resection improves survival. Arch Surg. 2006;141(10):1000–4. discussion 1005.
51. Landry CS, Scoggins CR, McMasters KM, Martin 2nd RC. Management of hepatic metastasis of gastrointestinal carcinoid tumors. J Surg Oncol. 2008;97(3):253–8.
52. Sarmiento JM, Heywood G, Rubin J, Ilstrup DM, Nagorney DM, Que FG. Surgical treatment of neuroendocrine metastases to the liver: a plea for resection to increase survival. J Am Coll Surg. 2003;197(1):29–37.
53. Le Treut YP, Delpero JR, Dousset B, et al. Results of liver transplantation in the treatment of metastatic neuroendocrine tumors. A 31-case French multicentric report. Ann Surg. 1997;225(4):355–64.

54. Nobin A, Mansson B, Lunderquist A. Evaluation of temporary liver dearterialization and embolization in patients with metastatic carcinoid tumour. Acta Oncol. 1989;28(3):419–24.
55. Carrasco CH, Charnsangavej C, Ajani J, Samaan NA, Richli W, Wallace S. The carcinoid syndrome: palliation by hepatic artery embolization. AJR Am J Roentgenol. 1986;147(1):149–54.
56. Eriksson BK, Larsson EG, Skogseid BM, Lofberg AM, Lorelius LE, Oberg KE. Liver embolizations of patients with malignant neuroendocrine gastrointestinal tumors. Cancer. 1998;83(11):2293–301.
57. Ensminger WD, Gyves JW. Clinical pharmacology of hepatic arterial chemotherapy. Semin Oncol. 1983;10(2):176–82.
58. Sigurdson ER, Ridge JA, Kemeny N, Daly JM. Tumor and liver drug uptake following hepatic artery and portal vein infusion. J Clin Oncol. 1987;5(11):1836–40.
59. Gupta S, Johnson MM, Murthy R, et al. Hepatic arterial embolization and chemoembolization for the treatment of patients with metastatic neuroendocrine tumors: variables affecting response rates and survival. Cancer. 2005;104(8):1590–602.
60. Perry LJ, Stuart K, Stokes KR, Clouse ME. Hepatic arterial chemoembolization for metastatic neuroendocrine tumors. Surgery. 1994;116(6):1111–6. discussion 1116–1117.
61. Ho AS, Picus J, Darcy MD, et al. Long-term outcome after chemoembolization and embolization of hepatic metastatic lesions from neuroendocrine tumors. AJR Am J Roentgenol. 2007;188(5):1201–7.
62. Moertel CG, Johnson CM, McKusick MA, et al. The management of patients with advanced carcinoid tumors and islet cell carcinomas. Ann Intern Med. 1994;120(4):302–9.
63. Nave H, Mossinger E, Feist H, Lang H, Raab H. Surgery as primary treatment in patients with liver metastases from carcinoid tumors: a retrospective, unicentric study over 13 years. Surgery. 2001;129(2):170–5.
64. Pape UF, Bohmig M, Berndt U, Tiling N, Wiedenmann B, Plockinger U. Survival and clinical outcome of patients with neuroendocrine tumors of the gastroenteropancreatic tract in a german referral center. Ann N Y Acad Sci. 2004;1014:222–33.
65. Henn AR, Levine EA, McNulty W, Zagoria RJ. Percutaneous radiofrequency ablation of hepatic metastases for symptomatic relief of neuroendocrine syndromes. AJR Am J Roentgenol. 2003;181(4):1005–10.
66. Berber E, Flesher N, Siperstein AE. Laparoscopic radiofrequency ablation of neuroendocrine liver metastases. World J Surg. 2002;26(8):985–90.
67. Hellman P, Ladjevardi S, Skogseid B, Akerstrom G, Elvin A. Radiofrequency tissue ablation using cooled tip for liver metastases of endocrine tumors. World J Surg. 2002;26(8):1052–6.
68. Edge SB, Byrd DR, Compton CC, Fritz AG, Greene FL, Trotti A, editors. AJCC Cancer Staging Manual. 7th ed. New York: Springer; 2009.
69. Bilimoria KY, Bentrem DJ, Merkow RP, et al. Application of the pancreatic adenocarcinoma staging system to pancreatic neuroendocrine tumors. J Am Coll Surg. 2007;205(4):558–63.

Chapter 7
Management of Neuroendocrine Tumor Hormonal Syndromes

Jonathan Strosberg

Abstract Tumors originating in the diffuse neuroendocrine system are characterized by a propensity to secrete a variety of peptide hormones, biogenic amines, and other vasoactive substances. These circulating factors can give rise to a remarkable array of clinical signs and symptoms including flushing, diarrhea, diabetes, hypoglycemia, rash, bronchospasm, and valvular heart disease. Neuroendocrine tumors which produce pathologically elevated hormone levels associated with a corresponding clinical syndrome are termed "functioning" whereas tumors lacking any association with a hormonal syndrome are considered "nonfunctioning."

During the past three decades, the development of somatostatin analogs has revolutionized the treatment of several hormonal syndromes, notably the carcinoid syndrome, as well as rarer syndromes associated with hypersecretion of glucagon and vasoactive intestinal peptide (VIP). Accumulating evidence suggests that somatostatin analogs may also function as inhibitors of tumor growth. The proton pump inhibitors have had a remarkably favorable impact on the natural history of patients with the Zollinger–Ellison syndrome.

This chapter focuses on interventions which are specifically designed to ameliorate hormonal symptoms associated with carcinoid and pancreatic endocrine tumors. It is important, however, for clinicians to recognize that any therapy which effectively treats the underlying malignancy is likely to palliate the associated hormonal syndrome.

Keywords Somatostatin analogs • Carcinoid syndrome • Zollinger–Ellison syndrome • Pancreatic endocrine tumors • Cytoreductive surgery, hepatic artery embolization • Cytotoxic chemotherapy • Vascular endothelial growth factor • Mammalian target of rapamycin

J. Strosberg (✉)
Department of Gastrointestinal Oncology, H. Lee Moffitt Cancer Center and Research Institute,Tampa, FL 33612, USA
e-mail: Jonathan.strosberg@moffitt.org

J.C. Yao et al. (eds.), *Neuroendocrine Tumors*, Current Clinical Oncology,
DOI 10.1007/978-1-60327-997-0_7, © Springer Science+Business Media, LLC 2011

Introduction

Tumors originating in the diffuse neuroendocrine system are characterized by a propensity to secrete a variety of peptide hormones, biogenic amines, and other vasoactive substances. These circulating factors can give rise to a remarkable array of clinical signs and symptoms including flushing, diarrhea, diabetes, hypoglycemia, rash, bronchospasm, and valvular heart disease. Neuroendocrine tumors which produce pathologically elevated hormone levels associated with a corresponding clinical syndrome are termed "functioning," whereas tumors lacking any association with a hormonal syndrome are considered "nonfunctioning."

During the past three decades, the development of somatostatin analogs has revolutionized the treatment of several hormonal syndromes, notably the carcinoid syndrome, as well as rarer syndromes associated with hypersecretion of glucagon and vasoactive intestinal peptide (VIP). Accumulating evidence suggests that somatostatin analogs may also function as inhibitors of tumor growth. The proton pump inhibitors have had a remarkably favorable impact on the natural history of patients with the Zollinger–Ellison syndrome.

This chapter focuses on interventions which are specifically designed to ameliorate hormonal symptoms associated with carcinoid and pancreatic endocrine tumors. It is important, however, for clinicians to recognize that any therapy which effectively treats the underlying malignancy is likely to palliate the associated hormonal syndrome. Cytoreductive surgery, for example, can effectively control symptoms of hormone hypersecretion in cases where a significant reduction in tumor burden is achieved. Likewise, hepatic artery embolization should be considered in patients with surgically unresectable hormone-producing liver metastases. Cytotoxic chemotherapy appears to be particularly active in patients with pancreatic endocrine tumors. Radiolabled somatostatin analogs effectively target somatostatin-receptor expressing tumors. A rising number of novel agents, including inhibitors of vascular endothelial growth factor (VEGF) and mammalian target of rapamycin (mTOR) will likely play a future role in management of metastatic neuroendocrine tumors and palliation of hormonal syndromes.

The Carcinoid Syndrome

The clinical carcinoid syndrome was first elucidated in 1954 by Thorson and colleagues who drew an association between a metastatic carcinoid tumor of the small intestine and a constellation of unusual sings and symptoms. These included right heart valvular disease, peripheral vasomotor symptoms, bronchoconstriction, and "an unusual type of cyanosis" [1]. Bean and colleagues further elaborated on the flushing phenomenon, describing an ephemeral erythematous rash "resembling in clinical miniature the fickle phantasmagory of the Aurora Borealis" [2]. One year earlier, serotonin (5-hydroxytryptamine) was extracted from a carcinoid tumor and identified as the primary hormonal factor responsible for the carcinoid syndrome [3, 4]. Serotonin is derived from the amino acid tryptophan, and is enzymatically inactivated in the liver into 5-hydroxyindoleacetic acid (5-HIAA), a urinary metabolite. Consequently, the carcinoid syndrome occurs primarily in patients with metastatic carcinoid tumors that secrete serotonin directly into the systemic (rather than portal) circulation. Other vasoactive substances elaborated by carcinoid tumors include biogenic amines (such as histamine, dopamine, and hydroxytryptophan), tachykinins (kallikriein, substance P) and prostaglandins [5–8].

The carcinoid syndrome is associated in nearly all cases with metastatic carcinoid tumors of the distal small intestine and proximal colon (midgut) [9–11]. Carcinoid tumors of the distal colon and rectum (hindgut) are not associated with a hormonal syndrome [12]. Foregut carcinoid tumors (pulmonary, gastric, and duodenal) and pancreatic endocrine tumors infrequently secrete serotonin. An atypical carcinoid syndrome has been described in patients with foregut carcinoid tumors which secrete the serotonin precursor 5-hydroxytryptophan (5-HTP) due to diminished intracellular levels of amino-acid decarboxylase [13].

In an analysis of 91 patients with the carcinoid syndrome, diarrhea and flushing were the most commonly observed symptoms, occurring in 73% and 65% of patients, respectively. Carcinoid heart disease was detected in 10% of cases and bronchospasm in 8% [14]. A variety of hormones contribute to development of diarrhea and abdominal pain, including serotonin, substance P, prostaglandins, histamines, and tachikinins [15, 16]. Serotonin is thought to directly stimulate peristalsis, resulting in significantly reduced colonic transit times [17]. It may also affect intestinal electrolyte and fluid secretion via 5-HT2A receptors [18]. The flushing phenomenon is attributable to multiple vasoactive substances including protaglandins, kinins, and serotonin [16, 19–21]. Flushing typically involves the face, neck, and upper torso, and may be precipitated by stress, alcohol, food containing tyramines or spicy foods [22]. Patients with chronic flushing may develop chronic facial telangiectasias resembling rosacea (Fig. 7.1). Carcinoid heart disease typically occurs in patients with extreme elevations of circulating serotonin [23, 24]. Characteristic thickening and fibrosis of right-sided cardiac valves produces tricuspid regurgitation and pulmonic valve stenosis [25]. The right heart is invariably affected due to its direct exposure to serotonin secreted by liver metastases. Left heart valves are clinically involved in only 10% of cases. The underlying mechanism of fibroblast proliferation in the cardiac valves is uncertain [26, 27].

Management of the Carcinoid Syndrome

The introduction of somatostatin analogs has had a dramatic impact on management of the carcinoid syndrome. Native human somatostatin is a cyclic peptide hormone ubiquitously distributed in the body. It has an inhibitory effect on gastrointestinal motility, secretion, and absorption of nutrients. It also inhibits the release of other neuroendocrine hormones. Its actions are mediated through five somatostain receptor subtypes (SSTRs 1-5) belonging to a family of G-protein coupled receptors.

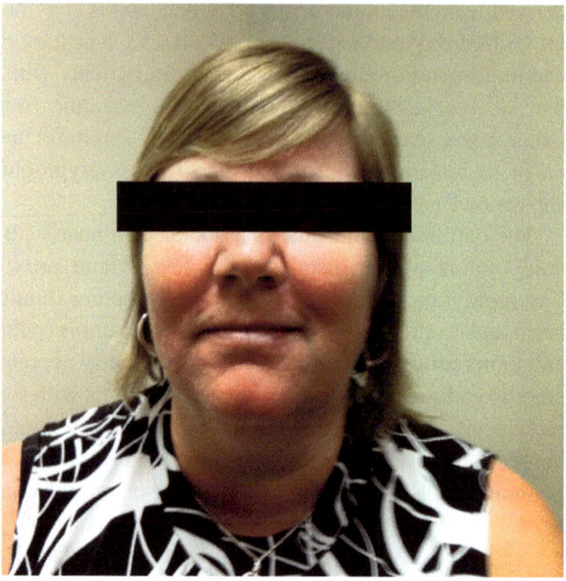

Fig. 7.1 Chronic skin changes caused by persistent flushing in a patient with advanced carcinoid syndrome

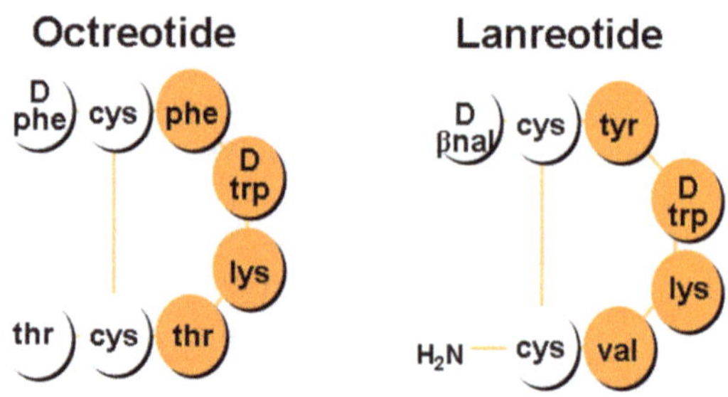

Fig. 7.2 Chemical structure of the synthetic somatostatin analogs octreotide and lanreotide. Adapted from Susini et al. [28]

The clinical use of native human somatostatin is impeded by its short half-life of approximately 2 min.

The somatostatin analogs octreotide and lanreotide were developed by shortening the somatostatin polypeptide chain, eliminating enzymatic cleavage sites but conserving binding sites (Fig. 7.2) [28, 29]. As a result, the two octapeptides have a half-life which exceeds 2 h and an avid binding affinity to SSTR2 [30]. Kvols et al. conducted the first clinical trial of octreotide in patients with the carcinoid syndrome, reporting amelioration of flushing and diarrhea in 88% of patients, and major reductions in urinary 5-HIAA in 72% [31]. Numerous additional studies have validated the powerful antisecretory activity of octreotide at doses of 100–500 μg administered subcutaneously 2–3 times daily [32–34]. Side effects, which are generally mild, include nausea, bloating, and steatorrhea. An increased rate of biliary stone and sludge formation is observed due to inhibitory effects of octreotide on gallbladder contractility. Therefore, prophylactic cholecystectomy should be performed on patients undergoing abdominal surgery.

A longer acting, depot formulation of octreotide (Sandostatin LAR®) has been available for the past decade, enabling monthly dosing and greatly enhancing patient comfort [35]. Intramuscular administration of 20–30 mg every 4 weeks represents a standard dose schedule. Patients who experience exacerbation of symptoms towards the end of each treatment cycle may benefit from increased frequency of administration (every 2–3 weeks). Likewise, higher doses of up to 60 mg every 3–4 weeks may be administered for patients with refractory symptoms [33]. Doses exceeding 60 mg are unlikely to be of additional palliative benefit given saturation of somatostatin receptors [36]. Supplemental dosing with subcutaneous octreotide is occasionally of benefit to patients with breakthrough symptoms.

A long-acting formulation of lanreotide (Somatuline Autogel®) is administered as a deep subcutaneous injection at doses of 90–120 mg every 4 weeks [37]. It has similar somatostatin-binding properties, clinical activity, and side-effect profile. A new somatostatin analog in development, pasireotide, binds avidly to four of the five somatostatin receptors (SSTRs 1, 2, 3, and 5) [38]. Clinical trials are currently testing its ability to palliate flushing and diarrhea in patients who are refractory to Sandostatin LAR.

Other Anti-Diarrheal Agents

Patients whose diarrhea persists despite somatostatin analog therapy may benefit from loperamide and/or diphenoxylate/atropine (Lomotil). For more severe or refractory diarrhea, the opiates paregoric and tincture of opium may be prescribed. Patients who have undergone resection of the distal small bowel frequently develop bile malabsorption which can be treated with bile acid sequestrants such as cholestyramine or colestipol [39]. Somatostatin analog therapy infrequently causes symptomatic fat malabsorption and steatorrhea which may respond to pancreatic enzyme supplementation. Several studies demonstrate that serotonin receptor antagonists, such as ondansetron, can palliate diarrhea in patients with the carcinoid syndrome, however the magnitude of benefit is small [40, 41].

Nutritional Measures

Niacin deficiency occurs due to diversion of tryptophan catabolism toward serotonin production. Pellagra, a disease associated with severe niacin deficiency, manifests as a clinical triad of dermatitis, diarrhea, and dementia and tends to resolve with niacin supplementation. While pellagra is observed rarely in patients with carcinoid tumors [42], subclinical niacin deficiency may occur more often; however, it is unclear whether routine screening of patients for subclinical niacin deficiency is of benefit [43].

It is important to note that foods containing high levels of serotonin appear to have no influence on the carcinoid syndrome. They need only be avoided during 24-h urine collections for 5-HIAA as they can lead to false-positive results. Other triggers of flushing, such as alcohol or spicy foods, vary among patients who generally learn to modify their diet as needed.

Treatment and Prophylaxis of the Carcinoid Crisis

The term "carcinoid crisis" refers to an episode of circulatory collapse and/or bronchospasm caused by an acute release of serotonin and other vasoactive substances into the circulation [44, 45]. Triggers include general anesthesia and epinephrine. Carcinoid syndrome patients who undergo an invasive procedure should receive a supplementary dose of octreotide 250–500 μg subcutaneously or intravenously 1–2 h prior to the procedure. Patients who develop intra-operative hypotension should receive bolus intravenous doses of 500–1,000 μg until control of symptoms is achieved. Alternatively, continuous intravenous infusion of 50–200 μg/h may be given after a bolus dose.

The Insulinoma Syndrome

Insulinomas are characterized by fasting hypoglycemia associated with neuroglycopenic symptoms such as dizziness, lethargy, diplopia, confusion, palpitations, and diaphoresis. The classical diagnostic "Whipple triad" consists of symptomatic hypoglycemia, low plasma glucose levels (<40 mg/dL), and relief of symptoms with glucose administration [46]. Most often, diagnosis is established during a monitored fast where serum glucose is measured along with insulin, proinsulin, and c-peptide in order to demonstrate hypoglycemia associated with inappropriate insulin elevation [47].

Approximately 90% of insulinomas are localized to the pancreas and considered benign [48]. Because the majority of insulinomas are surgically curable, long-term medical treatment of hypoglycemia is rarely required. Among patients with metastatic, unresectable insulinomas, dietary adjustments may help to prevent hypoglycemic attacks. Recommended measures include scheduled snacks of complex carbohydrates in between meals. During acute hypoglycemic episodes, rapidly absorbed carbohydrates (such as fruit juices) should be available. Continuous intravenous infusion of glucose may be necessary for patients with severe refractory hypoglycemia.

The benefits of somatostatin analog therapy for management of hypoglycemia are inconsistent. Only 50% of insulinomas express high levels of somatostatin receptors which bind to currently available somatostatin analogs [49]. While several studies have described palliation of hypoglycemia with somatostatin analog therapy [50–52], others have reported exacerbation of symptoms [53] due to suppression of counter regulatory hormones, including glucagon and growth hormone. Consequently, a monitored trial of short-acting octreotide, measuring effects on serum glucose and insulin, is recommended prior to initiation of long-acting somatostatin analog therapy.

The sulphonamide diazoxide counteracts hypoglycemia by directly affecting pancreatic beta-cell potassium channels [54] and by stimulating gluconeogenesis [55]. Commonly prescribed doses range from 100 to 600 mg/day [56]. Dose-limiting side effects include fluid retention and hirsutism. Diazoxide has not been studied in a well-controlled fashion and responses vary.

Everolimus, an oral inhibitor of mTOR, has demonstrated promising activity in pancreatic endocrine carcinomas [57]. Amongst its reported side effects is hyperglycemia, a phenomenon that may be related to suppression of insulin production or induction of peripheral insulin resistance. In one published summary of four cases of malignant insulinoma, treatment with everolimus resulted in rapid improvement in glycemic control [58]. This effect was observed even in two patients who did not experience any radiologic tumor regression, supporting the hypothesis that everolimus may exert a direct hyperglycemic effect in insulinoma patients.

The Gastrinoma (Zollinger–Ellison) Syndrome

The gastrinoma syndrome, characterized by peptic ulceration, dyspepsia, and diarrhea [59], was first described in 1955 by Zollinger and Ellison [60]. The syndrome is caused by hypersecretion of gastrin, a peptide hormone which stimulates the parietal cells of the stomach to produce excess gastric acid. Peptic ulcerations primarily impact the first part of the duodenum, but can also affect atypical locations such as the distal duodenum and upper jejunum [61, 62]. Ulcer perforation is a presenting symptom in up to 7% of cases [63]. Severe and persistent diarrhea may occur due to the passage of excess gastric acid into the small intestine, neutralizing pancreatic bicarbonate secretion and causing malabsorption. Precipitation of bile acids due to the low pH environment may also contribute to diarrhea [62].

Gastrinomas usually originate within the proximal duodenum or the head of the pancreas [61, 64]. Approximately 20% of gastrinomas arise in the context of multiple endocrine neoplasia type 1 (MEN1), an autosomal dominant hereditary condition [65]. The diagnosis of gastrinoma can be strongly suspected in patients who present with typical symptoms whose serum gastrin levels exceed ten times the upper limit of normal (i.e., >1,000 pg/ml). In cases where the diagnosis is equivocal, a positive secretin stimulation (>200 pg/ml increase in serum gastrin over baseline) is considered diagnostic [66]. Other typical characteristics are a basal gastric acid output of >15 mEq/h, or a gastric pH less than 2.5 among patients who are not on acid-suppressing medications. Useful imaging studies include CT scans, MRIs, ^{111}In-pentetreotide scintigraphy [67], and endoscopic ultrasonography [68]. Surgical duodenal transillumination can identify small duodenal gastrinomas [69].

Prior to the advent of H_2-receptor antagonists and proton pump inhibitors, the Zollinger–Ellison syndrome was a highly morbid condition necessitating palliative gastrectomy and vagotomy [70]. Today, high-dose proton pump inhibitors effectively control symptoms in the large majority of cases [66, 71]. The typical recommended starting dose of omeprazole is 60 mg per day; however, some patients require doses as high as 120 mg per day for optimal control of acid output [72]. Other proton pump inhibitors are equally safe and efficacious [73, 74]. Relief of symptoms may be an unreliable measure of acid suppression [75], and some studies recommend titration of proton-pump inhibitors to achieve an optimal gastric acid secretion rate of <10 mEq/h [76].

Because proton-pump inhibitors have been so effective at controlling the Zollinger–Ellison syndrome, there is little information on the role of somatostatin analogs in symptom management. Studies of octreotide and lanreotide demonstrate the ability of somatostatin analogs to reduce levels of serum gastrin [77–79]. Moreover, accumulating data on the antiproliferative role of somatostatin analogs suggests that they may play an important role in control of tumor growth [80, 81].

Surgical resection should always be considered for localized, sporadic tumors, or in metastatic cases where surgical cytoreduction can be performed with a curative or near-curative intent [82]. The potential benefits of surgery are not as well established in MEN1, in which pancreaticoduodenal tumors are invariably multifocal. One study employed transhepatic portal venous sampling for gastrin, followed by surgical exploration of patients with regionalized gastrin secretion, in order to normalize serum gastrin levels [83]. However, this approach remains controversial [84]. It is interesting to note that patients with MEN1 and hypercalcemia may experience palliation of the Zollinger–Ellison Syndrome after correction of hypercalcemia via parathyroid surgery.

The Vipoma (Verner–Morrison) Syndrome

In 1958, Verner and Morrison described an association between islet cell tumors and a syndrome consisting of profuse watery diarrhea and hypokalemia [85]. It was not until 1973 that the peptide hormone, VIP was implicated as the causative factor [86]. VIPomas are exceedingly rare, with an estimated incidence of approximately 1 in 10 million [87]. VIP stimulates intestinal secretion and inhibits electrolyte and water absorption in the bowel, leading to secretory diarrhea and hypokalemia. It also inhibits gastric acid secretion (causing achlorhydria) and induces vasodilation (causing flushing) [88]. The volume of watery diarrhea (which often exceeds 3 l/day despite fasting) has led some to describe this syndrome as "pancreatic cholera." Hypercalcemia and hyperglycemia are rare manifestations [87].

Patients who present with severe diarrheal symptoms may require intensive intravenous fluids and correction of electrolyte abnormalities. Somatostatin-analog therapy can result in substantial palliation of symptoms in the majority of cases [78, 89]. Symptomatic responses may be disproportionate to reductions in plasma concentrations of VIP, suggesting that direct inhibition of gastrointestinal secretion contributes to symptom palliation [90].

The Glucagonoma Syndrome

Glucagonomas are rare tumors arising from the alpha cells of the pancreas [91], with an estimated incidence of 1 in 20 million [92]. The majority are considered malignant. Clinical manifestations are protean, and may include hyperglycemia, anorexia, weight loss, venous thromboses, anemia, angular stomatitis, glossitis, neuropsychiatric symptoms, and an unusual rash called necrolytic migratory erythema (NME) [93]. NME characteristically manifests as painful, weeping erythematous papules or plaques primarily involving the lower extremities, perineum, and perioral region (Fig. 7.3) [94]. The lesions may wax and wane, leaving bronze-colored indurated scars. The underlying mechanism of NME is uncertain, but may be related to deficiency of amino acids and/or zinc. Hyperglycemia can develop when excess serum glucagon overwhelms the counter-regulatory effects of insulin. Cachexia can be attributed to the catabolic effects of glucagon. The etiology of deep venous thrombosis (which can occur in approximately 30% of cases) [95] is uncertain.

The glucagonoma syndrome is particularly sensitive to somatostatin analog therapy [93, 96]. In one retrospective study, somatostatin analogs led to major reductions in serum glucagon in 9 of 13 patients, resulting in complete remission of NME in eight patients and major reductions in insulin requirements in four patients [93]. Neuropsychiatric symptoms can likewise resolve with somatostatin-analog therapy [97]. Hyperglycemia appears to be less responsive to somatostatin analogs, but can be managed with insulin or oral hypoglycemic agents [98]. Nutritional support, including total parenteral nutrition, may be considered in patients with uncontrolled cachexia. Two case studies have documented improvement in NME after infusion of amino acids and correction of amino-acid deficiency [99, 100]. Another case study reported resolution of NME after zinc supplementation [101]. Due to the increased incidence of venous thrombosis, prophylactic anticoagulation should be considered.

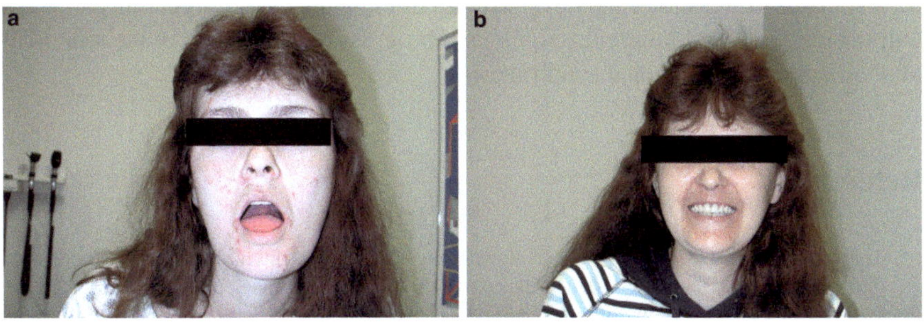

Fig. 7.3 Facial rash and angular stomatitis associated with neocrolytic migratory erythema (**a**). Resolution of rash 3 months after initiation of octreotide therapy (**b**)

Cushing's Syndrome

Cushing's syndrome resulting from ectopic production of ACTH is a rare manifestation of bronchopulmonary carcinoid tumors, occurring in approximately 2% of cases [102]. Among the rare patients who develop thymic carcinoid tumors, the incidence of ectopic Cushing syndrome appears to be substantially higher, ranging from 8 to 35%. Pancreatic endocrine tumors can also rarely secrete ACTH. Cushing syndrome should be suspected in patients who develop typical symptoms including central obesity, moon facies, dorsocervical fat deposition ("buffalo hump"), abdominal striae, proximal muscle weakness and atrophy, neuropsychiatric symptoms, hypertension, hyperglycemia, and osteoporosis [103]. Elevated levels of serum or urinary cortisol and serum ACTH can establish the diagnosis in most cases.

Because fulminant Cushing's syndrome can be fatal, bilateral adrenalectomy should be considered in cases where control of the underlying ACTH-secreting tumor is unlikely [104]. This can often be performed laparoscopically [105]. Oral medications which can aid in suppression of cortisol secretion include ketoconazole, metyrapone, and aminoglutethimide [106]. Both ketoconazole and metyrapone block the final step of cortisol synthesis, 11β hydroxylation of 11-deoxycortisol. Ketoconazole also inhibits the initial step in cortisol synthesis, cholesterol side-chain cleavage. Responses to somatostatin analog therapy are rare in ectopic ACTH. Down-regulation of somatostatin receptors by cortisol may contribute to resistance [107].

Conclusions

Recognition of endocrine syndromes and their appropriate therapies is essential for clinicians treating patients with neuroendocrine tumors. Somatostatin analogs represent a cornerstone of hormonal therapy due to their potent antisecretory effects and tolerable side-effect profile. Other agents, such proton pump inhibitors or opiate antidiarrheal drugs, can ameliorate the effects of elevated circulating hormones on their target tissues. Medical or surgical treatment of the underlying neuroendocrine neoplasm is often the most effective strategy for palliating hormonal syndromes. New somatostatin analogs and novel agents targeting oncogenic signaling pathways will undoubtedly build upon the significant progress already made in the treatment of neuroendocrine hormonal syndromes.

References

1. Thorson A, Biorck G, Bjorkman G, Waldenstrom J. Malignant carcinoid of the small intestine with metastases to the liver, valvular disease of the right side of the heart (pulmonary stenosis and tricuspid regurgitation without septal defects), peripheral vasomotor symptoms, bronchoconstriction, and an unusual type of cyanosis; a clinical and pathologic syndrome. Am Heart J. 1954;47(5):795–817.

2. Bean WB, Olch D, Weinberg HB. The syndrome of carcinoid and acquired valve lesions of the right side of the heart. Circulation. 1955;12(1):1–6.
3. Lembeck F. Detection of 5-hydroxytryptamine in carcinoid metastases. Naunyn Schmiedebergs Arch Exp Pathol Pharmakol. 1954;221(1):50–66.
4. Erspamer V, Asero B. Identification of enteramine, the specific hormone of the enterochromaffin cell system, as 5-hydroxytryptamine. Nature. 1952;169(4306):800–1.
5. Feldman JM. Increased dopamine production in patients with carcinoid tumors. Metabolism. 1985;34(3):255–60.
6. Sandler M, Karim SM, Williams ED. Prostaglandins in amine-peptide-secreting tumours. Lancet. 1968;2(7577):1053–4.
7. Lucas KJ, Feldman JM. Flushing in the carcinoid syndrome and plasma kallikrein. Cancer. 1986;58(10):2290–3.
8. Skrabanek P, Cannon D, Kirrane J, Powell D. Substance P secretion by carcinoid tumours. Ir J Med Sci. 1978;147(2):47–9.
9. Kvols LK. The carcinoid syndrome: a treatable malignant disease. Oncology (Huntingt). 1988;2(2):33–41.
10. Moertel CG, Sauer WG, Dockerty MB, Baggenstoss AH. Life history of the carcinoid tumor of the small intestine. Cancer. 1961;14:901–12.
11. Moertel CG. Karnofsky memorial lecture. An odyssey in the land of small tumors. J Clin Oncol. 1987;5(10):1502–22.
12. Caldarola VT, Jackman RJ, Moertel CG, Dockerty MB. Carcinoid tumors of the rectum. Am J Surg. 1964;107:844–9.
13. Sandler M, Snow PJ. An atypical carcinoid tumour secreting 5-hydroxytryptophan. Lancet. 1958;1(7012):137–9.
14. Davis Z, Moertel CG, McIlrath DC. The malignant carcinoid syndrome. Surg Gynecol Obstet. 1973;137(4):637–44.
15. Jensen RT. Overview of chronic diarrhea caused by functional neuroendocrine neoplasms. Semin Gastrointest Dis. 1999;10(4):156–72.
16. Cunningham JL, Janson ET, Agarwal S, Grimelius L, Stridsberg M. Tachykinins in endocrine tumors and the carcinoid syndrome. Eur J Endocrinol. 2008;159(3):275–82.
17. von der Ohe MR, Camilleri M, Kvols LK, Thomforde GM. Motor dysfunction of the small bowel and colon in patients with the carcinoid syndrome and diarrhea. N Engl J Med. 1993;329(15):1073–8.
18. Feldman JM. Carcinoid tumors and syndrome. Semin Oncol. 1987;14(3):237–46.
19. Matuchansky C, Launay JM. Serotonin, catecholamines, and spontaneous midgut carcinoid flush: plasma studies from flushing and nonflushing sites. Gastroenterology. 1995;108(3):743–51.
20. Vinik AI, Gonin J, England BG, Jackson T, McLeod MK, Cho K. Plasma substance-P in neuroendocrine tumors and idiopathic flushing: the value of pentagastrin stimulation tests and the effects of somatostatin analog. J Clin Endocrinol Metab. 1990;70(6):1702–9.
21. Smith AG, Greaves MW. Blood prostaglandin activity associated with noradrenaline-provoked flush in the carcinoid syndrome. Br J Dermatol. 1974;90(5):547–51.
22. Kvols LK. Metastatic carcinoid tumors and the malignant carcinoid syndrome. Ann N Y Acad Sci. 1994;733:464–70.
23. Lundin L, Norheim I, Landelius J, Oberg K, Theodorsson-Norheim E. Carcinoid heart disease: relationship of circulating vasoactive substances to ultrasound-detectable cardiac abnormalities. Circulation. 1988;77(2):264–9.
24. Robiolio PA, Rigolin VH, Wilson JS, et al. Carcinoid heart disease. Correlation of high serotonin levels with valvular abnormalities detected by cardiac catheterization and echocardiography. Circulation. 1995;92(4):790–5.
25. Pellikka PA, Tajik AJ, Khandheria BK, et al. Carcinoid heart disease. Clinical and echocardiographic spectrum in 74 patients. Circulation. 1993;87(4):1188–96.
26. Waltenberger J, Lundin L, Oberg K, et al. Involvement of transforming growth factor-beta in the formation of fibrotic lesions in carcinoid heart disease. Am J Pathol. 1993;142(1):71–8.

27. Beauchamp RD, Coffey Jr RJ, Lyons RM, Perkett EA, Townsend Jr CM, Moses HL. Human carcinoid cell production of paracrine growth factors that can stimulate fibroblast and endothelial cell growth. Cancer Res. 1991;51(19):5253–60.
28. Susini C, Buscail L. Rationale for the use of somatostatin analogs as antitumor agents. Ann Oncol. 2006;17(12):1733–42.
29. Bauer W, Briner U, Doepfner W, et al. SMS 201-995: a very potent and selective octapeptide analogue of somatostatin with prolonged action. Life Sci. 1982;31(11):1133–40.
30. Pless J, Bauer W, Briner U, et al. Chemistry and pharmacology of SMS 201-995, a long-acting octapeptide analogue of somatostatin. Scand J Gastroenterol Suppl. 1986;119:54–64.
31. Kvols LK, Moertel CG, O'Connell MJ, Schutt AJ, Rubin J, Hahn RG. Treatment of the malignant carcinoid syndrome. Evaluation of a long-acting somatostatin analogue. N Engl J Med. 1986;315(11):663–6.
32. Kvols LK. Therapy of the malignant carcinoid syndrome. Endocrinol Metab Clin North Am. 1989;18(2):557–68.
33. Oberg K, Kvols L, Caplin M, et al. Consensus report on the use of somatostatin analogs for the management of neuroendocrine tumors of the gastroenteropancreatic system. Ann Oncol. 2004;15(6):966–73.
34. di Bartolomeo M, Bajetta E, Buzzoni R, et al. Clinical efficacy of octreotide in the treatment of metastatic neuroendocrine tumors. A study by the Italian Trials in Medical Oncology Group. Cancer. 1996;77(2):402–8.
35. Rubin J, Ajani J, Schirmer W, et al. Octreotide acetate long-acting formulation versus open-label subcutaneous octreotide acetate in malignant carcinoid syndrome. J Clin Oncol. 1999;17(2):600–6.
36. Woltering EA, Mamikunian PM, Zietz S, et al. Effect of octreotide LAR dose and weight on octreotide blood levels in patients with neuroendocrine tumors. Pancreas. 2005;31(4):392–400.
37. Ruszniewski P, Ish-Shalom S, Wymenga M, et al. Rapid and sustained relief from the symptoms of carcinoid syndrome: results from an open 6-month study of the 28-day prolonged-release formulation of lanreotide. Neuroendocrinology. 2004;80(4):244–51.
38. Schmid HA. Pasireotide (SOM230): development, mechanism of action and potential applications. Mol Cell Endocrinol. 2008;286(1–2):69–74.
39. Westergaard H. Bile acid malabsorption. Curr Treat Options Gastroenterol. 2007;10(1):28–33.
40. Saslow SB, Scolapio JS, Camilleri M, et al. Medium-term effects of a new 5HT3 antagonist, alosetron, in patients with carcinoid diarrhoea. Gut. 1998;42(5):628–34.
41. Wymenga AN, de Vries EG, Leijsma MK, Kema IP, Kleibeuker JH. Effects of ondansetron on gastrointestinal symptoms in carcinoid syndrome. Eur J Cancer. 1998;34(8):1293–4.
42. Fleischmajer R, Hyman AB. Clinical significance of derangements of tryptophan metabolism. A review of pellagra, carcinoid and H disease. Arch Dermatol. 1961;84:563–73.
43. Shah GM, Shah RG, Veillette H, Kirkland JB, Pasieka JL, Warner RR. Biochemical assessment of niacin deficiency among carcinoid cancer patients. Am J Gastroenterol. 2005;100(10):2307–14.
44. Kvols LK. Therapeutic considerations for the malignant carcinoid syndrome. Acta Oncol. 1989;28(3):433–8.
45. Kahil ME, Brown H, Fred HL. The carcinoid crisis. Arch Intern Med. 1964;114:26–8.
46. Whipple AO, Frantz VK. Adenoma of islet cells with hyperinsulinism: a review. Ann Surg. 1935;101(6):1299–335.
47. Service FJ, Dale AJ, Elveback LR, Jiang NS. Insulinoma: clinical and diagnostic features of 60 consecutive cases. Mayo Clin Proc. 1976;51(7):417–29.
48. Service FJ, McMahon MM, O'Brien PC, Ballard DJ. Functioning insulinoma–incidence, recurrence, and long-term survival of patients: a 60-year study. Mayo Clin Proc. 1991;66(7):711–9.
49. Service FJ. Insulinoma and other islet-cell tumors. Cancer Treat Res. 1997;89:335–46.
50. Izumiyama H, Gotyo N, Fukai N, et al. Glucose-responsive and octreotide-sensitive insulinoma. Intern Med. 2006;45(8):519–24.
51. Usukura M, Yoneda T, Oda N, et al. Medical treatment of benign insulinoma using octreotide LAR: a case report. Endocr J. 2007;54(1):95–101.

52. Vezzosi D, Bennet A, Rochaix P, et al. Octreotide in insulinoma patients: efficacy on hypoglycemia, relationships with Octreoscan scintigraphy and immunostaining with anti-sst2A and anti-sst5 antibodies. Eur J Endocrinol. 2005;152(5):757–67.
53. Healy ML, Dawson SJ, Murray RM, Zalcberg J, Jefford M. Severe hypoglycaemia after long-acting octreotide in a patient with an unrecognized malignant insulinoma. Intern Med J. 2007;37(6):406–9.
54. Flatt PR, Shibier O, Szecowka J, Berggren PO. New perspectives on the actions of sulphonylureas and hyperglycaemic sulphonamides on the pancreatic beta-cell. Diabete Metab. 1994;20(2):157–62.
55. Fajans SS, Floyd Jr JC, Thiffault CA, Knopf RF, Harrison TS, Conn JW. Further studies on diazoxide suppression of insulin release from abnormal and normal islet tissue in man. Ann N Y Acad Sci. 1968;150(2):261–80.
56. Gill GV, Rauf O, MacFarlane IA. Diazoxide treatment for insulinoma: a national UK survey. Postgrad Med J. 1997;73(864):640–1.
57. Yao JC, Phan AT, Chang DZ, et al. Phase II study of RAD001 (everolimus) and depot octreotide (Sandostatin LAR) in patients with advanced low grade neuroendocrine carcinoma (LGNET). J Clin Oncol. 2006; 24(18S): 4042.
58. Kulke MH, Bergsland EK, Yao JC. Glycemic control in patients with insulinoma treated with everolimus. N Engl J Med. 2009;360(2):195–7.
59. Roy PK, Venzon DJ, Shojamanesh H, et al. Zollinger-Ellison syndrome. Clinical presentation in 261 patients. Medicine (Baltimore). 2000;79(6):379–411.
60. Zollinger RM, Ellison EH. Primary peptic ulcerations of the jejunum associated with islet cell tumors of the pancreas. Ann Surg. 1955;142(4):709–23. discussion, 724-708.
61. Jensen RT. Gastrointestinal endocrine tumours. Gastrinoma. Baillieres Clin Gastroenterol. 1996;10(4):603–43.
62. Meko JB, Norton JA. Management of patients with Zollinger-Ellison syndrome. Annu Rev Med. 1995;46:395–411.
63. Waxman I, Gardner JD, Jensen RT, Maton PN. Peptic ulcer perforation as the presentation of Zollinger-Ellison syndrome. Dig Dis Sci. 1991;36(1):19–24.
64. Norton JA. Surgical treatment and prognosis of gastrinoma. Best Pract Res Clin Gastroenterol. 2005;19(5):799–805.
65. Gibril F, Jensen RT. Zollinger-Ellison syndrome revisited: diagnosis, biologic markers, associated inherited disorders, and acid hypersecretion. Curr Gastroenterol Rep. 2004;6(6):454–63.
66. Berna MJ, Hoffmann KM, Long SH, Serrano J, Gibril F, Jensen RT. Serum gastrin in Zollinger-Ellison syndrome: II. Prospective study of gastrin provocative testing in 293 patients from the National Institutes of Health and comparison with 537 cases from the literature. evaluation of diagnostic criteria, proposal of new criteria, and correlations with clinical and tumoral features. *Medicine (Baltimore).* Nov 2006;85(6):331-364.
67. Jensen RT, Gibril F. Somatostatin receptor scintigraphy in gastrinomas. Ital J Gastroenterol Hepatol. 1999;31 Suppl 2:S179–85.
68. Varas Lorenzo MJ, Miquel Collell JM, Maluenda Colomer MD, Boix Valverde J, Armengol Miro JR. Preoperative detection of gastrointestinal neuroendocrine tumors using endoscopic ultrasonography. Rev Esp Enferm Dig. 2006;98(11):828–36.
69. Frucht H, Norton JA, London JF, et al. Detection of duodenal gastrinomas by operative endoscopic transillumination. A prospective study. Gastroenterology. 1990;99(6):1622–7.
70. Zollinger RM, Ellison EC, Fabri PJ, Johnson J, Sparks J, Carey LC. Primary peptic ulcerations of the jejunum associated with islet cell tumors. Twenty-five-year appraisal. Ann Surg. 1980;192(3):422–30.
71. Lamberts R, Creutzfeldt W, Struber HG, Brunner G, Solcia E. Long-term omeprazole therapy in peptic ulcer disease: gastrin, endocrine cell growth, and gastritis. Gastroenterology. 1993;104(5):1356–70.
72. Maton PN, Vinayek R, Frucht H, et al. Long-term efficacy and safety of omeprazole in patients with Zollinger-Ellison syndrome: a prospective study. Gastroenterology. 1989;97(4):827–36.

73. Hirschowitz BI, Simmons J, Mohnen J. Long-term lansoprazole control of gastric acid and pepsin secretion in ZE and non-ZE hypersecretors: a prospective 10-year study. Aliment Pharmacol Ther. 2001;15(11):1795–806.
74. Metz DC, Comer GM, Soffer E, et al. Three-year oral pantoprazole administration is effective for patients with Zollinger-Ellison syndrome and other hypersecretory conditions. Aliment Pharmacol Ther. 2006;23(3):437–44.
75. Raufman JP, Collins SM, Pandol SJ, et al. Reliability of symptoms in assessing control of gastric acid secretion in patients with Zollinger-Ellison syndrome. Gastroenterology. 1983;84(1):108–13.
76. Wolfe MM, Jensen RT. Zollinger-Ellison syndrome. Current concepts in diagnosis and management. N Engl J Med. 1987;317(19):1200–9.
77. Wymenga AN, Eriksson B, Salmela PI, et al. Efficacy and safety of prolonged-release lanreotide in patients with gastrointestinal neuroendocrine tumors and hormone-related symptoms. J Clin Oncol. 1999;17(4):1111.
78. Maton PN, Gardner JD, Jensen RT. Use of long-acting somatostatin analog SMS 201-995 in patients with pancreatic islet cell tumors. Dig Dis Sci. 1989;34(3 Suppl):28S–39.
79. Kvols LK, Buck M, Moertel CG, et al. Treatment of metastatic islet cell carcinoma with a somatostatin analogue (SMS 201-995). Ann Intern Med. 1987;107(2):162–8.
80. Arnold R, Trautmann ME, Creutzfeldt W, et al. Somatostatin analogue octreotide and inhibition of tumour growth in metastatic endocrine gastroenteropancreatic tumours. Gut. 1996;38(3): 430–8.
81. Saijo F, Naito H, Funayama Y, et al. Octreotide in control of multiple liver metastases from gastrinoma. J Gastroenterol. 2003;38(9):905–8.
82. Norton JA, Fraker DL, Alexander HR, et al. Surgery to cure the Zollinger-Ellison syndrome. N Engl J Med. 1999;341(9):635–44.
83. Thompson NW. Surgical treatment of the endocrine pancreas and Zollinger-Ellison syndrome in the MEN 1 syndrome. Henry Ford Hosp Med J. 1992;40(3–4):195–8.
84. Norton JA, Jensen RT. Resolved and unresolved controversies in the surgical management of patients with Zollinger-Ellison syndrome. Ann Surg. 2004;240(5):757–73.
85. Verner JV, Morrison AB. Islet cell tumor and a syndrome of refractory watery diarrhea and hypokalemia. Am J Med. 1958;25(3):374–80.
86. Bloom SR, Polak JM, Pearse AG. Vasoactive intestinal peptide and watery-diarrhoea syndrome. Lancet. 1973;2(7819):14–6.
87. Smith SL, Branton SA, Avino AJ, et al. Vasoactive intestinal polypeptide secreting islet cell tumors: a 15-year experience and review of the literature. Surgery. 1998;124(6):1050–5.
88. Marks IN, Bank S, Louw JH. Islet cell tumor of the pancreas with reversible watery diarrhea and achylorhydraia. Gastroenterology. 1967;52(4):695–708.
89. O'Dorisio TM, Gaginella TS, Mekhjian HS, Rao B, O'Dorisio MS. Somatostatin and analogues in the treatment of VIPoma. Ann N Y Acad Sci. 1988;527:528–35.
90. Oberg K, Eriksson B. Endocrine tumours of the pancreas. Best Pract Res Clin Gastroenterol. 2005;19(5):753–81.
91. McGavran MH, Unger RH, Recant L, Polk HC, Kilo C, Levin ME. A glucagon-secreting alpha-cell carcinoma of the pancreas. N Engl J Med. 1966;274(25):1408–13.
92. Boden G. Glucagonomas and insulinomas. Gastroenterol Clin North Am. 1989;18(4):831–45.
93. Wermer RA, Fatourechi V, Wynne AG, Kvols LK, Lloyd RV. The glucagonoma syndrome. Clinical and pathologic features in 21 patients. Medicine (Baltimore). 1996;75(2):53–63.
94. Wilkinson DS. Necrolytic migratory erythema with carcinoma of the pancreas. Trans St Johns Hosp Dermatol Soc. 1973;59(2):244–50.
95. Stacpoole PW. The glucagonoma syndrome: clinical features, diagnosis, and treatment. Endocr Rev. 1981;2(3):347–61.
96. Boden G, Ryan IG, Eisenschmid BL, Shelmet JJ, Owen OE. Treatment of inoperable glucagonoma with the long-acting somatostatin analogue SMS 201-995. N Engl J Med. 1986;314(26): 1686–9.

97. Holmes A, Kilpatrick C, Proietto J, Green MD. Reversal of a neurologic paraneoplastic syndrome with octreotide (Sandostatin) in a patient with glucagonoma. Am J Med. 1991;91(4):434–6.
98. Bloom SR, Polak JM. Glucagonoma syndrome. Am J Med. 1987;82(5B):25–36.
99. Norton JA, Kahn CR, Schiebinger R, Gorschboth C, Brennan MF. Amino acid deficiency and the skin rash associated with glucagonoma. Ann Intern Med. 1979;91(2):213–5.
100. Alexander EK, Robinson M, Staniec M, Dluhy RG. Peripheral amino acid and fatty acid infusion for the treatment of necrolytic migratory erythema in the glucagonoma syndrome. Clin Endocrinol (Oxf). 2002;57(6):827–31.
101. Sinclair SA, Reynolds NJ. Necrolytic migratory erythema and zinc deficiency. Br J Dermatol. 1997;136(5):783–5.
102. Limper AH, Carpenter PC, Scheithauer B, Staats BA. The Cushing syndrome induced by bronchial carcinoid tumors. Ann Intern Med. 1992;117(3):209–14.
103. Howlett TA, Rees LH, Besser GM. Cushing's syndrome. Clin Endocrinol Metab. 1985;14(4):911–45.
104. Porterfield JR, Thompson GB, Young Jr WF, et al. Surgery for Cushing's syndrome: an historical review and recent ten-year experience. World J Surg. 2008;32(5):659–77.
105. Young Jr WF, Thompson GB. Role for laparoscopic adrenalectomy in patients with Cushing's syndrome. Arq Bras Endocrinol Metabol. 2007;51(8):1349–54.
106. Nieman LK. Medical therapy of Cushing's disease. Pituitary. 2002;5(2):77–82.
107. de Herder WW, Lamberts SW. Is there a role for somatostatin and its analogs in Cushing's syndrome? Metabolism. 1996;45(8 Suppl 1):83–5.

Chapter 8
Management of Metastatic Carcinoid Tumors

Matthew H. Kulke

Abstract For patients with localized carcinoid tumors, surgical resection alone is often curative. Patients with metastatic disease, on the other hand, often present a therapeutic challenge. While somatostatin analogs are highly effective in controlling symptoms of hormonal secretion, they are only rarely associated with tumor regression. Selected patients with hepatic metastases may benefit from surgical debulking, embolization, or other ablative therapies. The clinical benefit associated with the administration of systemic agents such as alpha interferon or cytotoxic chemotherapy is less clear, and the widespread use of such regimens has been limited by their relatively modest anti-tumor activity as well as concerns regarding their potential toxicity. New treatment approaches for patients with metastatic carcinoid tumors are being actively explored.

Keywords Carcinoid tumors • Metastatic disease • Somatostatin analogs • Ablative therapies • Cytotoxic chemotherapy

Introduction

For patients with localized carcinoid tumors, surgical resection alone is often curative. Patients with metastatic disease, on the other hand, often present a therapeutic challenge. While somatostatin analogs are highly effective in controlling symptoms of hormonal secretion, they are only rarely associated with tumor regression. Selected patients with hepatic metastases may benefit from surgical debulking, embolization, or other ablative therapies. The clinical benefit associated with the

M.H. Kulke (✉)
Medical Oncology, Dana-Farber Cancer Institute, Harvard Medical School,
44 Binney Street, Boston, MA 02115, USA
e-mail: matthew_kulke@dfci.harvard.edu

J.C. Yao et al. (eds.), *Neuroendocrine Tumors*, Current Clinical Oncology,
DOI 10.1007/978-1-60327-997-0_8, © Springer Science+Business Media, LLC 2011

administration of systemic agents such as alpha interferon (IFN-α) or cytotoxic chemotherapy is less clear, and the widespread use of such regimens has been limited by their relatively modest anti-tumor activity as well as concerns regarding their potential toxicity. New treatment approaches for patients with metastatic carcinoid tumors are being actively explored.

Carcinoid Tumor Subtypes

The clinical presentation and clinical course of patients with carcinoid tumors can vary depending upon the tumor site of origin. Carcinoid tumors may arise from nearly any organ. A commonly used classification scheme groups carcinoid tumors according to their presumed derivation from the embryonic gut: foregut (bronchial and gastric), midgut (small intestine and appendiceal), and hindgut (rectal) (Table 8.1).

Bronchial Carcinoid Tumors

Bronchial carcinoids comprise approximately 2% of primary lung tumors [1, 2]. Typical carcinoids, also classified as well-differentiated pulmonary neuroendocrine tumors, are most often central in location, causing symptoms of cough, wheezing, hemoptysis, and recurrent post-obstructive pneumonia [3, 4]. They are only rarely associated with the classic carcinoid syndrome; they have, however, been associated with ectopic ACTH secretion resulting in Cushing's syndrome [3, 5–7]. Approximately one-third of bronchial carcinoids demonstrate "atypical" histologic features [1, 4, 6, 8]. Atypical carcinoids are characterized

Table 8.1 Initial clinical presentation of carcinoid tumors

Tumor	Symptom
Foregut	
Bronchial carcinoids	Cough, hemoptysis, post-obstructive pneumonia, Cushing's syndrome. Carcinoid syndrome rare
Gastric carcinoids	Usually asymptomatic and found incidentally
Midgut	
Small intestine carcinoids	Intermittent bowel obstruction or mesenteric ischemia. Carcinoid syndrome common when metastatic
Appendiceal carcinoids	Usually found incidentally. May cause carcinoid syndrome when metastatic
Hindgut	
Rectal carcinoids	Either found incidentally or discovered due to bleeding, pain, and constipation. Rarely cause hormonal symptoms, even when metastatic

by the presence of frequent mitoses or areas of necrosis. Whereas typical carcinoid tumors are generally indolent, with metastases reported in less than 15% of cases, atypical carcinoids pursue an aggressive clinical course [3, 6, 7, 9]. Accordingly, long-term survival rates for patients with typical carcinoid tumors following surgical resection generally exceed 85%, but are significantly less for patients who undergo resection for atypical carcinoids.

Gastric Carcinoid Tumors

Gastric carcinoid tumors can be subclassifed into three distinct groups: those associated with chronic atrophic gastritis (type 1), those associated with the Zollinger–Ellison syndrome (type 2), and sporadic gastric carcinoids (type 3). Type 1 and type 2 carcinoids generally pursue an indolent course and can be resected endoscopically, with subsequent interval follow-up. Between 15 and 25% of gastric carcinoids are sporadic. In contrast to type I and type II carcinoids, these lesions develop in the absence of hypergastrinemia, are usually greater than 1 cm in size, and tend to pursue an aggressive clinical course. Because of the aggressive nature of these lesions, most are treated with gastrectomy if not already metastatic [10, 11].

Small Intestine Carcinoid Tumors

Small bowel carcinoid tumors comprise approximately one third of small bowel tumors in surgical series [12]. Approximately 5–7% will present with the carcinoid syndrome, at which time hepatic metastases are usually also present [13, 14]. Tumor size is an unreliable predictor of metastatic disease, and metastases have been reported even from tumors measuring less than 0.5 cm [15]. Mesenteric fibrosis and associated ischemia, caused by a characteristic desmoplastic reaction, is often present in association with small bowel carcinoids. These tumors are also frequently associated with "buckling" or tethering of the intestine due to extensive mesenteric involvement [13, 16]. Resection of the small bowel primary tumor, together with associated mesenteric metastases, leads to significant reduction in tumor-related symptoms of pain and obstruction, and can be reasonably recommended in symptomatic patients with known metastatic disease [17].

Appendiceal Carcinoid Tumors

Patients with appendiceal carcinoid tumors generally present at relatively young age, the mean age at presentation in the recent SEER database analysis was 49 years, and in older series is even younger [18, 19]. The clinical behavior of appendiceal carcinoid tumors can be predicted based on the size of the tumor. Over 95% of appendiceal carcinoid tumors are less than 2 cm in diameter [20, 21]. The incidence of metastatic disease in such patients is extraordinarily low, although rare cases have been reported in the literature [21–26]. In contrast, approximately one-third of patients with appendiceal carcinoid tumors measuring more than 2 cm in diameter have either nodal or distant metastases [20]. Based on the low incidence of metastases in patients whose tumors measure less than 2 cm, simple appendectomy is felt to be sufficient in such cases. In contrast, the higher incidence of metastases in patients whose tumors measure more than 2 cm in diameter has led to the recommendation for complete right hemicolectomy if more distant metastatic spread is not already present [20].

Rectal Carcinoid Tumors

Approximately 50% of rectal carcinoid tumors are asymptomatic and found on routine endoscopy [27]. As with appendiceal lesions, the size of the primary lesion correlates closely with the probability of metastases, which occur in less than 5% of tumors measuring less than 1 cm, but in the majority of lesions greater than 2 cm [28, 29]. Two-thirds of rectal carcinoid tumors are less than 1 cm and are successfully treated with local excision. The management of tumors measuring 1–2 cm is controversial. Although most tumors of this size can be managed with local excision, several authors have suggested that the presence of muscular invasion, symptoms at diagnosis, or ulceration are poor prognostic factors that warrant more extensive surgical procedures [27–29]. Tumors measuring greater than 2 cm have traditionally been managed with low anterior resection or abdominoperineal resection, although the presence of more distant disease in many such cases may make the clinical benefit of such procedures questionable.

Initial Evaluation of Patients with Metastatic Carcinoid Tumors

While the biology and clinical course of metastatic carcinoid disease may vary according to the primary site of the original tumor, patients with metastatic disease are in most cases evaluated and treated in a similar fashion regardless of primary site.

Imaging Techniques

Patients in whom metastatic disease is suspected are generally first evaluated with an abdominal CT scan to rule out liver metastases. Liver function tests are an unreliable indicator of tumor involvement, and the serum alkaline phosphatase is frequently normal despite extensive liver involvement by carcinoid tumor. Carcinoid liver metastases are often hypervascular, and may become isodense relative to the liver with the administration of intravenous contrast. Multiphasic CT scans should thus be performed both before and after the administration of intravenous contrast agents [30, 31]. Magnetic resonance imaging may be helpful in cases where CT findings are equivocal.

Over 90% of carcinoid tumors, contain high concentrations of somatostatin receptors, and can be imaged with a radiolabeled form of the somatostatin analog octreotide (111-indium pentetreotide) [32–34]. The uptake of radiolabeled octreotide is also predictive of clinical response to therapy with somatostatin analogs. The sensitivity of this technique appears to be higher for extrahepatic than for hepatic lesions, presumably because of heterogeneous octreotide uptake in normal liver [35, 36]. In one series, for example, octreotide scintigraphy detected 12 of 12 known extra-hepatic lesions, but only 12 of 24 hepatic lesions [35]. Greater sensitivity for hepatic lesions may be achieved by the use of single photon emission computed tomography (SPECT) imaging [37, 38].

Tumor Markers

Because of the often indolent nature of carcinoid tumors, patients with metastatic disease who are asymptomatic can sometimes be closely monitored without treatment. The serial measurement of tumor markers may be helpful in these cases to monitor disease progression, and also to subsequently monitor treatment response. The serial measurement of the serotonin metabolite 5-hydroxyindoleacetic acid (HIAA) in 24-h urine collections has been commonly used for monitoring of patients with metastatic carcinoid tumors. Although elevated urinary 5-HIAA levels are highly specific for carcinoid tumors, they are not particularly sensitive: in one study, only 73% of patients with metastatic carcinoid tumors had elevated levels [39]. Furthermore, 5-HIAA levels are generally elevated in patients with primary midgut carcinoid tumors, but are not useful in patients with either foregut (bronchial, gastric) or hindgut (rectal) carcinoid tumors, which do not secrete serotonin. The use of urinary 5-HIAA levels can also be limited by false positives. The normal rate of 5-HIAA excretion ranges from 2 to 8 mg/day (10–42 μmol/day). Values of up to 30 mg/day (157 μmol/day) may be found in patients with malabsorption syndromes such as celiac and Whipple's disease, as well as after the ingestion of large amounts of tryptophan-rich foods. Although some patients with the carcinoid syndrome have similar modest elevations, most have values for urinary 5-HIAA excretion above 100 mg/day (523 μmol/day) [40].

Another tumor marker, chromogranin A (CGA) is a 49-kD protein that is contained in the neurosecretory vesicles of neuroendocrine tumor cells, and is detectable in the plasma of patients with endocrine neoplasms. Because it does not rely on serotonin secretion, serum chromogranin A is a more sensitive and broadly applicable marker than urinary 5-HIAA, and may be used not only in patients with metastatic small bowel and appendiceal carcinoid tumors, but also in patients with bronchial and rectal carcinoid tumors in whom urinary 5-HIAA levels are less likely to be elevated [41, 42]. Plasma CGA levels have also been shown to correlate with treatment response, and may also have prognostic value: in one series of 71 patients with metastatic carcinoid tumors, CGA levels of more than 5,000 μg/mL were independently associated with poor prognosis [42].

Surgical Considerations in Patients with Metastatic Carcinoid

Carcinoid Heart Disease

Carcinoid heart disease occurs in approximately two-thirds of patients with the carcinoid syndrome [43]. Carcinoid heart lesions are characterized by plaque-like, fibrous endocardial thickening that classically involves the right side of the heart, and often causes retraction and fixation of the leaflets of the tricuspid and pulmonary valves. Tricuspid regurgitation is a nearly universal feature of carcinoid heart disease; tricuspid stenosis, pulmonary regurgitation, and pulmonary stenosis may also occur [44]. Left-sided heart disease occurs in less than 10% of patients [45, 46].

The preponderance of lesions in the right heart suggests that carcinoid heart disease is related to factors secreted by liver metastases into the hepatic vein. Among patients with carcinoid syndrome, patients with heart disease exhibit higher levels of serum serotonin and urinary 5-HIAA excretion than patients without heart disease [43, 45–48]. Other investigators have suggested that high atrial natriuretic peptide may also contribute to the pathogenesis of this disease. Whether these factors are directly responsible for the cardiac lesions, however, is unclear. Treatment with somatostatin analogs resulting in decreased serotonin secretion may not prevent the development of carcinoid heart disease and does not result in regression of cardiac lesions [46, 47].

The indolent nature of metastatic carcinoid, combined with the availability of effective treatments for carcinoid syndrome, has led to interest in valve replacement surgery for selected patients. Right-sided heart failure in such patients may lead to significant morbidity and mortality. In early series, valvular replacement in patients with symptomatic carcinoid heart disease has been associated with relatively high perioperative morbidity [45, 49]. Surviving patients, however, appear to achieve significant symptomatic improvement, and more advanced techniques may facilitate the future use of valve replacement surgery in carcinoid patients [50].

Surgical Resection of Hepatic Metastases

The predominant site of metastatic spread in patients with neuroendocrine tumors involving the GI tract is the liver. In patients with a limited number of hepatic metastases, surgical resection has resulted in both long-term survival and in significant palliation of symptoms [51–53]. In one series of 74 patients undergoing hepatic resection for metastatic disease, over 90% experienced symptomatic relief, and the 4-year survival rate exceeded 70% [51]. The number of patients with liver-isolated metastatic disease in whom liver transplantation (OLT) has been attempted is small, and its role in such patients remains unclear [54–56]. Most series have reported high rates of both perioperative mortality and early tumor recurrence. One multicenter European study reported a 5-year survival rate of 36% among highly selected patients with metastatic carcinoid tumors [55]. However, because many patients with metastatic carcinoid may have indolent disease and encouraging 5-year survival rates without treatment, it is difficult to assess the impact of hepatic transplantation in this population.

Hepatic Artery Embolization

Hepatic arterial embolization may be used as a palliative technique in patients with hepatic metastases who are not candidates for surgical resection. Hepatic artery embolization is based on the principle that tumors in the liver derive most of their blood supply from the hepatic artery, whereas healthy hepatocytes derive most of their blood supply from the portal vein. Embolization of the hepatic arterial blood supply can be performed with or without the concurrent injection of chemotherapy. The response rates associated with embolization, as measured either by decrease in hormonal secretion or by radiographic regression, are generally greater than 50% [57–66]. However, the duration of response can be brief, ranging from 4 to 24 months in uncontrolled series [58, 61]. In one of the largest series of 81 patients undergoing embolization or chemoembolization for carcinoid tumor, the median duration of response was 17 months, and the probability of progression-free survival at 1, 2, and 3 years was 75, 35, and 11%, respectively [61]. More recently, radioembolization has also shown promise. In a retrospective series of 148 neuroendocrine tumor patients treated with $^{(90)}$Y microspheres, partial or complete responses were observed in 63% of patients, with only mild associated toxicity [67]. Partial radiologic responses were observed in 50% of patients in a prospective study, in which 32 patients were treated with $^{(90)}$Y microspheres [68]. While early studies reported a significant incidence of post-embolization complications, improved techniques have, in recent years, reduced the incidence of such complications, making embolization an important and generally safe treatment option for patients with neuroendocrine tumors [61].

RFA and Cryoablation

Other approaches to the treatment of hepatic metastases have included the use of radiofrequency ablation (RFA) and cryoablation, either alone or in conjunction with surgical debulking. These approaches can be performed using a percutaneous or laparoscopic approach. While they appear to be less morbid than either resection or hepatic artery embolization, their long-term efficacy, particularly in patients with large volume hepatic disease is not clearly established. Most published reports are small case studies of fewer than 40 patients [69]. In one series, 31 symptomatic patients with metastatic carcinoid, islet cell tumor, or medullary thyroid cancer, underwent resection, cryosurgery, and/or RFA [70]. Symptoms were eliminated in 27 (87%), and 16 had progressive or recurrence disease with a median follow-up of 26 months.

Systemic Therapy for Metastatic Carcinoid

Somatostatin Analogs and Alpha Interferon

Often, patients first become symptomatic from symptoms of hormonal hypersecretion rather than from symptoms related to tumor bulk. This is especially true for patients with small bowel or appendiceal carcinoid tumors, in whom symptoms are typically absent until hepatic metastases supervene, and the secretion of serotonin and other vasoactive substances into the systemic circulation results in the carcinoid syndrome. This syndrome is characterized by episodic flushing, secretory diarrhea, and the development of wheezing and right-sided valvular heart disease.

The carcinoid syndrome, as well as other hormonal syndromes associated with neuroendocrine tumors, can often be well controlled with somatostatin analogs. Somatostatin is a 14-amino acid peptide that inhibits the secretion of a broad range of hormones, and acts by binding to somatostatin receptors, which are expressed on the majority of neuroendocrine tumors [71]. In an initial study, the subcutaneous administration of the somatostatin analog octreotide, administered at a dosage of 150 ucg three times a day, improved the symptoms of carcinoid syndrome in 88% of patients [72]. More recently, the use of a long-acting depot form of octreotide, which can be administered on a monthly basis, has largely obviated the need for patients to inject themselves on a daily basis. Long-acting octreotide is typically initiated at a dose of 20 mg IM after a brief trial of the short-acting formulation, with gradual escalation of the dose as needed for optimal control of symptoms [73]. Patients may, in addition, use additional short-acting octreotide for breakthrough symptoms. Lanreotide is another somatostatin analog that has been used for the management of carcinoid syndrome [74–78]. A randomized study of lanreotide SR vs. octreotide in 33 patients with carcinoid syndrome demonstrated equivalent efficacy for symptom control and reduction in tumor cell markers [76].

The addition of IFN-α to therapy with somatostatin analogs has also been reported to be effective in controlling symptoms in patients with the carcinoid syndrome who may be resistant to somatostatin analogs alone [79, 80]. The ability of IFN-α to stimulate T-cell function and to control the secretion of tumor products led to its initial use in patients with the carcinoid syndrome [81]. Therapy with low-dose IFN-α has been reported to result in biochemical responses in approximately 40% of patients with metastatic neuroendocrine tumors [82]. In clinical trials, doses of IFN-α have ranged from 3 to 9 MU subcutaneously (SC), administered from 3 to 7 times/week. IFN-α is somewhat myelosuppressive, and the dose is often titrated in individual patients to achieve a total leukocyte count of 3,000/μL. The more widespread acceptance of IFN-α in the treatment of metastatic neuroendocrine tumors has been limited by studies challenging its efficacy as well as the potential for side effects, which may include myelosuppression, fatigue, and depression [83].

Recent evidence suggest that somatostatin analogs either with or without IFN, may also have a direct antineoplastic effect. The comparable efficacy of lantreotide, IFN-α, or combined therapy was evaluated in a prospective randomized trial involving 80 therapy-naive patients with documented progressive metastatic neuroendocrine tumors [78]. The rates of objective partial response (4, 4, and 7% for lanreotide, IFN, and combined therapy, respectively) were low in all three groups; however, treatment resulted in apparent disease stabilization in a higher proportion of patients (28, 26, and 18%, respectively). In a recent randomized study, 85 patients with unresectable or metastatic midgut neuroendocrine tumors were randomized to receive treatment with octreotide LAR or placebo. Patients randomized to the octreotide arm had a significantly longer progression-free survival duration (14.3 vs. 6 months; $p=0.0037$), which led to early termination of the study [84]. A randomized trial evaluating the effect of lanreotide vs. placebo on progression-free survival is ongoing.

Cytotoxic Chemotherapy

Cytotoxic chemotherapy has contributed in only a limited fashion to the treatment of patients with metastatic carcinoid tumors (Table 8.2). Studies of single-agent therapy with 5-fluorouracil, streptozocin, or doxorubicin have shown that these agents are associated with response rates of approximately 20% [85]. Combination chemotherapy does not appear to be significantly superior to single-agent therapy in the treatment of patients with metastatic carcinoid tumors. In an initial trial, the Eastern Oncology Cooperative Group (ECOG) randomized 118 patients to receive streptozocin combined with either 5-fluorouracil or cyclophosphamide [86]. Response rates, as measured either by tumor regression or a decrease in urinary 5-HIAA levels, were 33% for strepotozicin/5-fluorouracil and 26% for streptozocin/cyclophosphamide. There was no difference in survival between the two groups, and both regimens were associated with significant toxicity. In an attempt to decrease the toxicity associated with 5-fluorouracil and streptozocin, the ECOG in a subsequent trial increased the dosing interval between cycles of streptocin/5-fluorouracil and compared this regimen to doxorubicin alone [87]. Although these regimens were better tolerated, the response rate for streptozocin and 5-fluorouracil dropped to 22%, as compared to only 21% for doxorubicin alone. The median survival duration

Table 8.2 Selected trials of cytotoxic chemotherapy regimens in patients with advanced carcinoid tumors

Regimen	Patients[a]	Radiological tumor response rate (%)	PFS/TTP	Median overall survival (months)	References
Phase II trials					
Dacarbazine (DTIC)	56	16	NR		Bukowski et al. [89]
DTIC	61	8	NR		Sun et al. [88]
Temozolomide + thalidomide	14	7	NR		Kulke et al. [105]
Etoposide	17	12	NR		Kelsen et al. [106]
Paclitaxel	24	8	3.2 Months		Ansell et al. [93]
Docetaxel	21	0	10 Months		Kulke et al. [95]
Gemcitabine	18	0	8.3 Months		Kulke et al. [94]
Streptozocin + fluorouracil + doxorubicin + cyclophosphamide	56	30	NR		Bukowski et al. [107]
Randomized trials					
Streptozocin + cyclophosphamide	47	26	NR	12.5	
Streptozocin + fluorouracil	42	33	NR	11.2	Moertel and Hanley [86]
Doxorubicin	81	21	NR	11.1	
Streptozocin + fluorouracil	80	22	NR	14.9	Engstrom et al. [87]
Doxorubicin + fluorouracil	88	15.9%	4.5 Months	15.7	
Streptozocin + fluorouracil	88	16	5.3 Months	24.3	Sun et al. [88]

[a]Number of patients evaluable for efficacy endpoints are listed

for patients randomized to streptozocin and 5-fluourouracil was 14 months as compared to 11 months for patients randomized to doxorubicin. This survival difference was not statistically significant. Most recently, streptozocin/5-FU was compared to 5-FU/doxorubicin in a randomized trial in which 249 patients were enrolled and 176 were evaluable. The response rate associated with the two regimens were similar (16% vs. 15.9%), although there was a slight survival benefit associated with streptozocin/5-FU [88].

Dacarbazine (DTIC) has been evaluated as a potential alternative to streptozocin-based therapy in carcinoid tumors. A Southwest Oncology Group study reported that treatment with DTIC was associated with an objective radiologic response rate of 16% in 56 patients with metastatic carcinoid tumors [89]. In an ECOG study evaluating the efficacy of DTIC in patients who had failed either streptozocin/5-FU or streptozocin/doxorubicin, the overall response rate was 8%. The addition to 5-fluorouracil and epirubicin to DTIC (FDE) does not appear to further enhance antitumor activity beyond that seen with DTIC alone, and has been associated with an objective response rate of 25% in a heterogeneous group of patients with advanced neuroendocrine tumors [90].

Patients with poorly differentiated neuroendocrine tumors have been previously reported to be more responsive to cytotoxic chemotherapy than patients with well-differentiated tumors. In an initial study, a combination of cisplatin and etoposide commonly used for small cell lung cancer was associated with an overall tumor response rate of 67% in 18 patients with "anaplastic" neuroendocrine tumors (presumably analogous to poorly differentiated neuroendocrine tumors), but had little activity in more well-differentiated tumor subtypes [91]. In a subsequent study of 36 patients with advanced neuroendocrine tumors, treatment with cisplatin and etoposide was associated with an overall radiologic response rate of 36% and a median survival time of 19 months. All patients enrolled in this study had either poorly differentiated histology or a rapidly progressing clinical course, suggesting that few, if any of these patients had more classic, indolent carcinoid or pancreatic endocrine tumors [92].

Newer chemotherapeutic agents have, to date, proved relatively inactive in neuroendocrine tumors. High-dose paclitaxel, administered with granulocyte-colony stimulating factor, was evaluated in 24 patients with metastatic carcinoid and islet cell tumors [93]. Significant hematologic toxicity was observed, and the objective radiologic response rate was only 8%. Treatment with docetaxel was associated with biochemical responses but no radiologic responses in a recent phase II trial of 21 patients with carcinoid tumors [94]. No responses were observed in 19 neuroendocrine tumor patients treated with gemcitabine [95].

Novel Treatment Approaches for Metastatic Carcinoid Tumors

The modest efficacy of current systemic treatment regimens has led to interest in the development of novel therapeutic approaches for patients with advanced neuroendocrine tumors. Such approaches include the use of radiolabeled somatostatin analogs, as well as regimens incorporating angiogenesis inhibitors and small molecule tyrosine kinase inhibitors.

Peptide Receptor Radio-Therapy

The high rate of somatostatin receptor expression in neuroendocrine tumors provides the rationale for use of radionuclide therapy for patients with inoperable or metastatic disease. The available radiolabeled somatostatin analogs differ from one another in their affinity for the various somatostatin receptor subtypes and in the radionuclides to which they are conjugated. The most frequently used radionuclides for targeted radiotherapy have included indium (^{111}In), yttrium (^{90}Y), and lutecium (^{177}Lu), which differ from one another in terms of emitted particles, particle energy, and tissue penetration (Table 8.3) [96]. [^{177}Lu-DOTA, Tyr3]octreotate has been used in the treatment of 504 patients with neuroendocrine tumors strongly expressing somatostatin receptors. Efficacy results for this retrospective series, reported for 310 of the 504 patients, suggest an overall tumor response rate of up to 30% [97].

Table 8.3 Therapeutic efficacy of radiolabeled somatostatin analogs in neuroendocrine tumors

Agents	Patients	Tumor response rate (%)	References
[^{111}In-DTPA]Octreotide	26	0	Valkema et al. [108]
	26	8	Anthony et al. [109]
[^{90}Y-DOTA,Tyr3]Octreotide	29	7	Otte et al. [110]
	30	23	Paganelli et al. [111]
	41	24	Waldherr et al. [112]
	39	34	Waldherr et al. [113]
	32	9	DeJong et al. [114]
	75	37	Teunissen et al. [115]
	90	4.4	Bushnell et al. [98]
[^{90}Y-DOTA]Lanreotide	39	20	Virgolini et al. [116]
[^{177}Lu-DOTA,Tyr3]Octreotate	125	28	Kwekkeboom et al. [117]
	310	30	Kwekkeboom et al. [97]

Relatively few prospective trials of radiopeptide therapy have been reported. In one such study, ^{90}Y-DOTA-Tyr3-octreotide was evaluated in 90 patients, who received three cycles of therapy once every 6 weeks. Although objective tumor response rates were modest (4.4%), over 50% of patients for whom symptoms were evaluable reported improvement [98]. No prospective, randomized data yet exists for radiopeptide therapy in neuroendocrine tumors.

VEGF Pathway Inhibitors

Neuroendocrine tumors are highly vascular, and overexpression of the growth factor, vascular endothelial growth factor (VEGF) has been observed in carcinoid tumors [99]. Therapies targeting VEGF (bevacizumab) and the VEGF receptor (sorafenib, sunitinib) have been evaluated in the phase II setting in patients with advanced carcinoid disease (Table 8.4).

Bevacizumab was evaluated in a phase II trial, in which 44 patients with advanced carcinoid tumors who were receiving a stable dose of octreotide were randomly assigned to treatment with either bevacizumab or pegylated IFN-α-2b [100]. Four of twenty-two (18%) bevacizumab-treated patients achieved confirmed radiographic partial responses, as compared with no responses among patients treated with pegylated IFN-α-2b. Additionally, after 18 weeks, 96% of bevacizumab-treated patients remained progression-free, as compared to 68% of the IFN-α-2b–treated patients. These encouraging results have led to the development of an ongoing study, led by the Southwest Oncology Group, in which patients are randomized to receive either IFN-α-2b or bevacizumab in addition to octreotide, with a primary end point of progression-free survival.

The small molecule tyrosine kinase inhibitor sorafenib was evaluated in 50 patients with carcinoid and 43 patients with pancreatic neuroendocrine tumors. In a preliminary analysis, responses were observed in 7% of the carcinoid patients and

Table 8.4 Phase II trials of biologically targeted agents in carcinoid tumors

Agent	Molecular target(s)	Patients	Tumor subtype	Tumor response rate (%)	Median PFS/TTP (months)	References
Imatinib	PDGFR-α, -β; KIT; Bcr-Abl	27	Carcinoid	4	5.5	Yao et al. [118]
Bevacizumab + octreotide	Vascular endothelial growth factor (VEGF)	22	Carcinoid	18	Not reported	Yao et al. [100]
Sunitinib	VEGFR, PDGFR, C-Kit, RET, FLT3	41	Carcinoid	2	10.2	Kulke et al. [102]
		66	Pancreatic endocrine	16	7.7	
Sorafenib	VEGFR, B-Raf	50	Carcinoid	7	Not reported	Hobday et al. [101]
		43	Pancreatic endocrine	11	Not reported	
Gefitinib	EGFR	40	Carcinoid	3	Not reported	Hobday et al. [119]
		31	Pancreatic endocrine	6	Not reported	
Temsirolimus	Mammalian target of rapamycin (mTOR)	21	Carcinoid	5	6.0	Duran et al. [103]
		15	Pancreatic endocrine	7	10.6	
Everolimus (RAD001) + octreotide	mTOR	30	Carcinoid	17	14.5	Yao et al. [104]
		30	Pancreatic endocrine	27	11.5	

11% of the pancreatic NET patients [101]. In another phase II study, 109 patients with advanced neuroendocrine tumors received repeated 6-week treatment cycles of sunitinib, administered orally at 50 mg once daily for 4 weeks, followed by 2 weeks off treatment [102]. While RECIST-defined partial responses were observed in only 2% of the carcinoid cohort, 44% of the carcinoid patients in the study experienced at least some degree of tumor shrinkage.

mTOR Inhibitors

The mammalian target of rapamycin (mTOR) is a serine-threonine kinase that participates in the regulation of cell growth, proliferation, and apoptosis through modulation of the cell cycle. mTOR also mediates downstream signaling from a number of pathways, including the VEGF and insulin-like growth factor (IGF) signaling implicated in neuroendocrine tumor growth. Two rapamycin derivatives have been evaluated recently in neuroendocrine tumors: temsirolimus and everolimus (RAD001).

In an initial multicenter study, 37 patients with advanced progressive neuroendocrine tumors were treated with weekly intravenous temsirolimus. The intent-to-treat response rate for the cohort was 5.6%. Outcomes were similar between patients with carcinoid and pancreatic neuroendocrine tumors [103]. In a second phase II study, 30 patients with carcinoid tumors and 30 with pancreatic neuroendocrine tumors were treated with a combination of the mTOR inhibitor everolimus, 5–10 mg/day, and depot octreotide (30 mg every 4 weeks). The overall tumor response rate in evaluable patients was 17% in the carcinoid cohort [104]. Evaluation of the activity and safety of everolimus in patients with neuroendocrine tumors is ongoing.

Conclusions

Patients with carcinoid tumors have diverse clinical presentations, related to both the tumor site of origin and the potential for hormone secretion. The non-specific nature of many of these symptoms unfortunately often leads to a late diagnosis, after metastatic disease has developed. Patients with metastatic disease may nevertheless benefit from a number of different therapeutic options. Somatostatin analogs are highly effective in ameliorating the symptoms of flushing and diarrhea associated with carcinoid syndrome. Recent evidence also suggests that somatostatin analogs also have a direct antiproliferative effect in patients with metastatic carcinoid tumors of midgut origin.

A tendency for carcinoid tumors to metastasize to the liver presents an opportunity for hepatic directed therapy in appropriately selected patients. In patients who are not candidates for hepatic resection, hepatic artery embolization may result in clinical benefit.

Additional systemic treatment approaches to patients with advanced carcinoid are rapidly evolving. While patients with poorly differentiated or high-grade tumors may respond well to platinum-based regimens, the majority of patients with well-differentiated, low-grade tumors unfortunately appear to be resistant to traditional cytotoxic agents. IFN-α may have some efficacy in patients with low-grade tumors, although the experience with this drug has been mixed.

Encouragingly, however, preliminary data suggest that novel treatment approaches may hold significant promise for patients with advanced carcinoid tumors. The clinical experience with peptide receptor radiotherapy suggests that this modality may be beneficial, particularly in patients whose tumors are highly octreotide avid. Therapeutic agents targeting the VEGF and mTOR signaling pathways have also been associated with antitumor activity in early stage clinical trials, and confirmatory studies are currently underway. The early evidence of activity observed with these agents suggests that inhibition of these pathways with additional drugs or drug combinations may be a promising way forward in the treatment of this unique disease.

References

1. Harpole D, Feldman J, Buchanan S, et al. Bronchial carcinoid tumors: a retrospective analysis of 126 patients. Ann Thorac Surg. 1992;54:50–5.
2. Vadasz P, Palffy G, Egervary M, et al. Diagnosis and treatment of bronchial carcinoid tumors: clinical and pathological review of 120 operated patients. Eur J Cardiothorac Surg. 1993;7:8–11.
3. Okike N, Bernatz P, Woolner L. Carcinoid tumors of the lung. Ann Thorac Surg. 1976;22:270–7.
4. Fink G, Krelbaum T, Yellin A, et al. Pulmonary carcinoid: presentation, diagnosis, and outcome in 142 cases in Israel and review of 640 cases from literature. Chest. 2001;119:1647–51.
5. Oberg K, Alm G, Magnusson A, et al. Treatment of malignant carcinoid tumors with recombinant interferon alfa-2b: development of neutralizing interferon antibodies and possible loss of antitumor activity. J Natl Cancer Inst. 1989;81:531–5.
6. McCaughan B, Martini N, Bains M. Bronchial carcinoids: review of 124 cases. J Thorac Cardiovasc Surg. 1985;89:8–17.
7. Chughtai T, Morin J, Sheiner N, et al. Bronchial carcinoid-twenty years' experience defines a selective surgical approach. Surgery. 1997;122:801–8.
8. Skuladottir H, Hirsch F, Hansen H, et al. Pulmonary neuroendocrine tumors: incidence and prognosis of histological subtypes. A population-based study in Denmark. Lung Cancer. 2002;37:127–35.
9. Torre M, Barberis M, Barbieri B, et al. Typical and atypical bronchial carcinoids. Respir Med. 1989;83:305–8.
10. Rindi G, Luinetti O, Cornaggia M, et al. Three subtypes of gastric argyrophil carcinoid and the gastric neuroendocrine carcinoma: a clinicopathologic study. Gastroenterology. 1993;104:994–1006.
11. Rindi G, Bordi C, Rappel S, et al. Gastric carcinoids and neuroendocrine carcinomas: pathogenesis, pathology, and behavior. World J Surg. 1996;20:168–72.
12. Barclay T, Schapira D. Malignant tumors of the small intestine. Cancer. 1983;51:878–81.

13. Moertel C, Sauer W, Dockerty M, et al. Life history of the carcinoid tumor of the small intestine. Cancer. 1961;14:901–12.
14. Burke AP, Thomas RM, Elsayed AM, et al. Carcinoids of the jejunum and ileum: an immunohistochemical and clinicopathologic study of 167 cases. Cancer. 1997;79:1086–93.
15. Makridis C, Oberg K, Juhlin C, et al. Surgical treatment of mid-gut carcinoid tumors. World J Surg. 1990;14:377–85.
16. Eckhauser FE, Argenta LC, Strodel WE, et al. Mesenteric angiopathy, intestinal gangrene, and midgut carcinoids. Surgery. 1981;90:720–8.
17. Hellman P, Lundstrom T, Ohrvall U, et al. Effect of surgery on the outcome of midgut carcinoid disease with lymph node and liver metastases. World J Surg. 2002;26:991–7.
18. Moertel C, Dockerty M, Judd E. Carcinoid tumors of the vermiform appendix. Cancer. 1968;21:270–8.
19. Modlin IM, Lye KD, Kidd M. A 5-decade analysis of 13,715 carcinoid tumors. Cancer. 2003;97:934–59.
20. Moertel CG, Weiland LH, Nagorney DM, et al. Carcinoid tumor of the appendix: treatment and prognosis. N Engl J Med. 1987;317:1699–701.
21. Anderson J, Wilson B. Carcinoid tumors of the appendix. Br J Surg. 1985;72:545–6.
22. Syracuse D, Perzin K, Weidel P, et al. Carcinoid tumors of the appendix: mesoappendiceal extension and nodal metastases. Ann Surg. 1979;190:58–63.
23. Bowman G, Rosenthal D. Carcinoid tumors of the appendix. Am J Surg. 1983;146:700–3.
24. Thirlby R, Kasper C, Jones R. Metastatic carcinoid tumor of the appendix: report of a case and review of the literature. Dis Colon Rectum. 1984;27:42–6.
25. MacGillivray D, Heaton R, Rushin J, et al. Distant metastases from a carcinoid tumor of the appendix less than one centimeter in size. Surgery. 1992;111:466–71.
26. Pearlman D, Srinivasan K. Malignant carcinoid of the appendix: metastases from a small primary tumor which appeared as appendiceal intussusception. N Y State J Med. 1971;71:1529–31.
27. Jetmore A, Ray J, Gathright J, et al. Rectal carcinoids: the most frequent carcinoid tumor. Dis Colon Rectum. 1992;35:717–25.
28. Soga J. Carcinoids of the rectum: tumors of the carcinoid family-urgut endocrinomas. Acta Med Biol. 1982;29:157–201.
29. Naunheim K, Zeitels J, Kaplan E, et al. Rectal carcinoid tumors – treatment and prognosis. Surgery. 1983;94:670–6.
30. Woodard P, Feldman J, Paine S, et al. Midgut carcinoid tumors: CT findings and biochemical profiles. J Comput Assist Tomogr. 1995;19:400–5.
31. Sugimoto E, Lorelius L, Eriksson B, et al. Midgut carcinoid tumors: CT appearance. Radiologica. 1995;36:367–71.
32. Lamberts S, Bakker W, Reubi J, et al. Somatostatin receptor imaging in the localization of endocrine tumors. N Engl J Med. 1990;323:1246–9.
33. Kvols LK, Brown ML, O'Connor MK, et al. Evaluation of a radiolabeled somatostatin analog (I-123 octreotide) in the detection and localization of carcinoid and islet cell tumors. Radiology. 1993;187:129–33.
34. Kaltsas G, Korbonits M, Heintz E, et al. Comparison of somatostatin analog and meta-iodobenzylguanidine radionuclites in the diagnosis and localization of advanced neuroendocrine tumors. J Clin Endocrinol Metab. 2001;86:895–902.
35. Krenning E, Kwekkeboom D, Bakker W, et al. Somatostatin receptor scintigraphy with [111In-DTPA-D-Phe1] - and [123-Tyr3]-octreotide: the Rotterdam experience with more than 1000 patients. Eur J Nucl Med. 1993;20:716–31.
36. Schillaci O, Scopinaro F, Danieli R, et al. Single photon emission computerized tomography increases the sensitivity of indium-111-pentetreotide scintigraphy in detecting abdominal carcinoids. Anticancer Res. 1997;17:1753–6.
37. Schillaci O, Corleto V, Annibale B, et al. Single photon emission computed tomography procedure improves accuracy of somatostatin receptor scintigraphy in gastro-entero pancreatic tumours. Ital J Gastroenterol Hepatol. 1999;31 Suppl 2:S186–9.

38. Gibril F, Reynolds J, Doppman J, et al. Somatostatin receptor scintigraphy: its sensitivity compared to that of other imaging methods in detection of primary and metastatic gastrinomas. A prospective study. Ann Intern Med. 1996;125:26–34.
39. Feldman JM, O'Dorisio TM. Role of neuropeptides and serotonin in the diagnosis of carcinoid tumors. Am J Med. 1986;81:41–8.
40. Meko JB, Norton JA. Management of patients with Zollinger-Ellison syndrome. Annu Rev Med. 1995;46:395–411.
41. Eriksson B, Oberg K, Stridsberg M. Tumor markers in neuroendocrine tumors. Digestion. 2000;62 Suppl 1:33–8.
42. Janson E, Holmberg L, Stridsberg M, et al. Carcinoid tumors: analysis of prognostic factors and survival in 301 patients from a referral center. Ann Oncol. 1997;8:685–90.
43. Lundin L, Norheim I, Landelius J, et al. Carcinoid heart disease: relationship of circulating vasoactive substances to ultrasound-detectable cardiac abnormalities. Circulation. 1988;77:264–9.
44. Simula D, Edwards W, Tazelaar H, et al. Surgical pathology of carcinoid heart disease: a study of 139 valves from 75 patients spanning 20 years. Mayo Clin Proc. 2002;77:139–47.
45. Robiolio P, Rigolin V, Wilson J, et al. Carcinoid heart disease: correlation of high serotonin levels with valvular abnormalities detected by cardiac catherterization and echocardiography. Circulation. 1995;77:264–9.
46. Pellikka P, Tajik A, Khandheria B, et al. Carcinoid heart disease: clinical and echocardiographic spectrum in 74 patients. Circulation. 1993;87:1188–96.
47. Moller J, Connolly H, Rubin J, et al. Factors associated with progression of carcinoid heart disease. N Engl J Med. 2003;348:1005–15.
48. Zuetenhorst J, Bonfrer J, Korse C, et al. Carcinoid heart disease: the role of urinary 5-hydroxyindoleacetic acid excretion and plasma levels of atrial antriuretic peptide, transforming growth factor beta and fibroblast growth factor. Cancer. 2003;97:1609–15.
49. Connolly H, Nishimura R, Smith H, et al. Outcome of cardiac surgery for carcinoid heart disease. J Am Coll Cardiol. 1995;25:410–6.
50. Voigt P, Braun J, Teng O, et al. Double bioprosthetic valve replacement in right sided carcinoid heart disease. Ann Thorac Surg. 2005;79:2147–9.
51. Que F, Nagorney D, Batts K, et al. Hepatic resection for metastatic neuroendocrine carcinomas. Am J Surg. 1995;169:36–43.
52. McEntee G, Nagorney D, Kvols L, et al. Cytoreductive hepatic surgery for neuroendocrine tumors. Surgery. 1990;108:1091–6.
53. Norton J, Warren R, Kelly M, et al. Aggressive surgery for metastatic liver neuroendocrine tumors. Surgery. 2003;134:1057–65.
54. Alsina A, Bartus S, Hull D, et al. Liver transplant for metastatic neuroendocrine tumor. J Clin Gastroenterol. 1990;12:533–7.
55. LeTreut Y, Delpero J, Dousset B. Results of liver transplantation in the treatment of metastatic neuroendocrine tumors: a 31 case French multicentric report. Ann Surg. 1997;225:355–64.
56. Lang H, Oldhafer K, Weimann A, et al. Liver transplantation for metastatic neuroendocrine tumors. Ann Surg. 1997;225:347–54.
57. Ajani J, Carrasco C, Charnsangavej C, et al. Islet cell tumors metastatic to the liver: effective palliation by sequential hepatic artery embolization. Ann Intern Med. 1988;108:340–4.
58. Moertel CG, Johnson CM, McKusick MA, et al. The management of patients with advanced carcinoid tumors and islet cell carcinomas. Ann Intern Med. 1994;120:302–9.
59. Ruszniewski P, Rougier P, Roche A, et al. Hepatic arterial chemoembolization in patients with liver metastases of endocrine tumors. A prospective phase II study in 24 patients. Cancer. 1993;71:2624–30.
60. Eriksson B, Larsson E, Skogseid B, et al. Liver embolizations of patients with malignant neuroendocrine gastrointestinal tumors. Cancer. 1998;83:2293–301.
61. Gupta S, Yao JC, Ahrar K, et al. Hepatic artery embolization and chemoembolization for treatment of patients with metastatic carcinoid tumors: the M.D. Anderson experience. Cancer J. 2003;9:261–7.

62. Dominguez S, Denys A, Madeira I, et al. Hepatic arterial chemoembolization with streptozotocin in patients with metastatic digestive endocrine tumours. Eur J Gastroenterol Hepatol. 2000;12:151–7.
63. Drougas JG, Anthony LB, Blair TK, et al. Hepatic artery chemoembolization for management of patients with advanced metastatic carcinoid tumors. Am J Surg. 1998;175:408–12.
64. Diamandidou E, Ajani JA, Yang DJ, et al. Two-phase study of hepatic artery vascular occlusion with microencapsulated cisplatin in patients with liver metastases from neuroendocrine tumors. AJR Am J Roentgenol. 1998;170:339–44.
65. Loewe C, Schindl M, Cejna M, et al. Permanent transarterial embolization of neuroendocrine metastases of the liver using cyanoacrylate and lipiodol: assessment of mid- and long-term results. AJR Am J Roentgenol. 2003;180:1379–84.
66. Brown KT, Koh BY, Brody LA, et al. Particle embolization of hepatic neuroendocrine metastases for control of pain and hormonal symptoms. J Vasc Interv Radiol. 1999;10:397–403.
67. Kennedy AS, Dezarn WA, McNeillie P, et al. Radioembolization for unresectable neuroendocrine hepatic metastases using resin 90Y-microspheres: early results in 148 patients. Am J Clin Oncol. 2008;31:271–9.
68. King J, Quinn R, Glenn DM, et al. Radioembolization with selective internal radiation microspheres for neuroendocrine liver metastases. Cancer. 2008;113:921–9.
69. Hellman P, Ladjevardi S, Skogseid B, et al. Radiofrequency tissue ablation using cooled tip for liver metastases of endocrine tumors. World J Surg. 2002;26:1052–6.
70. Chung MH, Pisegna J, Spirt M, et al. Hepatic cytoreduction followed by a novel long-acting somatostatin analog: a paradigm for intractable neuroendocrine tumors metastatic to the liver. Surgery. 2001;130:954–62.
71. Reubi J, Kvols L, Waser B, et al. Detection of somatostatin receptors in surgical and percutaneous needle biopsy samples of carcinoids and islet cell carcinomas. Cancer Res. 1990;50:5969–77.
72. Kvols L, Moertel C, O'Connell M, et al. Treatment of the malignant carcinoid syndrome: evaluation of a long-acting somatostatin analog. N Engl J Med. 1986;315:663–6.
73. Rubin J, Ajani J, Schirmer W, et al. Octreotide acetate long-acting formulation versus open-label subcutaneous octreotide acetate in malignant carcinoid syndrome. J Clin Oncol. 1999;17:600–6.
74. Faiss S, Rath U, Mansmann U, et al. Ultra-high-dose lanreotide treatment in patients with metastatic neuroendocrine gastroenteropancreatic tumors. Digestion. 1999;60:469–76.
75. Wymenga A, Eriksson B, Salmela P, et al. Efficacy and safety of prolonged-release lanreotide in patients with gastrointestinal neuroendocrine tumors and hormone-related symptoms. J Clin Oncol. 1999;17:1111.
76. O'Toole D, Ducreux M, Bommelaer G, et al. Treatment of carcinoid syndrome: a prospective crossover evaluation of lanreotide versus octreotide in terms of efficacy, patient acceptability, and tolerance. Cancer. 2000;88:770–6.
77. Ducreux M, Ruszniewski P, Chayvialle J, et al. The antitumoral effect of the long-acting somatostatin analog lanreotide, interferon alpha, and their combination for therapy of metastatic neuroendocrine gastroenteropancreatic tumors – the International Laureodtide and Interferon Alfa Study Group. Am J Gastroenterol. 2000;95:3276–81.
78. Faiss S, Pape UF, Bohmig M, et al. Prospective, randomized, multicenter trial on the antiproliferative effect of lanreotide, interferon alfa, and their combination for therapy of metastatic neuroendocrine gastroenteropancreatic tumors – the International Lanreotide and Interferon Alfa Study Group. J Clin Oncol. 2003;21:2689–96.
79. Janson ET, Kauppinen HL, Oberg K. Combined alpha- and gamma-interferon therapy for malignant midgut carcinoid tumors. A phase I-II trial. Acta Oncol. 1993;32:231–3.
80. Frank M, Klose K, Wied M, et al. Combination therapy with octreotide and alpha-interferon: effect on tumor growth in metastatic endocrine gastroenteropancreatic tumors. Am J Gastroenterol. 1999;94:1381–7.
81. Oberg K, Funa K, Alm G. Effects of leukocyte interferon on clinical symptoms and hormone levels in patients with mid-gut carcinoid tumors and carcinoid syndrome. N Engl J Med. 1983;309:129–33.

82. Oberg K, Eriksson B. The role of interferons in the management of carcinoid tumors. Acta Oncol. 1991;30:519–22.
83. Valimaki M, Jarvinen H, Salmela P, et al. Is the treatment of metastatic carcinoid tumor with interferon not as successful as suggested? Cancer. 1991;67:547–9.
84. Rinke A, Muller H, Schade-Brittinger C, et al. Placebo-controlled, double blind, prospective, randomized study on the effect of octreotide LAR in the control of tumor growth in patients with metastatic neuroendocrine midgut tumors: a report from the PROMID study group. J Clin Oncol. 2009;27:4656–63.
85. Moertel CG. Treatment of the carcinoid tumor and the malignant carcinoid syndrome. J Clin Oncol. 1983;1:727–40.
86. Moertel CG, Hanley JA. Combination chemotherapy trials in metastatic carcinoid tumor and the malignant carcinoid syndrome. Cancer Clin Trials. 1979;2:327–34.
87. Engstrom PF, Lavin PT, Moertel CG, et al. Streptozocin plus fluorouracil versus doxorubicin therapy for metastatic carcinoid tumor. J Clin Oncol. 1984;2:1255–9.
88. Sun W, Lipsitz S, Catalano P, et al. Phase II/III study of doxorubicin with fluorouracil compared with streptozocin with fluorouracil or dacarbazine in the treatment of advanced carcinoid tumors: Eastern Cooperative Oncology Group Study E1281. J Clin Oncol. 2005;23:4897–904.
89. Bukowski R, Tangen C, Peterson R, et al. Phase II trial of dimethyltriazenoimidazole carboxamide in patients with metastatic carcinoid. A Southwest Oncology Group study. Cancer. 1994;73:1505–8.
90. Bajetta E, Ferrari L, Procopio G, et al. Efficacy of a chemotherapy combination for the treatment of metastatic neuroendocrine tumors. Ann Oncol. 2002;13:614–21.
91. Moertel C, Kvols L, O'Connell M, et al. Treatment of neuroendocrine carcinomas with combined etoposide and cisplatin: evidence of major therapeutic activity in the anaplastic variants of these neoplasms. Cancer. 1991;68:227–32.
92. Fjallskog ML, Granberg DP, Welin SL, et al. Treatment with cisplatin and etoposide in patients with neuroendocrine tumors. Cancer. 2001;92:1101–7.
93. Ansell SM, Pitot HC, Burch PA, et al. A phase II study of high-dose paclitaxel in patients with advanced neuroendocrine tumors. Cancer. 2001;91:1543–8.
94. Kulke MH, Kim H, Clark JW, et al. A phase II trial of gemcitabine for metastatic neuroendocrine tumors. Cancer. 2004;101:934–9.
95. Kulke MH, Kim H, Stuart K, et al. A phase II study of docetaxel in patients with metastatic carcinoid tumors. Cancer Invest. 2004;22:353–9.
96. Kwekkeboom D, Bakker W, Kooij P, et al. 177Lu-DOTA, Tyr3 octreotate: comparison with [111In-DTPA] octreotide in patients. Eur J Nucl Med. 2001;28:1319–25.
97. Kwekkeboom DJ, de Herder WW, Kam BL, et al. Treatment with the radiolabeled somatostatin analog [177Lu-DOTA 0, Tyr3]octreotate: toxicity, efficacy, and survival. J Clin Oncol. 2008;26:2124–30.
98. Bushnell Jr DL, O'Dorisio TM, O'Dorisio MS, et al. 90Y-Edotreotide for metastatic carcinoid refractory to octreotide. J Clin Oncol. 2010;28:1652–9.
99. Terris B, Scoazec J, Rubbia L. Expression of vascular endothelial growth factor in digestive neuroendocrine tumors. Histopathology. 1998;32:133–8.
100. Yao JC, Phan A, Hoff PM, et al. Targeting vascular endothelial growth factor in advanced carcinoid tumor: a random assignment phase II study of depot octreotide with bevacizumab and pegylated interferon alpha-2b. J Clin Oncol. 2008;26:1316–23.
101. Hobday TJ, Rubin J, Holen K, et al. MC044h, a phase II trial of sorafenib in patients (pts) with metastatic neuroendocrine tumors (NET): a phase II consortium (P2C) study. J Clin Oncol. 2007;2007 ASCO Annual Meeting Proceedings Part I. 25:Abstract 4505.
102. Kulke MH, Lenz HJ, Meropol NJ, et al. Activity of sunitinib in patients with advanced neuroendocrine tumors. J Clin Oncol. 2008;26:3403–10.
103. Duran I, Kortmansky J, Singh D, et al. A phase II clinical and pharmacodynamic study of temsirolimus in advanced neuroendocrine carcinomas. Br J Cancer. 2006;95:1148–54.
104. Yao JC, Phan AT, Chang DZ, et al. Efficacy of RAD001 (everolimus) and octreotide LAR in advanced low- to intermediate-grade neuroendocrine tumors: results of a phase II study [erratum appears in J Clin Oncol. 2008;26(34):5660]. J Clin Oncol. 2008;26:4311–8.

105. Kulke MH, Stuart K, Enzinger PC, et al. Phase II study of temozolomide and thalidomide in patients with metastatic neuroendocrine tumors. J Clin Oncol. 2006;24:401–6.
106. Kelsen DP, Buckner J, Einzig A, et al. Phase II trial of cisplatin and etoposide in adenocarcinomas of the upper gastrointestinal tract. Cancer Treat Rep. 1987;71:329–30.
107. Bukowski RM, Johnson KG, Peterson RF, et al. A phase II trial of combination chemotherapy in patients with metastatic carcinoid tumors. A Southwest Oncology Group Study. Cancer. 1987;60:2891–5.
108. Valkema R, De Jong M, Bakker WH, et al. Phase I study of peptide receptor radionuclide therapy with [In-DTPA]octreotide: the Rotterdam experience. Semin Nucl Med. 2002;32:110–22.
109. Anthony LB, Woltering EA, Espenan GD, et al. Indium-111-pentetreotide prolongs survival in gastroenteropancreatic malignancies. Semin Nucl Med. 2002;32:123–32.
110. Otte A, Herrmann R, Macke HR, et al. Yttrium 90 DOTATOC: a new somatostatin analog for cancer therapy of neuroendocrine tumors. Schweiz Rundsch Med Prax. 1999; 88:1263–8.
111. Paganelli G, Zoboli S, Cremonesi M, et al. Receptor-mediated radiotherapy with 90Y-DOTA-D-Phe1-Tyr3-octreotide. Eur J Nucl Med. 2001;28:426–34.
112. Waldherr C, Pless M, Maecke HR, et al. The clinical value of [90Y-DOTA]-D-Phe1-Tyr3-octreotide (90Y-DOTATOC) in the treatment of neuroendocrine tumours: a clinical phase II study. Ann Oncol. 2001;12:941–5.
113. Waldherr C, Pless M, Maecke H, et al. Tumor response and clinical benefit in neuroendocrine tumors after 7.4 GBq 90Y-DOTATOC. J Nucl Med. 2002;43:610–6.
114. DeJong M, Valkema R, Jamar F, et al. Somatostatin-receptor targeted radionucleotide therapy of tumors: preclinical and clinical findings. Semin Nucl Med. 2002;32:133–40.
115. Teunissen JJ, Kwekkeboom DJ, de Jong M, et al. Endocrine tumours of the gastrointestinal tract. Peptide receptor radionuclide therapy. Best Pract Res Clin Gastroenterol. 2005; 19:595–616.
116. Virgolini I, Britton K, Buscombe J, et al. In- and Y-DOTA-lanreotide: results and implications of the MAURITIUS trial. Semin Nucl Med. 2002;32:148–55.
117. Kwekkeboom DJ, Teunissen JJ, Bakker WH, et al. Radiolabeled somatostatin analog [177Lu-DOTA0, Tyr3]octreotate in patients with endocrine gastroenteropancreatic tumors. J Clin Oncol. 2005;23:2754–62.
118. Yao JC, Zhang JX, Rashid A, et al. Clinical and in vitro studies of imatinib in advanced carcinoid tumors. Clin Cancer Res. 2007;13:234–40.
119. Hobday T, Holen K, Donehower R, et al. A phase II trial of gefitinib in patients with progressive metastatic neuroendocrine tumors: a phase II consortium study. J Clin Oncol. 2006;2006 ASCO Annual Meeting Proceedings 24:A4043.

Chapter 9
Medical Management of Islet Cell Carcinoma

Barbro Eriksson

Abstract Pancreatic endocrine tumors (PET), also often called islet cell tumors, are rare neoplasms thought to have an indolent natural course when compared to exocrine cancers of the pancreas. Their annual incidence is <1 per 100,000 person per year in the general population. Most tumors are sporadic but 15–30% can be part of multiple endocrine neoplasia type 1, von Hippel–Lindau's disease, neurofibromatosis 1, or tuberous sclerosis (TSC1/2). Due the indolent nature and unspecific symptoms of the tumors, there is usually a delay in diagnosis, from 1 to 6 years, and, hence, they are metastastic and unresectable, when the diagnosis is finally made. The prognosis of patients with endocrine pancreatic tumors is difficult to predict because the criteria of malignancy have been ambiguous. Recently, two new classification systems have been developed. The WHO-classification divides PETs into three general categories: (1) well differentiated endocrine tumors of *benign* behavior (confined to the pancreas, non-angioinvasive, no perineural invasion, <2 cm in diameter <2% Ki-67 positive cells) or *uncertain* behavior (confined to the pancreas and one or more of the following features: >2 cm in diameter, >2% Ki-67 positive cells, angioinvasion, perineural invasion), (2) well-differentiated endocrine carcinomas, low-grade malignant, with gross local invasion and/or metastases, and (3) poorly differentiated endocrine carcinomas, high-grade malignant. Recently, two tumor-node-metastasis (TNM) staging systems has been proposed, one by ENETS (Table 9.1), and another by the American Joint Committee on Cancer (AJCC) (Table 9.2), which will be used in the United States. Both the WHO and ENETS TNM-classifications are being adopted and validated by several groups.

Keywords Pancreatic endocrine tumors • Multiple endocrine neoplasia type 1 • von Hippel–Lindau's disease • Neurofibromatosis 1 • Tuberous sclerosis (TSC1/2)

B. Eriksson (✉)
Department of Medical Sciences, Uppsala University Hospital, Uppsala, Sweden
e-mail: barbro.eriksson@medsci.uu.se

J.C. Yao et al. (eds.), *Neuroendocrine Tumors*, Current Clinical Oncology,
DOI 10.1007/978-1-60327-997-0_9, © Springer Science+Business Media, LLC 2011

Introduction

Pancreatic endocrine tumors (PET), also often called islet cell tumors, are rare neoplasms thought to have an indolent natural course when compared to exocrine cancers of the pancreas. Their annual incidence is <1 per 100,000 person per year in the general population [1–3]. Most tumors are sporadic but 15–30% can be part of multiple endocrine neoplasia type 1, von Hippel–Lindau's disease, neurofibromatosis 1, or tuberous sclerosis (TSC1/2). Due the indolent nature and unspecific symptoms of the tumors, there is usually a delay in diagnosis, from 1 to 6 years, and, hence, they are metastastic and unresectable, when the diagnosis is finally made. The prognosis of patients with endocrine pancreatic tumors is difficult to predict because the criteria of malignancy have been ambiguous. Recently, two new classification systems have been developed. The WHO-classification divides PETs into three general categories [4]: (1) well-differentiated endocrine tumors of *benign* behavior (confined to the pancreas, non-angioinvasive, no perineural invasion, <2 cm in diameter <2% Ki-67 positive cells) or *uncertain* behavior (confined to the pancreas and one or more of the following features: >2 cm in diameter, >2% Ki-67 positive cells, angioinvasion, perineural invasion), (2) well-differentiated endocrine carcinomas, low-grade malignant, with gross local invasion and/or metastases, and (3) poorly differentiated endocrine carcinomas, high-grade malignant. Recently, two tumor-node-metastasis (TNM) staging systems has been proposed, one by ENETS (Table 9.1) [5], and another by the American Joint Committee on Cancer (AJCC) (Table 9.2) [6], which will be used in the United States. Both the WHO and ENETS TNM-classifications are being adopted and validated by several groups [7, 8].

By tradition, these tumors have been categorized on the basis of their clinical manifestations into functioning and non-functioning tumors. Functioning tumors are associated with distinct clinical syndromes caused by inappropriate secretion of biologically active substances. Within this group are insulinomas, gastrinomas, glucagonomas, VIPomas, and the more rare adrenocorticotropic-secreting tumors (ACTH-omas), GRF-omas, calcitonin-producing tumors, parathyroid hormone-related peptide tumors. Non-functioning or "non-syndromic" tumors are not associated with a distinct hormonal syndrome but still may show elevated biomarker levels in the blood. Immunohistochemically, non-functioning are indistinguishable from functioning tumors. The presentation of non-functioning tumor is usually due to an effect of tumor mass with local invasion and/or distant metastases with abdominal pain being the major presenting symptom. The proportion of these tumors is increasing in most centers dealing with these patients and nowadays constitutes >50% of the patient population.

The majority of PETs belong to WHO group 2, i.e. they are well-differentiated endocrine carcinomas [7], with the exception of insulinomas, which in more than 90% of cases belong to WHO group 1. Frequent sites of metastases are lymph nodes, and liver, with less common dissemination to bone, lung, and brain. The survival rates in different series depend on the patient population with regard to type of tumor, tumor differentiation, stage of the disease, age, and whether surgery has been performed [6]. The overall 5-year survival in some recent series has been in a range from 42 to 65%. [7, 9, 10].

Table 9.1 TNM staging system for neuroendocrine pancreatic tumors according to ENETS [5]

Table 9.1 Proposal for a TNM classification and disease staging for endocrine tumors of the pancreas

TNM			
T—primary tumor			
TX	Primary tumor cannot be assessed		
T0	No evidence of primary tumor		
T1	Tumor limited to the pancreas and size <2 cm		
T2	Tumor limited to the pancreas and size 2–4 cm		
T3	Tumor limited to the pancreas and size >4 cm or invading duodenum or bile duct		
T4	Tumor invading adjacent organs (stomach, spleen, colon, adrenal gland) or the wall of large vessels (celiac axis or superior mesenteric artery)		
	For any T, add (m) for multiple tumors		
N—regional lymph nodes			
NX	Regional lymph node cannot be assessed		
N0	No regional lymph node metastasis		
N1	Regional lymph node metastasis		
M—distant metastases			
MX	Distant metastasis cannot be assessed		
M0	No distant metastases		
M1[a]	Distant metastasis		
Stage			
Disease stages			
Stage I	T1	N0	M0
Stage IIa	T2	N0	M0
IIb	T3	N0	M0
Stage IIIa	T4	N0	M0
IIIb	Any T	N1	M0
Stage IV	Any T	Any N	M1

[a] M1 specific sites defined according to Sobin and Wittekind [29]

Management of patients with these multi-faceted tumors require a multidisciplinary approach. A characteristic of endocrine tumors is their relatively high rate of resectability in comparison with adenocarcinomas of the pancreas. Local extension beyond the capsule of the pancreas, regional lymph nodal metastases, and liver metastases are not absolute contraindications to surgery [11, 12]. Patients with tumors amenable to surgical treatment should undergo the appropriate type of resection. However, in the majority of patients with neuroendocrine pancreatic tumors, curative surgery is rarely possible and, hence, other approaches are necessary.

Because PETs (except insulinomas) are metastatic in more than 50% of cases, treatment must be directed at both tumor growth and hormonal symptoms. With the development of symptomatic medical therapies (proton pump inhibitors, somatostatin analogs – SAs) that can control hormonal symptoms, the most common cause of death is currently tumor progression and liver failure; hence, antitumoral treatment has become relatively more important to prolong survival [13]. The institution of systemic medical treatment can be controversial because of the slow growth of the tumors and the fact that only palliative treatment is available. When palliative treatment is offered it is extremely important to weigh the expected side-effects and quality of life against the expected response to treatment. Because of the heterogeneity

Table 9.2 TNM staging system for exocrine and endocrine pancreas, according to AJCC

PANCREAS STAGING FORM

CLINICAL Extent of disease before any treatment	STAGE CATEGORY DEFINITIONS	PATHOLOGIC Extent of disease through completion of definitive surgery
☐ y clinical – staging completed after neoadjuvant therapy but before subsequent surgery	TUMOR SIZE: ____________	☐ y pathologic – staging completed after neoadjuvant therapy AND subsequent surgery
	PRIMARY TUMOR (T)	
☐ TX	Primary tumor cannot be assessed	☐ TX
☐ T0	No evidence of primary tumor	☐ T0
☐ Tis	Carcinoma *in situ**	☐ Tis
☐ T1	Tumor limited to the pancreas, 2 cm or less in greatest dimension	☐ T1
☐ T2	Tumor limited to the pancreas, more than 2 cm in greatest dimension	☐ T2
☐ T3	Tumor extends beyond the pancreas but without involvement of the celiac axis or the superior mesenteric artery	☐ T3
☐ T4	Tumor involves the celiac axis or the superior mesenteric artery (unresectable primary tumor)	☐ T4
	*Note: This also includes the "PanInIII" classification	
	REGIONAL LYMPH NODES (N)	
☐ NX	Regional lymph nodes cannot be assessed	☐ NX
☐ N0	No regional lymph node metastasis	☐ N0
☐ N1	Regional lymph node metastasis	☐ N1
	DISTANT METASTASIS (M)	
☐ M0	No distant metastasis (no pathologic M0; use clinical M to complete stage group)	
☐ M1	Distant metastasis	☐ M1

ANATOMIC STAGE • PROGNOSTIC GROUPS

CLINICAL GROUP	T	N	M	PATHOLOGIC GROUP	T	N	M
☐ 0	Tis	N0	M0	☐ 0	Tis	N0	M0
☐ IA	T1	N0	M0	☐ IA	T1	N0	M0
☐ IB	T2	N0	M0	☐ IB	T2	N0	M0
☐ IIA	T3	N0	M0	☐ IIA	T3	N0	M0
☐ IIB	T1	N1	M0	☐ IIB	T1	N1	M0
	T2	N1	M0		T2	N1	M0
	T3	N1	M0		T3	N1	M0
☐ III	T4	Any N	M0	☐ III	T4	Any N	M0
☐ IV	Any T	Any N	M1	☐ IV	Any T	Any N	M1
☐ Stage unknown				☐ Stage unknown			

HOSPITAL NAME/ADDRESS	PATIENT NAME/INFORMATION

Adapted from Edge et al. [97]

and the varying degree of aggressiveness, there is no standard approach to medical management. Furthermore, most of the published studies have been single center, retrospective series, using inconsistent response criteria, including neuroendocrine tumors with different primary sites and histopathology.

Response Criteria

In earlier studies of chemotherapeutic agents, the following so-called WHO-criteria were used to evaluate the therapeutic effects of chemotherapy and other agents [14]: *complete remission (CR)* was defined as a complete disappearance of tumor lesions on conventional imaging, *objective or partial remission (OR or PR)* was defined as a decrease of more than 50% in tumor size. Tumor size was defined as the product of the maximum diameter and its perpendicular. *Stable disease* was defined as a decrease of less than 50% in tumor size. *Progressive disease* was defined as an increase of more than 25% in tumor size, or the appearance of new metastases. The WHO-criteria are still being used in routine clinical management.

In most clinical trials currently performed, the so-called Response Evaluation Criteria in Solid Tumors [15], are being employed. They differ somewhat from the WHO-criteria; *partial remission (PR)* is defined as a reduction of at least 30% in the tumor load estimated as the sum of the longest diameters of all measurable lesions, taking as the reference the baseline sum of the longest diameter. *Progressive disease (PD)* is defined as at least a 20% increase in the tumor load, taking as a reference the smallest sum of longest diameter recorded since the treatment started or the development of new lesions. *Stable disease (SD)* is defined as a less 30% decrease or less than 20% increase in the sum of longest diameters. Recently, a modification (RECIST 1.1) has been introduced [16].

If one compares the WHO- and RECIST-criteria, PR with both methods will require approximately the same tumor volume reduction, whereas PD will require a much greater increase in tumor volume with RECIST than with WHO-criteria. This fact has to be kept in mind when the results of clinical trials are compared.

With the development of new biological and molecular targeted therapies, that may exert cytostatic rather than cytotoxic effects on tumors, the concept of "disease control" is becoming more accepted, whereby stable disease (as opposed to tumor shrinkage) is considered to be a positive response to treatment. Therapy may also produce symptomatic relief and biochemical reduction of hormone secretion and there is an on-going debate, whether biochemical response should be an end-point and evaluated in addition to tumor size. Changes is health-related quality of life as a result of treatment need also to be assessed to optimize management. A patient-specific European Organization for Research and Treatment of Cancer (EORTC) QLQ-GINET21 instrument has been developed [17].

Chemotherapy

Systemic chemotherapy, the cornerstone for non-surgical treatment over the last 50 years, represents a rather selective treatment for patients with metastatic disease of well-differentiated PET. Strategies when to start treatment are sometimes difficult but patients with bulky, progressive tumors are candidates for treatment. Not all patients will respond and patient selection is essential to increase the chance of response and minimize unnecessary side-effects. Tumor differentiation determines the response to cytotoxic chemotherapy and therefore correct histological characterization should be applied using strict World Health Organization (WHO) criteria and Ki-67 indexes [4]. It has, however, not yet been established at which Ki-67 index different chemotherapy protocols should be given. If this proliferation marker is above 15–20%, then the tumor is poorly differentiated, and platinum-base chemotherapeutic regimens should be chosen. For low- and moderately proliferate tumors, streptozotocin-based combinations have been used.

Single Agents

The nitrosurea compound, streptozotocin (STZ), has been in clinical use since 1967, and Murray-Lyon et al. reported improvement in hypoglycaemic episodes and tumor load in certain endocrine pancreatic tumors in 1968 [18]. The U.S. Food and Drug Administration approved the use of STZ for "islet-cell" carcinoma in 1982. Other old-generation cytotoxic DNA-damaging agents, 5-fluorouracil (5-FU), doxorubicin (Dox) [19], and dacarbazine (DTIC) [20] have been associated with low success rates as single agents and considerable systemic toxicity, mainly gastrointestinal and cumulative cardiotoxicity. Temozolomide (TMZ) is a relatively new chemotherapeutic agent, registered for treatment of malignant glioma [21]. It is an alkylating agent, sharing it's active metabolite with DTIC. The first patient with a NET, who received this drug in 1999 in our department had recurrent brain metastases of a thymic carcinoid after radiotherapy of the brain. The brain metastases as well as metastases in other locations decreased significantly in size and the response lasted for more than a year. Subsequently, a relatively large number of patients with different types of so-called foregut NE tumors, received TMZ as monotherapy as second to fourth line treatment and the results were published in 2007 [22]. Twelve patients with advanced PETs were included and PR was observed in one patient (8%), and SD was noted in eight (67%). The median duration of response was 7 months and TMZ was well tolerated.

Other "newer" cytotoxic agents, such as paclitaxel [23], capecitabine [24], gemcitabine [25], and topotecan [26] have all been shown to be more or less inactive as single agents in low to intermediate grade neuroendocrine tumors.

Combination Chemotherapy

The advantage of the combination of STZ plus 5-FU over STZ alone was first reported in a small randomized ECOG-study in 1980 [27]. The overall response rates (RR) were 63 and 36%, respectively. The same investigators then compared the two regimens, STZ plus doxorubicin (STZ/Dox) and STZ plus 5-FU (STZ/5FU) [28].

STZ/Dox was shown to be superior to STZ/5FU (69 vs. 45% overall RR) with median time to progression (20 vs. 6.9 months), and overall survival (2.2 vs. 1.4 years). The doxorubicin arm was, however, associated with more side-effects, including alopecia, myelosuppression, and cardiotoxicity. No group has since been able to reproduce or achieve the same response rates most likely because the response criteria used in the Moertel study included hormonal responses and clinical assessment of hepatomegaly. The most recent reports of outcome with STZ/Dox or STZ/Dox/5-FU describe RR of 6–39%, and these are exclusively radiological responses [29–31]. Our experience of the two combinations is that STZ plus 5-FU is as effective as STZ/Dox and that responses can be long-lasting, >3 years in some patients [32].

One problem with the Dox combination is the cardiotoxicity of Dox which necessitates the withdrawal for cumulative exposure. This means that the combination of STZ plus 5-FU may be used after maximum treatment with Dox. STZ can cause nausea and vomiting but these side-effects can be almost completely controlled by 5-HT3 antagonists. Renal dysfunction, including proteinuria and a decrease in creatinine clearance, occurs in 20–70% of patients, is the dose-limiting toxic effect. Long-term use of STZ requires careful monitoring of renal function with creatinine clearance before each course [32]. Dehydration after STZ treatment can cause irreversible renal damage, and therefore generous hydration, either orally or if necessary by intravenous infusion, is recommended.

Other chemotherapeutic combinations have been evaluated recently in phase II trials with almost equivalent response rates. Oxilaplatin combined with capecitabine achieved a 30% objective RR, 20% biochemical RR and 50% symptomatic RR in patients with well-differentiated NET [33]. Based on in vitro data indicating synergistic effects between TMZ and capecitabine in neuroendocrine tumor cell lines, the combination was given to PET patients. In two small retrospective series, the reported response rates have been high. In one such study among patients who have failed prior chemotherapy a response rate of 59% was reported [34]. In a separate report, with this combination as first-line treatment, an even higher response rate of 71% was reported [35].

Others have tested triplet chemotherapy regimen such as DTIC, 5-FU, plus epirubicin, or carboplatin, gemcitabine plus irinotecan without achieving better response rates and unacceptable toxicity [36–38].

STZ-based chemotherapy remains the gold standard for low to moderately proliferative unresectable PETs. It seems, however, that in the future chemotherapeutic management of malignant PET, STZ may be replaced by TMZ and 5-FU with capicitabine.

Chemotherapy for Poorly Differentiated NETs

The combination of cisplatin plus etoposide, a regimen effective in small cell lung cancer, was reported in Moertel's study from 1991, and was shown to produce high RR (67%) in patients with anaplastic NET [39]. In contrast, the activity was far less in patients with well-differentiated PET, only 14% responding. Our group gave this regimen with reduced etoposide doses as first-line treatment to aggressive foregut tumors with 50% RR, and as second-line treatment to STZ-resistant PETs and the RR for the latter group was only 25% [40]. The duration of response was <1 year. Toxicity with cisplatin-based regimens is significant with nephrotoxicity being dose-limiting. Substitution of cisplatin with carboplatin tends to make therapy more tolerable.

For this type of tumors, there is an urgent need for new chemotherapeutic regimens.

Biotherapy

Somatostatin Analogs

SAs have been registered world-wide for the treatment of functioning NET (carcinoids, VIP-omas, glucagonomas, etc.) but has not been approved as antitumoral agents. According to a relatively recent consensus report, the accepted indications for the use of SAs should include: patients with peptide-/amine-induced syndromes with clinical symptoms, and patients with progression of metastatic disease even without a syndrome [41]. The latter indication has been controversial.

Somatostatin and its analogues (SAs) exert their influence on endocrine tumor cells via various mechanisms. Somatostatin inhibits multiple functions, and its action is mediated via five G-protein-coupled membrane receptors (sst1-5) [42–44]. Natural somatostatin binds with high affinity to all five sst's, whereas the synthetic analogues bind with high affinity to sst2 and 5, and with lower affinity to sst3 [45]. Ligand binding inhibits adenylate cyclase activity, and reduces calcium channel activity, which blocks hormone synthesis and secretion. The inhibition of secretion appears to be largely mediated via sst2 and sst5 [46].

An inhibitory effect on proliferation via sst1, 2 and 5 may be due to the activation of phosphotyrosine phosphatases and the mitogen-activated protein kinase (MAPK) activity [47, 48]. Apoptosis has been shown to be mediated via sst2 and sst3 [49, 50]. Additional antiproliferative effects of SA may be exerted directly via the receptors or indirectly via inhibition of growth factors, stimulation of the immune system, or inhibition of angiogenesis [51].

The basis for use of SAs is the high expression of sst's in more than 80% of NET according to autoradiographic and scintigraphic studies [52, 53]. Octreotide scintigraphy is nowadays a routine diagnostic tool, providing staging for the patients and serving as a predictive test for sensitivity to treatment with unlabeled and labeled SA [53]. The density is higher in tumor tissue compared to normal tissue, which allows for specific tumor-targeted effects that should reduce the side-effects, i.e. the suppression of physiologically secreted hormones from normal tissues. However, the density of different subtypes of sst's varies considerably between different tumor types, among the same type of tumors and within a given tumor.

Two different analogs, octreotide and lanreotide, are regularly used in the clinic. They have a 1–2 h half-life and can be administered subcutaneously, intravenously and intramuscularly. The subcutaneous formulation of octreotide should be given 2–3 times daily, while slow release formulations (SAs complexed with polyDL-lacticed-co-glycolide) can be given every 2 weeks (somatuline long acting) or once per month (octreotide long-acting repeatable (LAR)) intramuscularly. The dispersion of lanreotide in water creates a gel, which can be injected subcutaneously once a month. These slow release formulations improve the quality of life for the patients by relieving them of the inconvenience of taking multiple daily injections.

Presently, the multireceptor SAs pasireotide or SOM 230, which binds to sst1, 2, 3 and 5, is being tested in clinical trials [54].

Antisecretory Effects

Octreotide administered subcutaneously (sc) at standard doses of 100–1,500 μg daily (individually adjusted) in two to four divided doses produces symptomatic responses in 70–90% of patients with small-bowel NETs and biochemical responses in up to 70% of patients with rapid reduction in urinary 5-hydroxyindole acetic acid (5HIAA) [55]. Similarly, in patients VIP-omas and glucagonomas, the symptomatic and biochemical effects are very prompt [56]. Because of the inhibitory effect of SA on normally produced glucagon and growth hormone, caution should be observed in patients with insulinomas. Benign insulinomas usually lack sst2 [45] and hypoglycaemia can be worsened – so for this subgroup of tumors, SAs are contraindicated. As a contrast, malignant insulinomas may express sst2 in a high percentage and a positive octreotide scintigraphy then could suggest that the patient could benefit from SAs treatment. Also patients with the more rare tumors producing ectopic ACTH, ectopic gonadotropin releasing factor (GNRH) and parathyroid hormone-related peptide (causing hypercalcemia) can respond biochemically. While SAs are effective in lowering the gastrin concentration and acid secretion in gastrinoma patients, effective symptomatic relief in these patients can be achieved by proton pump inhibition. Whether SAs should be used in non-functioning EPT has been a matter of debate. The consensus guidelines suggest that SAs are indicated in non-symtomatic (non-functioning) patients with progressive metastatic disease ([41] see above). The indication should preferably include the requirement of a positive octreotide scintigraphy and a low proliferation rate.

Long-acting formulations appear to be as effective in this respect and routinely most patients are transferred from short-acting octreotide (1–3 sc injections per day) to octreotide-LAR (20 or 30 mg), or put directly on Lanreotide Autogel (90 or 120 mg) [57]. The dose should then be adjusted individually according to symptomatic and biochemical responses. Short-acting octreotide may have to be added until steady-state conditions have been reached. The median duration of the anti-secretory effect has been reported to be between 2 and 18 months [56] but in many cases hormonal symptom can be controlled for extended time periods. Adverse events of SAs treatment have been rather mild due to the adaptation of normal pituitary and gastrointestinal functions to the drug. Apart from nausea, transient abdominal cramps, flatulence, diarrhea, and local reaction at the injection site, no important side-effects have been noted [56]. In 20–50% gallstones are formed de novo but these remain often asymptomatic [56].

Loss of response or tachyphylaxis is a well-known phenomenon, which still remains unexplained although it seems to be a post-receptor phenomenon. Some patients may respond to increased doses.

Antiproliferative Effects

Several groups have looked into the anti-proliferative effects of SAs [58–61] although significant tumor shrinkage can be demonstrated in less than 10% of patients with NET [56]. However, stabilization of tumor growth after CT-verified progression prior to treatment, occurs in 37–50% of patients with NET of various locations [58, 62]. The median duration of stabilization was 18–26.5 months [58, 63]. High-dose SA treatment (12 mg in four divided daily doses) given to patients failing on standard octreotide treatment, produced stabilization in 70% and PR in 5% and tumor biopsies showed increased apoptosis after 6 and 12 months [61] indicating an antitumoral effect.

The information about the antiproliferative effects of SAs in malignant PETs is scarce. Typically, small numbers of these patients have been included in other studies. Shojanmanesh and colleagues looked [64] into the antiproliferative efficacy of long-term treatment of octreotide in 15 patients with malignant gastrinoma with progressive hepatic metastases before start of treatment (verified by CT, MRI or US). Initial doses of octreotide were 200 μg twice per day and then maintenance with 20–30 mg octretoide-LAR every month was given. Tumors in 8 of 15 patients (53%) responded at 3 months with 7 of 15 (47%) demonstrating tumor stabilization and 1/15 decrease in tumor size (6%). The mean duration of response was 25.0 months (range 5.5–54.1 months). "Slow-growing tumors" (according to CT) were more likely to respond to treatment (86 vs. 0%) according to this report.

Whether SAs should be used to control tumor growth and dissemination has been controversial as mentioned. However, the PROMID study published in 2009 will strengthen the role for SAs as antitumor agents in NET [65]. This placebo-controlled study of 85 (intended to be 162) treatment-naïve metastatic well-differentiated midgut carcinoids (95.3% with low Ki-67 <2%), showed that otreotide-LAR significantly lengthened time to tumor progression (primary endpoint of the study) compared with placebo (15.6 vs. 5.9 months; $p=0.000072$). Stable disease was observed in 66.7% of patients treated with octreotide-LAR and in 37.2% of patients in the placebo group. Octreotide-LAR was effective in both functioning and non-functioning tumors, while those (>75%) with the smallest tumor burden in the liver (<10%) and resected primary experienced the greatest benefit (median 27.1 vs. 72 months; $p=0.0001$).

The PROMID study thus indicates an antiproliferative effect of SAs and confirms the controversial second indication in the ENETS consensus guidelines from 2004.

The results have now been included in the revised version of the NCCN guidelines for asymptomatic patients with metastatic carcinoid tumors and should then also be applied in low proliferative PETs (Ki-67 <2%), including non-functioning tumors.

Interferon

Interferon-alpha (IFN) was introduced in metastatic carcinoid tumors because of its immuno-stimulatory effects [66]. Subsequent studies have shown that IFN has several mechanisms of actions, including direct effects on tumor cells, which induces accumulation of tumor cells in the G0–G1-phase of the cell cycle, a process, in which p21 and p27 may be involved [67]. It has also been shown to reduce the expression of growth factors/receptors, including basic fibroblast growth factor (bFGF), and vascular endothelial growth factor (VEGF) [68]. IFN treatment, in addition, results in a reduction of the number of viable tumor cells within metastatic lesions followed by an increase in fibrotic tissue [69].

IFN has been registered in most European countries for treatment of metastatic carcinoid tumors. At doses of 3–9 million units of recombinant interferon given 3–7 days a week, symptomatic improvement of flush and diarrhea will be noticed in >50% of patients, a more than 50% reduction in biochemical markers will be seen in 40–50%, whereas a more than 50% reduction in tumor size occurs in <10% of patients [70]. The dosage should be individually titrated. Side-effects are dose-dependent and include flu-like symptoms initially. More severe adverse reactions include chronic fatigue, mental depression, and autoimmune phenomena [70].

The first report of the use of IFN in PETs was published by Öberg in 1985, in which two patients with VIP-oma (brothers with MEN1), failing on chemotherapy, responded dramatically with a reduction in VIP-levels and symptoms [71]. In a larger group of patients with chemotherapy-resistant PET, 47% of patients had a reduction in tumor markers (>50%), 12% a radiological response and the duration of response was 20 months [32]. Stabilization was seen in 25%. Patients with the VIP-omas syndrome appeared to respond better than the other types of PET. In current practice, IFN is most of the time combined with SA as treatment in low-proliferative PET [72], if STZ combinations can not be given, or if no other clinical trial is suitable.

Novel Molecular Targeted Therapy

Since none of the available systemic/medical therapies can cure patients with metastatic neuroendocrine disease, there has been a strong drive to identify molecular alterations that can be new potential targets for therapy. It is beyond the scope of this overview to go into molecular biology but it has been well established that NET show increased expression of numerous growth factors and their receptors.

Growth factors that have been implicated include bFGF, VEGF, platelet-derived growth factor (PDGF), transforming growth factor (TGF) alpha and beta, insulin-like growth factor (IGF-1), epidermal growth factor (EGF) receptor, and stem cell factor (c-kit) [73–77]. Several of the corresponding receptors have shown increased expression in NET, such as epidermal growth factor receptor (EGFR), PDGF-receptor, IGF-1-receptor, and VEGF-receptors (VEGF-FLK and VEGF-FLT).

Targeting Angiogenesis

Already at a small size, a tumor requires neovascularization to grow and metastasize. Well-differentiated neuroendocrine carcinomas are known to be well vascularized. Currently, there are a number of anti-angiogenic compounds undergoing clinical evaluation. They include: (1) the humanized monoclonal antibodies against VEGF, bevacizumab; (2) small molecules that interact with the tyrosine kinase signal transduction, such as sunitinib, sorafenib, pazopanib and imatinib; and (3) other angiogenesis inhibitors, such as thalidomide and endostatin.

Both well-differentiated carcinoids and pancreatic NET overexpress VEGF and its receptors [78, 79]. Yao et al. [80] reported evidence for clinical activity of bevacizumab in advanced carcinoid patients with stable disease on octreotide. In a phase II trial, 44 patients were randomized to receive octreotide combined with bevacizumab, or pegylated IFN. After 18 weeks, 95% of patients receiving bevacizumab remained progression-free, compared to 68% of those in the IFN arm ($p=0.02$). The toxicity was modest, mainly hypertension.

A phase II study with the combination of bevacizumab and TMZ in NET showed preliminary RR of 24% for pancreatic tumors although the efficacy of bevacizumab is difficult to evaluate from the design of the study [81]. Bevacizumab is presently being evaluated in several combination studies with chemotherapeutic agents (capecitabine, STZ, TMZ) and two studies with oxilaplatin-based regimens show promising results in both carcinoids and PET [82, 83].

Sunitinib, a broad spectrum tyrosine kinase inhibitor with activity against VEGFR, PDGFR, and c-kit, was evaluated in a phase II trial of 107 patients with NET (41 carcinoids and 66 with PETs) with documented tumor progression before inclusion in the study [84]. The overall RR was 17% in pancreatic tumors and 2% of carcinoids and stable disease was observed in 68 and 83%, respectively. These responses and time to tumor progression of 7.7 and 10.2 months, respectively, suggested some antitumor activity. An international phase III study of sunitinib (37.5 mg daily) versus placebo in patients with progressive advanced PET has then been conducted [85]. At interim analysis of the first 154 patients, the randomization was stopped, since the PFS was 11.7 months in patients treated with sunitinib compared to 5.5 months in the placebo group ($p<0.001$). Updated safety and efficiency results of this phase III trial were recently presented [86]. A total of 171 patients were included, 86 in the sunitinib arm and 85 in the placebo arm. There was a significant improvement in PFS:11.4 versus 5.5 months (hazard ratio 0.418, $p=0.001$).

Updated results showed no significant difference in overall survival. Treatment appears better tolerated at 37.5 mg than previous studies at using the 50 mg dose. Grade ¾ adverse events occurred in 49.4 and 43.9%, respectively, mainly neutropenia (12%), hypertension 9.6%, hand–foot syndrome (6%), and leukopenia (6%). One case of cardiac failure was noticed in the treatment arm.

Sorafenib is known to inhibit kinase activity associated with the VEGF and PDGF receptors. Data from a phase II trial of 93 NET patients, of which 43 were PETs, demonstrated RR in 10% of PETs [87]. This agent is presently evaluated in combination with cytotoxic agents.

Imatinib is another tyrosine kinase inhibitor with activity against ABL, PDGF, and c-kit, approved for treatment of chronic myelocytic leukemia and GIST-tumors. The results in NETs have been rather disappointing with very few responses [88, 89].

Thalidomide is an old immuno-modulatory drug, which possesses anti-angiogenic properties due to its interaction with bFGF and VEGF. Kulke et al. reported of the combination of thalidomide with TMZ in advanced NET patients, of which 11 had pancreatic tumors [90]. There was a 50% decrease in CgA in 40% of patients, whereas the radiological response was 25% in the whole group and 44% in PETs. The median duration was 13.5 months, and side-effects were significant with grade 3–4 lymphopenia occurring in 69% and opportunistic infections in 10%.

Endostatin, another anti-angiogenic compound, has been evaluated in early phase I and phase II trials in NETs. Of 40 patients with advanced GEP-NET, none showed any radiological response although stabilization occurred in a relatively high percentage [91].

mTOR Inhibitors

Dysregulation of the intracellular protein mammalian target of rapamycin (mTOR) and its pathways is quite common in a variety of tumors and it also plays an important role in angiogenesis. Mechanisms that are affected involve signaling via growth factors (IGF-1), activating mutations of pathway kinases, or loss of tumor suppressor genes such as PTEN, TSC1/2-complexes [92].

A phase II study of temsirolimus, an mTOR-inhibitor, in advanced progressive NET was published in 2007 [93] demonstrating two PR and SD in 54% with time to progression of 6 months as a median.

The first phase II study of everolimus (RAD001) was reported by Yao et al., including 30 patients with carcinoid and 30 patients with PETs given the combination of octreotide-LAR 30 mg every 4 weeks and everolimus at 5 and 10 mg daily [94]. RR were 17 and 27% with a progression-free survival of 63 and 50 weeks, respectively. Patients treated with 10 mg of everolimus obtained a higher RR (30 vs. 13%) and prolonged median progression-free survival (72 vs. 50 weeks). A biochemical RR of 70% was noted in the 37 patients with elevated CgA levels.

A phase II study (RADIANT1), evaluated everolimus alone or in combination with octreotide-LAR in progressive chemoresistant pancreatic NET [95]. The first stratum (115 patients) received everolimus at 10 mg daily, the second stratum (45 patients) received octreotide-LAR plus everolimus 10 mg daily. The overall RR plus stabilization was higher with the combination (84 vs. 77%), as was median progression-free survival (16.7 vs. 9.7 months). A greater than 50% reduction in CgA was achieved in 56 and 49% of patients, respectively. In addition, there was a correlation between the decrease in CgA and median progression free survival. The treatment was well tolerated with few grade 3–4 events, mainly fatigue, diarrhea, and stomatitis. A confirmatory phase III study (RADIANT-3) comparing best supportive care plus everolimus or placebo has been performed [96]. Altogether 410 patients were included, 207 in the everolimus arm and 203 in the placebo arm. The majority of patients had well-differentiated PET, 82 and 84%, respectively, 17 and 15% moderately differentiated. Fifty-eight percent in each group had received prior treatment. Everolimus prolonged median PFS from 4.6 to 11 months and demonstrated a 65% risk reduction for progression compared to placebo (hazard ratio = 0.35, $p < 0.0001$). The safety profile was acceptable and similar to the what have been observed with everolimus in other indication. Aphthous ulceration/stomatitis is the most common event occurring in 53% of patients. However, grade ¾ stomatitis occurred only in 5% of patients.

Conclusion

Approximately two-thirds of malignant PETs are metastatic at discovery. Even though the indications for surgery have been broadened during the last two decades to include aggressive surgery of locally advanced disease and cytoreductive procedures to reduce the tumor burden in the liver, the majority of patients will require additional medical/systemic treatment.

As opposed to NETs of other origin, PETs with low-to-moderate proliferative activity have been shown to respond to STZ-based combinations, either STZ plus doxorubicin or STZ plus 5-FU, have been the gold standard for treatment of patients with symptomatic, bulky or progressive PETs. Adverse events have to be monitored carefully. In the cytotoxic arena/arsenal, two new peroral compounds have emerged and been tested in phase II studies: TMZ which may replace STZ and capecitabine which can replace 5-FU. Mode of administrative and low toxicity are advantageous for the patients. Further studies are, however, needed.

SAs are excellent in the control of most functional NETs and this is also the case in PETs. The very few side effects of SAs make them suitable for long-term use. Long-acting formulations appear to be as effective as standard subcutaneous daily injections. As recently shown in the PROMID study, SAs have antiproliferative or tumoristatic properties. It should however, be noted that, as indicated in the study, single agents SA treatment should be reserved for patients with low proliferative tumors (Ki-67 <2%). In tumors with a higher proliferation rate, SA should be complemented or combined with other therapeutic modalities, e.g., chemotherapy, liver embolizations, IFN, etc.

Antitumoral activity of new targeted therapies is modest but still promising according to phase III trials. Both everolimus and sunitinib appear to have antiproliferative effects in PETs as single agents and their toxicity profiles are favorable, which means that these two new drugs have been added to the therapeutic arsenal of PETs.

References

1. Buchanan KD, Johnston CF, O'Hare MM, et al. Neuroendocrine tumors. A European view. Am J Mcd. 1986;81:14–22.
2. Eriksson B, Öberg K. Neuroendocrine pancreatic tumors. Clinical findings in a prospective study of 84 patients. Acta Oncol. 1989;28:373–7.
3. Halfdanarson T, Rubin J, Farnell M, et al. Pancreatic endocrine neoplasms: epidemiology and prognosis of pancreatic endocrine tumors. Endocr-Relat Cancer. 2008;15:409–74.
4. Solcia E, Klppel G, Sorbin L. Histological typing of endocrine tumors. In: World Health Organization international histological classification of endocrine tumours. 2nd ed. New York: Springer; 2000. p. 56–8.
5. Rindi G, Klöppel G, Ahlman H, et al. TNM staging of foregut neuroendocrine tumors: a consensus proposal including a grading system. Virchows Arch. 2006;449:395–401.
6. Edge SE, Byrd DR, Carducci MA, Compton CA. eds AJCC Cancer Staging Manual. 7th ed. New Yourk, NY: Springer; 2010.
7. Ekeblad S, Skogseid B, Öberg K, et al. Pancreatic endocrine tumors: survival and prognostic factors. Clin Cancer Res. 2008;14:7798–803.
8. Pape V, Jann H, Müller-Nordhorn J. Prognostic relevance of a novel TNM classification system for upper gastroenteropancreatic neuroendocrine tumors. Cancer. 2008;113(2):256–65.
9. Lepage C, Boncier AM, Phelip JM, et al. Incidence and management of malignant digestive endocrine tumours in a well defined French population. Gut. 2004;53(4):549–53
10. House MG, Cameron JL, Lillemoe KD, et al. Differences in survival for patients with resectable versus unresectable metastases from pancreatic islet cell cancer. J Gastrointest Surg. 2006;10:138–45.
11. Sarmiento JM, Farnell MB, Que FG, et al. Pancreatoduodenectomy for islet cell tumors of the head of the pancreas: long-term survival analysis. World J Surg. 2002;26:1267–71.
12. Musunuru S, Chen H, Rajpal S, et al. Metastatic neuroendocrine hepatic tumors; resection improves survival. Arch Surg. 2006;141:1000–5.
13. Eriksson B, Skogseid B, Lundqvist G, et al. Medical treatment and long-term survival in a prospective study of 84 patients with endocrine pancreatic tumors. Cancer. 1990;65:1883–90.
14. Miller AB, Hoogstraten B, Staquet M, et al. Reporting results of cancer treatment. J Natl Cancer Inst. 1981;47:207–14.
15. Therasse P, Arback SG, Esienhauer EA, et al. New guidelines to evaluate the response to treatment in solid tumors: European Organization for Research and Treatment of Cancer, National Cancer Institute of Canada. J Natl Cancer Inst. 2000;92:205–16.
16. Eisenhauer EA, Therasse P, Bogaerts J, et al. New response evaluation criteria in solid tumours: revised RECIST guideline (version 1.1). Eur J Cancer. 2009;45:228–47.
17. Davies AH, Larsson G, Arndill J, et al. Development of a disease specific Quality of Life questionnaire module for patients with gastrointestinal neuroendocrine tumours. Eur J Cancer. 2006;42:477–84.
18. Murray-Lyon IM, Eddleston AL, Williams R, et al. Treatment of multiple-hormone-producing malignant islet-cell tumor with streptozotocin. Lancet. 1968;2:895–8.
19. Moertel CG, Lavin PT, Hahn RG. Phase II trial of doxorubicin for advanced islet cell carcinoma. Cancer. 1982;61:1567–9.

20. Altimari A, Badrinath K, Reisel H, et al. DTIC therapy in patients with malignant intraabdominal neuroendocrine tumors. Surgery. 1987;102:1009–17.
21. Stupp R, Mason W, van den Bent M, et al. Radiotherapy plus concombinant temozolomide for glioblastoma. N Engl J Med. 2005;352:987–96.
22. Ekeblad S, Sundin A, Janson ET, et al. Temozolomide as monotherapy is effective in advanced malignant neuroendocrine tumors. Clin Cancer Res. 2007;12:2986–91.
23. Ansell SM, Pitot HC, Burch PA, et al. A phase II study of high-dose paclitaxel in patients with advanced neuroendocrine tumors. Cancer. 2001;91:1543–8.
24. Krzyzanowska MK, Tsao MS, Oza AM, et al. Capecitabine plus rofecoxib show no activity in patients with metastatic neuroendocrine tumors. Clin Oncol. 2006;18:88–9.
25. Kulke MH, Kim H, Clark JW, et al. A phase II trial of gemcitabine for metastatic neuroendocrine tumors. Cancer. 2004;101:934–9.
26. Ansell SM, Mahoney MR, Green EM, et al. Topotecan in patients with advanced neuroendocrine tumours; a phase II study with significant hematologic toxicity. Am J Clin Oncol. 2004;27:232–5.
27. Moertel CG, Hanley JA, Johnson LA. Streptozotocin alone compared with streptozotocin plus fluorouracil in the treatment of advanced islet-cell carcinoma. N Engl J Med. 1980;303:1189–95.
28. Moertel CG, Lefkopoulo M, Lipiz S, et al. Streptozotocin-doxorubicin, streptozotocin-fluorouracil, or chlorozotocin in the treatment of advanced islet-cell carcinoma. N Engl J Med. 1992;326:519–23.
29. Cheng PN, Salty LB. Failure to confirm major objective antitumor activity for streptozotocin and doxorubicin in the treatment of patients with advanced islet-cell carcinoma. Cancer. 1999;86:944–8.
30. Kouvaraki MA, Ajani JA, Hoff P, et al. Fluorouracil, doxorubicin, and streptozotocin in the treatment of patients with locally advanced and metastatic pancreatic endocrine carcinomas. J Clin Oncol. 2004;22:4762–71.
31. McCollum AD, Kulke MH, Ryan DP, et al. Lack of efficacy of streptozotocin and doxorubicin in patients with advanced pancreatic endocrine tumors. J Clin Oncol. 2004;27:485–8.
32. Eriksson B, Öberg K. An update of the medical treatment of malignant endocrine pancreatic tumors. Acta Oncol. 1993;32:203–8.
33. Bajetta E, Catena L, Procopiv G, et al. Are capecitabine and oxilaplatin (XELOX) suitable treatments for progressing low-grade and high-grade neuroendocrine tumors? Cancer Chemother Pharmacol. 2007;59:637–42.
34. Isacoff WH, Moss RA, Pecora AL, et al. Temozolomide/capecitabine therapy for metastatic neuroendocrine tumors of the pancreas. A retrospective review. J Clin Oncol (2006 ASCO Meeting Proceedings). 2006;24:abstract 14023.
35. Strosberg JR, Gardner N, Kvols L. First-line treatment of metastatic pancreatic endocrine carcinoma with capecitabine and temozolomide (abstract). J Clin Oncol. 2008;26:241.
36. Bajetta E, Rimassa L, Carnaghi C, et al. 5-fluorouracil, dacarbazine, epirubicin in the treatment of patients with neuroendocrine tumours. Cancer. 1998;83:372–8.
37. de Lima Lopes Jr G, Chiappori A, Simon G, et al. Phase I study of carboplatin in combination with gemcitabine and irinotecan in patients with solid tumors; preliminary evidence of activity in small cell and neuroendocrine carcinomas. Cancer. 2007;109:1413–9.
38. Ollivier S, Fonck M, Becouarn Y, et al. Dacarbazin, fluorouracil, and leucovorin in patients with advanced neuroendocrine tumors: a phase II trial. Am J Clin Oncol. 1998;21:237–40.
39. Moertel CG, Kvols LK, O'Connell MJ, et al. Treatment of neuroendocrine carcinomas with combined etoposide and cisplatin. Evidence of major therapeutic activity in the anaplastic variants of these neoplasms. Cancer. 1991;68:227–32.
40. Fjällskog ML, Granberg DP, Welin SL, et al. Treatment with cisplatin and etoposide in patients with neuroendocrine tumours. Cancer. 2001;92:1101–7.
41. Öberg K, Kvols L, Caplin M, et al. Consensus report of the use of somatostatin analogs for the management of neuroendocrine tumors of the gastroenteropancreatic system. Ann Oncol. 2004;15:966–73.

42. Yamada Y, Post SR, Wang K, et al. Cloning and functional characterization of a family of human and mouse somatostatin receptors expressed in brain, gastrointestinal tract, and kidney. Proc Natl Acad Sci. 1992;89:251–5.
43. Yamada Y, Reisine T, Law SF, et al. Somatostatin receptors, an expanding gene family: cloning and functional characterization of human SSTR2, a protein coupled to adenylyl cyclase. Mol Endocrinol. 1993;6:2136–42.
44. Yamada Y, Kagimoto S, Kubota A, et al. Cloning, functional expression and pharmacological characterization of a fourth (SSTR4) and fifth (SSTR5) human somatostatin receptor subtype. Biochem Biophys Res Commun. 1993;195:844–52.
45. Lamberts SW, van der Lely AJ, de Herder VW, et al. Octreotide. N Engl J Med. 1996;334:226–54.
46. Chen C, Vincent JD, Clarke JP. Ion channels and the signal transduction pathways in the regulation of growth hormone secretion. Trends Endocrinol Metab. 1994;5:227–33.
47. Buscail L, Delesque N, Estève JP, et al. Stimulation of tyrosine phosphatase and inhibition of call proliferation by somatostatin analogues: mediation by human somatostatin receptor subtypes SSTR1 and SSTR2. PNAS. 1994;91:2315–9.
48. Susini C. Buscail; Rationale for the use of somatostatin analogs as antitumor agents. Ann Oncol. 2006;17:1733–42.
49. Sharma K, Patel YC, Srikant CB. Subtype selective induction of wild-type p53 and apoptosis, but not cell cycle arrest by human somatostatin receptor subtype 3. Mol Endocrinol. 1996;10:1688–96.
50. Teijeiro R, Rios R, Costoya JA, et al. Activation of human somatostatin receptor 2 promotes apoptosis through a mechanism that is independent from induction of p53. Cell Physiol Biochem. 2002;12:31–8.
51. Dasgupta P. Somatostatin analogues: multiple roles in cellular proliferation, neoplasia, and angiogenesis. Pharmacol Ther. 2004;102:61–85.
52. Reubi JC, Kvols LK, Waser B, et al. Detection of somatostatin receptors in surgical and percutaneous needle biopsy of carcinoids and islet cell carcinoma. Cancer Res. 1990;50:5969–77.
53. Krenning EP, Kwekkeboom DJ, Bakker W, et al. Somatostatin receptor scintigraphy with [^{111}In-DTPA-D-Phe1]- and [^{123}1-Tyr3]-octreotide: the Rotterdam experience with more than 1,000 patients. Eur J Nucl Med. 1993;20:716–31.
54. Bruns C, lewis, Briner U, et al, SOM230: a novel somatostatin peptidomimetic with broad somatostatin release inhibiting factor (SRIF) receptor binding and a unique antisecretory profile. Eur J Endocrinol. 2002;146:707–16.
55. Kvols LK, Moertel CG, O'Connell MJ, et al. Treatment of the malignant carcinoid syndrome. Evaluation of a long-acting somatostatin analogue. N Engl J Med. 1986;315:663–6.
56. Eriksson B, Öberg K. Summing up 15 years of somatostatin analog therapy in neuroendocrine tumors: future outlook. Ann Oncol. 1999;10:S31–8.
57. Rubin J, Ajani J, Schirmer W, et al. Octreotide acetate long-acting formulation versus open-label subcutaneous octreotide acetate in malignant carcinoid syndrome. J Clin Oncol. 1999;17:600–6.
58. Arnold R, Trautmann ME, Ceutzfeldt W, et al. Somatostatin analogue octreotide and inhibition and inhibition of tumor growth in metastatic endocrine gastroenteropancreatic tumours. Gut. 1996;38:430–8.
59. Aparicio T, Ducreux M, Bandin E, et al. Antitumour activity of somatostatin analogues in progressive metastatic neuroendocrine. Eur J Cancer. 2001;37:1014–9.
60. Ducreux M, Ruszniewski P, Chayvialle JA, et al. The antitumoral effect of long-acting somatostatin analog lanreotide in neuroendocrine tumours. Ann J Gastroenterol. 2000;95:3276–81.
61. Eriksson B, Renstrup J, Imam H, et al. High-dose treatment with lanreotide of patients with advanced neuroendocrine tumors: clinical and biological effects. Ann Oncol. 1997;8:1041–4.
62. Saltz L, Trochanowski B, Buckley M, et al. Octreotide as an antineoplastic agent in the treatment of functional and non-functional tumors. Cancer. 1993;72:244–8.

63. Panzuto F, Fonzo M, Iannicelli E, et al. Longterm clinical outcome of somatostatin analogues for treatment of progressive, metastatic well-differentiated enteropancreatic carcinoma. Ann Oncol. 2006;17:461–6.
64. Shojamanesh H, Gibril F, Adeline L, et al. Prospective study of the antitumor efficacy of long-term octreotide treatment in patients with progressive metastatic gastrinoma. Cancer. 2002;94:331–43.
65. Rinke A, Muller H, Schade-Brittinger C, et al. Placebo-controlled, double-blind, prospective, randomized study on the effect of octreotide-LAR in the control of tumor growth in patients with metastatic neuroendocrine midgut tumors: a report from the PROMID study group. J Clin Oncol. 2009;27:4656–63.
66. Öberg K, Funa K, Alm G. Effects of leukocyte interferon upon clinical symptoms and hormone levels in patients with midgut carcinoid tumors and the carcinoid syndromes. New Engl J Med. 1983;309:129–33.
67. Zhou Y, Wang S, Yue BG, et al. Effects of interferon alpha on the expression of p21cip1/waf1 and cell cycle distribution in carcinoid tumors. Cancer Invest. 2002;20:348–56.
68. Öberg K, Eriksson B, Janson ET. Interferons alone or in combination with chemotherapy or other biologicals in the treatment of neuroendocrine gut and pancreatic tumors. Digestion. 1994;55:64–9.
69. Andersson T, Wilander E, Eriksson B, et al. Effects of interferon on tumor tissue content in liver metastases of human carcinoid tumors. Cancer Res. 1990;50:3413–5.
70. Oberg K. Neuroendocrine gastrointestinal tumors. Ann Oncol. 1996;7:453–63.
71. Oberg K, Alm G, Lindstrom H, et al. Successful treatment of therapy-resistant pancreatic cholera with human leucocyte interferon. Lancet. 1985;1(8431):725–7.
72. Fjällskog ML, Sundin A, Westlin JE, et al. Treatment of malignant endocrine pancreatic tumors with a combination of α-interferon and somatostatin analogs. Med Oncol. 2002;19: 35–42.
73. Chandry A, Funa K, Öberg K. Expression of growth factor peptides and their receptors in neuroendocrine tumors of the digestive system. Acta Oncol. 1993;32:107–14.
74. Beauchamp RD, Coffey RJ, Lyons RM, et al. Human carcinoid production of paracrine growth factors that can stimulate fiberblast and endothelial cell growth. Cancer Res. 1991;51: 5253–60.
75. Terris B, Scoazec JY, Rubbia L, et al. Expression of vascular endothelial growth factor in digestive neuroendocrine tumours. Histopathology. 1998;78:233–9.
76. Nilsson O, Wängberg B, Theodorsson E, et al. Presence of IGF-1 in human midgut carcinoid tumors - an autocrine regulator of carcinoid tumor growth. Int J Cancer. 1992;51:195–203.
77. Krishnamurthy S, Dayal Y. Immunohistochemical expression of transforming growth factor alpha and epidermal growth factor receptor in gastrointestinal carcinoids. Am J Surg Pathol. 1997;21:327–33.
78. Christofori G, Naik P, Hanahan D. Vascular endothelial growth factor and its receptors, flt+1, flk-1, are expressed in normal pancreatic islets and throughout islet cell tumorgenesis. Mol Endocrinol. 1995;9:1760–70.
79. Couvelard A, O'Toole D, Turley H, et al. Microvascular density and hypoxia-inducible factor pathway in pancreatic endocrine tumours. Negative correlation of microvascular density and VEGF expression with tumour progression. Br J Cancer. 2005;92:94–101.
80. Yao JC, Phan PM, Hoss HX, et al. Targeting vascular endothelial growth factor in advanced carcinoid tumor: a random assignment phase II study of depot octreotide with bevacizumab and pegylated interferon alpha-2b. J Clin Oncol. 2008;26:1316–23.
81. Kulke MH, Earle CL, Bhargava P, et al. A phase II of temozolomide and bevacizumab in patients with advanced neuroendocrine tumors. Proc Am Soc Clin Oncol. 2006;24:4044.
82. Kunz PL, Kuo T, Kaiser HL, et al. A phase II study of capecitabine, oxilaplatin, and bevacizumab for metastatic or unresectable neuroendocrine tumors; preliminary results. Proc Am Soc Clin Oncol. 2008;26:15502.
83. Venook AP, Ko AH, Tempero MA, et al. Phase II trial of FOLFOX plus bevacizumab in advanced, progressive neuroendocrine tumors. Proc Am Soc Clin Oncol. 2008;26:15545.

84. Kulke MH, Lenz NJ, Meropol J, et al. Activity of sunitinib in patients with advanced neuroendocrine tumors. J Clin Oncol. 2008;26:3403–10.
85. Raymond E, Raoul JL, Niccoli P, et al. Phase III randomized, double-blind trial of sunitinib vs placebo in patients with progressive, well-differentiated malignant pancreatic islet cell tumours. World Congress on Gastrointestinal Cancer; 2009. p. 0013.
86. Niccioli P, Raoul JL, Young-Jue B, et al. Updated safety and efficiency results of this phase III trial sunitinib vs placebo for treatment of pancreatic neuroendocrine tumors (NET). Proc Am Soc Clin Oncol. 2010;28(15):400.
87. Hobday TJ, Rubin J, Holen K, et al. MCO44h, a phase II trial of sorafenib in patients (pts) with metastatic neuroendocrine tumors (NET): a phase II consortium (P2C) study. Proc Am Soc Clin Oncol. 2007;25:4504.
88. Yao JC, Zhang JX, Rashid A, et al. Clinical and in vitro studies of imatinib in advanced carcinoid tumors. Clin Cancer Res. 2007;13:234–40.
89. Kindmark H, Janson ET, Gustafsson B, et al. Five patients with malignant endocrine tumors treated with imatinib mesylate (Gleevec). Acta Oncologica. 2010;49(1):100–1.
90. Kulke MH, Stuart K, Enzinger PC, et al. Phase II study of temozolomide and thalidomide in patients with metastatic neuroendocrine tumors. J Clin Oncol. 2006;24:401–6.
91. Kulke MH, Bergsland DP, Ryan DP, et al. Phase II study of recombinant human endostatin in patients with advanced neuroendocrine tumors. J Clin Oncol. 2006;24:3555–61.
92. Guba M. v Breidenbuch P, Steinbaner M, et al; Rapamycin inhibits primary and metastatic tumor growth by antiangiogenesis: involvement of vascular endothelial growth factor. Nat Med. 2002;8:128–35.
93. Duran I, Kortmansky J, Singh D, et al. A phase II clinical and pharmacodynamic study of temsirolimus in advanced neuroendocrine carcinomas. Br J Cancer. 2007;95:1148–54.
94. Yao JC, Phan AT, Chang DZ, et al. Efficacy of RAD001 (everolimus) and octreotide LAR in advanced low-to intermediate-grade neuroendocrine tumors: results of a phase II study. J Clin Oncol. 2008;26:4311–8.
95. Yao JC, Lombard-Bohas C, Bandin E, et al. A phase II trial of daily oral RAD001 (everolimus) in patients with metastatic pancreatic neuroendocrine tumors (NET) after failure of cytotoxic chemotherapy. ASCO Gastrointestinal Cancer Symposium; 2009. p. 122.
96. Yao JC, Shah MH, Tetsuhide I, et al. Phase III randomized trial of everolimus (RAD 001) vs placebo in advanced pancreatic NET (RADIANT-3). Ann Oncol. 2010;21. doi:10.1093/annonc/mdq340.
97. Edge SB, Byrd DR, Compton CC, editors. Exocrine and endocrine pancreas, Chap. 24. In: AJCC cancer staging manual. 7th ed. New York, NY: Springer; 2010. p. 241–9.

Chapter 10
Poorly Differentiated Neuroendocrine Tumors

Joao E. Bezerra, Rachel P. Riechelmann, and Paulo M. Hoff

Abstract Extra-pulmonary PDNET comprise a heterogeneous and complex group of diseases. They are associated with a poor outcome, with median survival seldom achieving 1 year among patients with advanced disease. The treatment of PDNET follows the same principles of those for small cell carcinoma of the lung, with platinum-based chemotherapy reserved for metastatic disease and chemoradiation delivered to localized tumors. Because of its low frequency, the management of PDNET has relied on retrospective series. Multicenter, randomized clinical trials, preferably with collaborative groups, are warranted to help us determine the best therapeutic approach to this aggressive cancer.

Keywords Platinum-based chemotherapy • Chemoradiation • Small cell cancer of the lung

Introduction

Poorly differentiated neuroendocrine tumors (PDNET) represent a rare and heterogeneous entity. Its etiology is poorly understood and they can arise from many different organs. PDNET usually have a dismal prognosis and are best managed by multidisciplinary approach, including surgery, radiation, and systemic chemotherapy. In advanced disease, the principles of treatment for small cell lung cancer are often applied.

The present chapter aimed to review the current concepts on epidemiology, etiology, diagnosis, and management of different types of PDNET.

P.M. Hoff (✉)
Instituto do Cancer do Estado de São Paulo, Faculdade de Medicina da Universidade de São Paulo, Hospital Sirio Libanes, São Paulo, Brazil
e-mail: Paulo.hoff@icesp.org.br

J.C. Yao et al. (eds.), *Neuroendocrine Tumors*, Current Clinical Oncology,
DOI 10.1007/978-1-60327-997-0_10, © Springer Science+Business Media, LLC 2011

Epidemiology

Overall, poorly differentiated neuroendocrine carcinomas represent 0.1–0.4% of all cancer, with approximately 1,000 new cases diagnosed in the United States yearly [1]. Specific risk factors for PDNET have not been identified but appear to be similar to those predisposing to the development of other types of cancer in the same organs [2].

Despite their diverse anatomic origins, these carcinomas look and behave similarly, usually presenting with metastasis at the time of diagnosis and progressing very rapidly. The patient's median overall survival is usually less than 1 year, ranging from a few weeks to several months. Cure is usually only possible when the tumor is identified before the development of metastasis.

Clinical Presentation

PDNET cannot be suspected from the presenting symptoms, as these are similar to those of other histological types of tumors arising in the same site. Since most patients are diagnosed in advanced stage, constitutional symptoms, such as weight loss and anorexia, are common.

Paraneoplastic syndromes secondary to ectopic hormonal secretion are not uncommon [3]. Ectopic production of vasoactive intestinal peptide [4], calcitonin [5], adrenocorticotropic hormone [6], and antidiuretic hormone [7] have been described in the literature.

Staging and Work-Up

Because extra-pulmonary small cell carcinomas are uncommon, the diagnosis should first exclude a primary lung small cell carcinoma. After the histologic diagnosis is established, a complete evaluation should include an X-ray and a computed tomography (CT) scan of the chest. A bronchoscopy, to exclude an occult lung primary tumor, particularly in heavy smokers, may be considered [3]. The usual evaluation of the affected organ must be performed in addition to the specific tests required for small cell carcinoma CT scan of the brain, abdominal imaging with CT or magnetic resonance image (MRI), PET-CT, and others as clinically indicated.

In 2006 the first proposal TNM staging for neuroendocrine tumors was developed by European Neuroendocrine Tumors Society (ENETS). This classification comprises gastroenteropancreatic neuroendocrine tumors and was designed to be applicable to both well-differentiated and poorly differentiated tumors [8, 9]. In 2009 the seventh edition of the AJCC/UICC TNM classification of malignant tumors also included a new classification of the gastrointestinal and pancreatic neuroendocrine tumors but without covering the poorly differentiated neuroendocrine tumors subtype [10].

However, some authors still advocate using the same staging system used for small cell carcinoma of the lung, based on data from the Veterans Administration Lung Study Group, dividing cases in limited or extensive stage disease [3, 11].

Histologic Characteristics

PDNET encompass a variety of histological entities including extra-pulmonary small cell carcinoma, extra-pulmonary large-cell high-grade carcinoma neuroendocrine carcinoma, small cell carcinoma of the lung and large-cell high-grade neuroendocrine carcinoma of the lung.

The small cell histology is the most common form of presentation of extra-pulmonary PDNET. Small cell carcinoma from different organs cannot be differentiated by their histologic features, which are indistinguishable from features of small cell carcinoma of the lung [12–18]. The WHO categorizes small cell carcinoma of the lung into three groups: oat-cell carcinomas, intermediate-cell carcinoma, and combined carcinomas. Combined carcinomas are those in which another recognizable histologic feature is found along with the histologic characteristics of small cell carcinoma [19].

Typical oat-cell-type tumors have small cells, two to three times the size of a mature lymphocyte, a high nucleus–cytoplasm ratio and minimal nuclear clearing, inconspicuous nucleoli, and dispersed chromatin. The intermediate-type tumors have relatively large cells with vesicular nuclei, prominent nucleoli, and comparatively abundant cytoplasm, and they are actually intermediate entities between the typical carcinoids and the oat cell [14, 20].

The typical small cell tumor has membrane-bound, electron-dense neurosecretory cytoplasmic granules that can be seen on electron microscopy. The number of these granules correlates with the tumor's degree of differentiation [21].

On Grimelius staining, these cells are argyrophilic and react with chromogranin. Immunohistochemistry is important in establishing the diagnosis; most tumors test positive for synaptophysin, chromogranin A, Leu-7, and neuron-specific enolase (NSE) [22–25]. However, PDNET present significantly reduced chomogranin A expression and intense staining for synaptophysin compared with well-differentiated neuroendocrine carcinomas [9]. Immunoreactivity for carcinoembryonic antigen (CEA) is often positive. Thyroid transcription factor-1 (TTF-1) is commonly expressed in small cell carcinomas of the lung and was proposed as a marker for distinguishing small cell lung cancers from extra-pulmonary small cell carcinoma [26]. However, other studies have reported similar TTF-1 expression between pulmonary and extra-pulmonary small cell carcinomas [27–29]. Most small cell carcinoma stain for AE1:AE3 and Cam5.2. Staining for high molecular weight keratins identified by the antibody 34BE12 is almost always negative in small cell carcinomas and may be useful to distinguish basaloid squamous cell carcinoma, an entity that may be confused with small cell carcinoma [30, 31].

Consistent with their aggressive clinical course, small cell carcinomas have a high proliferative rate. The mitotic index, determined by number of mitoses per unit area of tumor, is the conventional method to characterize high-grade tumors. Nevertheless, the definition of high-grade tumor differs among some classification systems [9, 32, 33]. Abundant necrosis, either confluent or punctuate, is present. The Ki-67 proliferation index provides an accurate assessment of the proliferative rate and has been incorporated in the classification systems. PDNET present high Ki67 proliferation index, usually >40% (>20% per AJCC and ENETs criteria) [32].

The histogenesis of extra-pulmonary small cell carcinoma is controversial. The original theories were that small cell carcinoma arises from amine precursor uptake and decarboxylation (APUD) cells [34–37]. Since 1968, when Pearse [38], proposed the acronym APUD to describe a group of cells with similar features and presumed embryological origin, considerable controversy, varying from neuroectodermal [39] to endodermal origins [40, 41] has surrounded the embryogenesis of these cells. The observation that small cell carcinoma is frequently found "combined" with squamous cells and adenocarcinomas [42] led investigators to propose the origin as being a totipotent stem cell, which could subsequently differentiate into either epithelial or neuroendocrine carcinoma or both [15].

Molecular Characteristics

The molecular events leading to the development of extra-pulmonary small cell carcinoma have not yet been elucidated. Cytogenetic studies may be useful to differentiate "true" extra-pulmonary tumors from metastatic small cell carcinoma that arose from an occult lung primary. Deletion of the short arm of chromosome 3 has been identified in up to 85% of the lung small cell carcinomas [43] but not in extra-pulmonary small cell carcinoma [44, 45].

Overexpression of p53 [16, 17, 46], loss of Rb expression [16, 47], Bcl-2 positivity [16], loss of *p*16 [17, 47], and mutation of k-ras [17] have been reported as being associated in the extra-pulmonary small cell carcinoma. Evidence suggests that these finds play a central role in the carcinogenesis of lung small cell carcinoma and probably in extra-pulmonary small cell carcinomas [48].

General Treatment Guidelines

Because of the rarity of PDNET of extra-pulmonary origin, well-designed randomized controlled trials have not been performed. Treatment recommendations for advanced disease are based on single-institution case series or small phase II trials and follow the therapies for small cell lung cancer. Complete surgical resection is the only curative therapeutic approach for early-stage disease. In this case, platin-based regimens have been advocated by some authors as a form of adjuvant chemotherapy [49]. Local treatment might be prescribed as part of the treatment regimen for patients who have localized disease or to control local symptoms. In this setting, a patient–physician discussion about the risks and benefits of adjuvant treatment is imperative. Especially because of the lack of solid evidence supporting such approach.

Most patients present with advanced disease, often with liver and lymph node metastases. Systemic chemotherapy is indicated for inoperable, advanced disease in patients with good organ function and performance status [11, 50]. The role of systemic therapy in patients with poor clinical conditions has not been established. Similarly to small cell lung cancer, regimens commonly used include cisplatin/carboplatin and etoposide [51–58]. While well-differentiated NET respond poorly to systemic chemotherapy, combination chemotherapy has been historically effective in PDNET, with tumor responses ranging from 40 to 80%, depending on response criteria definition [59–61] but median survival rarely exceeds 1 year. Other common combinations include cyclophosphamide, doxorubicin, and vincristine (CAV) and cyclophosphamide, doxorubicin, vincristine, and etoposide (CAVE) [62]. A phase II trial of paclitaxel, carboplatin and oral etoposide (PCE) for 66 patients with extra-pulmonary PDNET produced a tumor response of 33% in intention-to-treat analyses; the median duration of response and median survival for 56 evaluable patients were 9 and 14.8 months, respectively [63]. Based on encouraging results from a retrospective series [64], a phase II trial of 20 PDNET patients treated with the combination of irinotecan and cisplatin demonstrated good safety profile and led to 58% of tumor responses [65]. Newer agents and regimens are being evaluated in patients with small cell carcinoma of the lung [66], but their role in extra-pulmonary small cell carcinoma is currently undefined. Unfortunately, although responses to chemotherapy are high, the rate of durable responses is low. Specific recommendations for treatment of small cell carcinoma for different organs are discussed in the following section.

Characteristics of and Treatment Recommendations for Extra-Pulmonary PDNET

PDNET of the Head and Neck

Small cell carcinoma of the larynx was first described by Olofsson and Van Nostrand in 1972 [67]. Since then several small reports recognized the larynx as the most frequent affected site for small cell carcinoma in the head and neck [34].

Laryngeal small cell carcinoma appears to have the same risk factors as other laryngeal tumors, like tobacco and alcohol consumption. There is a slight male predominance and most patients are diagnosed between the ages of 60 and 80 [68].

Clinical presentation is not different from other laryngeal tumors and most symptoms are related with the presence of a laryngeal mass. The most common presenting symptoms are hoarseness, mass in the neck, dysphagia, dyspneia, and cough. Cervical lymph node metastases are no rarely the first sign of the disease before hoarseness becomes apparent [69].

Laryngeal small cell carcinoma is indistinguishable by histology from other highly aggressive neuroendocrine tumors like small cell lung cancer. Large cell PDNET have also been described. Most tumors present with a pure small cell histology but some show elements of squamous cell carcinoma or adenocarcinoma [69, 70]. These finds might either suggest a totipotent stem cell as an origin of laryngeal small cell carcinoma or just reflect the common risk factors for larynx tumors.

The surgical treatment with total laryngectomy seems to control the primary tumor but is insufficient to cure most patients. The use of systemic chemotherapy can improve dramatically the long-term survival. Aguilar et al. [71] reported a great improvement in 2-year survival in patients treated with local therapy in combination with chemotherapy versus local therapy alone (52 vs. 10%). Baugh et al. [72] reported a median survival of 19 months compared to 11 months for patients treated with or without adjuvant chemotherapy after a local therapy. In the same report, local disease control was similar between radiotherapy and total laryngectomy, suggesting that surgery may be performed only in those patients who did not achieve complete response with radiation therapy.

Besides high rate of local treatment failure, most patients present distant metastases early in the follow-up [73]. Intracranial metastasis seems to be more common in laryngeal small cell carcinoma than in other extra-pulmonary small cell carcinoma. Moreover, brain metastasis was reported to be the only place of recurrence in up to 42% of patients in a single series [74].

Salivary glands are one of the most common places for small cell carcinoma in head and neck. It accounts for about 1–2% of all salivary gland tumors and the parotid gland is the most affected site [75]. Salivary gland small cell carcinoma has a great potential for local invasion and distant metastasis. However, patients with salivary gland small cell carcinoma seem to have better prognosis when compared with lung small cell carcinoma and larynx small cell carcinoma, with a 2- and 5-year survival rates of 70 and 46%, respectively, compared with 16 and 5% for laryngeal small cell carcinoma [2]. Therapy approach usually follow the recommendation for laryngeal small cell carcinoma with extensive surgical resection or radiation therapy being applied for local control always associated with systemic chemotherapy.

Neuroendocrine tumors also affect the paranasal sinuses, with highly aggressive forms composing most of the cases. Small cell carcinoma of the paranasal sinuses has been associated with either high rates of local failure and distant recurrence, despite the more frequent use of chemotherapy among these patients [76, 77]. Intracranial recurrence is a major problem and prophylactic cranial irradiation in those patients who respond well to the initial therapy has been advocated [76].

Esophageal PDNET

The esophagus is the most common site of extra-pulmonary small cell carcinoma of the GI tract. The reported incidence of small cell carcinoma in relation to the total number of esophageal cancers varies widely, ranging from as low as 0.05% among

1,918 patients with esophageal cancer [78] to as high as 15% [79]. Recent reports by investigators in the United States cite an incidence of approximately 1–2% of all cases of esophageal cancer [3, 80]. Because of the limited number of cases of esophageal small cell carcinoma, no definite risk factors can be described. A possible association with tobacco use has been suggested, but esophageal small cell carcinoma has also been described among nonsmokers [80]. This tumor has an anatomic preference for the middle and lower thirds of the esophagus [34, 80], with a slightly higher incidence in men than in women (3:2), and its onset usually occurs after the fifth decade of life [7, 80]. Common presenting symptoms include dysphagia, weight loss, chest pain, and abdominal pain [81–83].

If untreated, the prognosis is poor, with median survival duration measured in weeks and no long-term survivals [84]. Patients who are treated aggressively have median survival of approximately 7 months, and patients occasionally survive for over 2 years [80, 85]. Treatment with surgery and radiation alone was used in the past, but the results were disappointing. The recent use of aggressive combination chemotherapy regimens developed for small cell carcinoma of the lung has resulted in markedly improved but usually transient responses [50, 86]. A multimodality approach to treatment seems to be important. Craig and colleagues [87] combined subtotal esophagectomy with chemotherapy or radiotherapy for seven patients with localized disease, and reported a mean survival duration of 20 months. One patient treated with surgery and chemotherapy survived for more than 96 months. Data from several single-institution reports suggest that the optimal treatment for patients with localized disease is a multimodality regimen consisting of chemotherapy designed for lung small cell carcinoma, followed by local regional consolidation, and either surgical resection or radiotherapy [84, 88, 89]. It has been suggested that surgical resection improves long-term survival for limited; stage disease [90]. Patients with advanced disease should be treated with chemotherapy alone; if they respond, local regional therapy can be considered. Patients who have a poor performance status and cannot be treated aggressively or for whom treatment has failed may benefit from close follow-up and the palliative measures commonly used for patients with esophageal small cell carcinomas and adenocarcinomas, including supportive care, radiotherapy, laser therapy, and stenting.

Gastric PDNET

Small cell carcinoma of the stomach also occurs infrequently. The first well-documented case was reported in 1976 [91], and since then, fewer than 50 cases have been cited in the literature [5]. It is not surprising that the majority of cases, including the largest series [92], were reported by Japanese investigators, and this suggests that similar risk factors may be involved in gastric small cell carcinoma and adenocarcinoma.

A small cell carcinoma incidence of less than 1% has been reported in patients with gastric cancer [92], but the incidence may be as low as 0.01% [91]. Most gastric small cell carcinomas are intermediate-type tumors and are combined with other histologies with no predilection for location in the stomach. Men are at a twofold increased risk for gastric small cell carcinoma compared to women, and the most common presenting symptoms are epigastralgia, nausea, melena, anorexia, and weight loss. At diagnosis, the majority of patients have advanced disease. The liver is the most common site of distant metastasis but involvement of brain, lungs, bones, lymph nodes, and bone marrow have been reported [92].

The median survival duration is 9 months [5], and few studies have described long-term survivals [34, 91]. Combination chemotherapy may prolong survival, but too few cases are available for a definitive recommendation. Of interest, in 1950 Bernatz [93] reported a 5-year-survival rate of close to 70% in 72 patients with small cell carcinoma of the stomach who were treated with surgical resection. However, most of these cancers had a mixed histologic pattern, and, more importantly, patients with the diagnosis of lymphoma rather than small cell carcinoma may have been included in the series [3, 93, 94].

PDNET of the Colon and Rectum

Small cell carcinoma of the colon and rectum are aggressive carcinomas that appear and behave similarly to their counterparts in the lung [12]. Clery and associates [95] first described small cell carcinoma of the colon and rectum in 1961 and suggested that the incidence of this entity represented 0.2% of all colon cancers. Since then, fewer than 100 cases of small cell carcinoma of the colon and rectum have been reported. Slightly over a third of the cases occurred in the rectum, followed by the cecum, sigmoid, transverse colon, and ascending colon [21].

The clinical presentation of this cancer includes hematochezia, weight loss, fatigue, anorexia, abdominal pain, and changes in bowel habits [13, 96], but the symptoms are usually similar to those of adenocarcinoma at a similar anatomic location. No preference among the sexes has been identified, and most of these carcinomas are diagnosed in 60–70 years of age. No risk factors have been firmly identified, but a case report suggests that patients who have ulcerative colitis might have a higher risk [21]. In about 15% of patients, the disease is confined to the organ or to the regional nodes, but 85% of patients present with distant metastasis. The liver is the organ most commonly affected by metastasis; other organs include the lymph nodes, bones, bone marrow, and skin [97–99]. Although small cell carcinomas frequently show coexistent squamous and glandular differentiation, the metastases observed almost always have small cell histologic characteristics [14].

Despite earlier reports of long-term survivors among patients with resectable colorectal carcinomas [95], the median survival duration for patients with small cell carcinoma of the colorectal area remains less than 1 year [13, 98, 99]. Use of multiagent chemotherapy, including drugs that are effective against bronchogenic small cell carcinoma, has been recommended and documented in case reports, but because of the rarity of this tumor, no large clinical trials have been conducted [13, 14, 98].

Patients with localized disease may be offered a combined modality approach, including local treatment with surgery or radiotherapy and chemotherapy. For patients with advanced disease, the treatment should focus on chemotherapy [11, 14, 98].

PDNET of Anal Canal

These tumors constitute less than 1% of anal canal cancers and are highly aggressive. They can be of small cell type or large cell type, showing similar outcomes. The management of early-stage anal canal PDNET is multidisciplinary, with most patients being treated with surgery and local radiation and/or systemic platin-based chemotherapy. Patients with inoperable disease can be treated with systemic chemotherapy combined or not radiation therapy [100].

PDNET of the Pancreas

Small cell carcinoma of the pancreas was originally described in 1951 [101], and a large review series showed that 1–1.5% of all pancreatic cancers consistently have small cell histologic features [34, 102]. Only 19 cases have been reported in the literature [103]. The disease has no known risk factors, and its epidemiology is not well defined. Common presenting symptoms include jaundice and abdominal discomfort. Among 15 patients who did not receive chemotherapy, the median survival duration was 2 months [98, 104]. Of four patients treated with chemotherapy, one patient achieved a partial response and three obtained complete responses, although two of the three patients with complete responses relapsed and died within a year. The third patient, who had widely metastatic disease at diagnosis, was alive and free of disease 9 years after treatment with cisplatin and etoposide [59, 103, 105].

On the basis of limited information, the optimal treatment for small cell carcinoma of the pancreas includes chemotherapy with the same agents used in the treatment of lung small cell carcinoma, with radiotherapy as consolidation.

PDNET at Other GI Sites

Small cell carcinomas have also been documented in the ampulla of Vater and the small intestines. These tumors are so rare that only a few cases have been reported. Toker [104] cited the only well-documented case of small cell carcinoma of the jejunum, which occurred in a 17-year-old girl. Treated with surgery, she had a prolonged disease-free survival. Six cases of small cell carcinoma of the ampulla of Vater have been described in the literature since the first report by Swanson et al. in 1986 [22, 106]. The patients, consisted of five men and one woman, tended to be of older age. The median survival duration was 10 months, with no long-term survivals [22, 107]. The usual presentation of this tumor includes signs of biliary obstruction and rapid development of metastases. Patients with good performance status should be offered chemotherapy as with small cell carcinoma of the lung, but no definitive data are available regarding the effectiveness of chemotherapy for this setting.

PDNET of the Prostate

Poorly differentiated neuroendocrine carcinoma accounts for less than 1% of de novo prostate cancers and slightly more than 1% of hormone refractory prostate cancers. They usually present characteristic small cell undifferentiated morphology under light microscopy and neuroendocrine differentiation similar to small cell lung cancer, although some of them may express specific markers of prostate cancer [108].

Small cell carcinoma of prostate was first described by Wenk et al. [109] in 1977. The etiology of prostatic small cell carcinoma is still on debate with either neuroendocrine APUD cells, totipotent stem cells or dedifferentiation of adenocarcinoma cells being postulated as the original clone. It may coexist in patients after a history of prostatic adenocarcinoma, particularly after long-term use of androgen deprivation therapy [110, 111].

Autopsy studies have identified small cell carcinoma in 10–20% of patients who died of prostate adenocarcinoma [110, 112, 113]. Focal neuroendocrine differentiation can often be seen by immunohistochemistry in samples of usual adenocarcinoma of the prostate and does not indicate the occurrence of a de novo small cell carcinoma [112, 114, 115]. In a single center study of 95 prostatic small cell carcinomas samples, pure small cell histology was seen in 57% of cases with the remaining cases mixed with adenocarcinoma. Moreover, in the mixed cases, small cell predominated over the adenocarcinoma with a median of 80% of the total tumor occupied by small cell component [116].

The clinical presentation of small cell carcinoma does not differ from other prostate tumors and correlates with the degree of urinary flow obstruction. Most patients complain of rapid onset dysuria and urinary retention. About 10% present with systemic constitutional symptoms including weight loss, anorexia, neurological symptoms, back pain, and hepatic dysfunction, reflecting early spreading of the disease. Paraneoplastic syndromes such as peripheral neuropathy, Eaton–Lambert syndrome, Cushing's syndrome, membranous nephropath, and hypercalcemia without bone metastases have been reported [117–119].

The use of serum tumor marker is of limited benefit. Prostate specific antigen (PSA) levels are usually low with values typically less than 2 ng/mL [117]. Elevated levels of serum chromogranin A, a powerful universal marker of neuroendocrine tissues, has been reported in patients with hormone-resistant prostatic adenocarcinoma and losses its specificity. High levels of CEA has also been reported but is non-specific and has not been demonstrated to be an independent predictor of disease outcomes

[120, 121]. Low serum albumin and elevated serum lactate deshydrogenase (LDH) has been associated with poor outcome [122, 123].

The diagnosis of prostatic small cell carcinoma usually relies on morphologic features. However, differentiation from Gleason pattern 5 adenocarcinoma is of major importance and sometimes might not be done without a comprehensive immunohistochemistry panel [26].

The most common sites of distant metastases are bone, retroperitoneal lymph nodes, liver, and lungs [117, 122, 124]. Furthermore, similar to other PDNET, brain metastases seem to be more common in patients with prostate small cell carcinoma than prostatic adenocarcinoma. In a retrospective study at M.D. Anderson Cancer Center, 16,280 patients with prostatic cancer were analyzed and brain metastases were significantly more common in prostatic small cell carcinoma than in prostate adenocarcinoma (16 vs. 0.8%) [125]. Although some authors advocate prophylactic cranial irradiation in high-risk patient with prostate small cell carcinoma, no data on efficacy is available and its routine use is not indicated by most [2, 125, 126].

Prostatic metastases from lung small cell carcinoma might occur but it is rare. However, primary small cell lung cancer should be excluded and a complete evaluation of the disease extension should be performed before treatment. PDNET of the prostate is aggressive and usually diagnosed at advanced clinical stage. Early-stage disease reports are uncommon and although there are few reports of long-term survivors, most patients develop metastases and die of the disease [122]. Unfortunately, most of treatment reports are based in retrospective case series, restraining the conclusions about the most effective treatment of the disease. Indeed, treatment decisions are generally guided by the experience on small cell lung cancer studies. Prostatectomy should be evaluated in selected patients with non-metastatic small cell carcinoma of the prostate because it has been associated with better local control and potential survival benefit in some series [122, 127, 128]. The role of adjuvant radiotherapy is uncertain, since treatment usually fails as a distant metastasis. However, in situations with increased risk of local recurrence (e.g., T2 disease or exiguous surgical margins), chemoradiotherapy is indicated. Platinum-based chemotherapy is usually offered either in adjuvant setting or combined with radiotherapy as definitive therapy. When diagnosed as a locally advanced disease, concurrent chemoradiation is usually the favored treatment employed. When disseminated metastases are present, a cisplatin-based systemic therapy is indicated. However, the optimal regimen has not been established.

Bladder PDNET

Poorly differentiated neuroendocrine carcinoma of the urinary bladder is a rare disease. It was first well documented by Cramer et al. [129] in 1981 and accounts for less than 1% of all bladder tumors. It is often found in conjunction with other tumors, most frequently transitional cell carcinoma and adenocarcinoma [130]. Unlike PDNET of the prostate, a history of other prior bladder malignancy is uncommon.

While PDNET of the bladder present morphologic features of small cell undifferentiated carcinoma, similar to small cell of the lung, a molecular study of bladder tumors suggested that both small cell carcinoma and urothelial cell cancer derive from the same clone population [131]. These evidences suggest a primitive multipotent cell as the origin of small cell bladder carcinoma rather than a specific neuroendocrine cell.

Symptoms due to the primary tumor are indistinguishable from other bladder tumors. The tumor usually infiltrates the bladder wall causing dysuria and hematuria. In large series, the average age of presentation is approximately 67 years and men are at almost a fourfold increased risk compared to women [130, 132, 133].

Small cell carcinoma of the bladder is highly aggressive and most patients present with locally advanced or metastatic disease. It tends to follow the metastatic trend of transitional cell carcinoma, with the most common sites being regional and distant lymph nodes, liver, and bone. At the diagnosis, more than a half of patients present at advanced stage, with up to 43% patients with stage IV [133]. Because no randomized clinical trial is available, most of the recommendations derive from retrospective series. For patient diagnosed with limited disease, treatment options include surgery, chemotherapy, and concurrent chemoradiation. Since relapses outside the radiation field are common, radiotherapy seems to have no role in the adjuvant treatment. Single institution studies have shown that some patients can achieve durable complete remissions with surgery alone. Choong et al. [132] reported a 5-year survival rate of 64% in patients with stage II disease after radical cystectomy, suggesting that adjuvant treatment might not be necessary in early disease. Siefker-Radtke et al. [134] in a retrospective report of 88 small cell carcinomas of the bladder from M.D. Anderson Cancer Center, patients treated with initial cystectomy had a 5-year survival rate of 36 versus 78% for patients receiving preoperative chemotherapy; survival between patients who did and did not receive adjuvant chemotherapy was similar.

Radiotherapy has been used as an alternative to cystectomy at many centers. In one study, 17 patients treated with sequential chemoradiation were retrospectively analyzed. All patients were treated with platinum-based chemotherapy followed by radiotherapy. A complete clinical response was achieved in 15 patients, with seven patients remained disease-free. The median overall survival was 33 months [135]. In a retrospective analysis of ten British Columbia Cancer Agency patients treated for bladder small cell carcinoma with concurrent chemoradiation, Lohrisch et al. [136] reported 70% 2-year and 44% 5-year overall survival, while disease-free survival was 70% at 2 and 5 years. Cheng et al. [130] analyzed 64 patients retrospectively and found no significant difference in overall survival between those patients who underwent or not cystectomy for local treatment, suggesting that definitive chemoradiation is an option for these patients

Distant metastatic disease is treated with chemotherapy. The most common regimen, based on small cell carcinoma of the lung, is cisplatin or carboplatin and etoposide. Others regimens have been used but have similar response rate. Metastatic bladder small cell carcinoma is highly responsive to chemotherapy but these responses are generally transient. Median survival of 2–8 months has been described [132, 137, 138].

Although prophylactic brain irradiation decreases the incidence of brain metastases and prolongs survival in patients with lung small cell carcinoma, there are no data in patients with bladder small cell carcinoma. The incidence of brain metastases, however, seems to be lower in bladder small cell carcinoma than in small cell carcinoma of the lung, therefore routine use of prophylactic cranial irradiation is not recommended [130, 134, 139, 140].

PDNET of the Uterine Cervix

Small cell carcinoma of the female genital tract is an uncommon disease and constitutes less than 2% of all gynecological malignancies. It may originate in the endometrium, ovary, fallopian tube, vagina, and vulva, but most frequently in the cervix [141]. Small cell cervical carcinoma corresponds to less than 3% of all cervical cancers, with a mean annual incidence around 0.06 per 100,000 women in the United States. The median age of presentation is 42 years (range, 20–87 years). Vaginal bleeding is the most common complain followed by pelvic pain.

Unlike the majority of PDNET arising from other organs, many patients with cervical PDNET have localized disease at the moment of diagnosis and are eligible for curative treatment. Nevertheless, cervix small cell carcinoma is an aggressive disease and carries a worse prognosis compared to squamous cell carcinoma of the cervix. In a matched case–control study, Lee et al. [142] reported a significantly shorter median progression-free survival (16.9 vs. 30.6 months) but similar median overall survival (47.7 vs. 49.1 months) for the small cell carcinoma group than for the squamous cell carcinoma.

Although there is no consensus about the optimal management for PDNET of the cervix, hysterectomy alone seems to be inadequate as a single modality of therapy in a curative setting. Sheets et al. [143] reported a median survival of 13.5 months among patients with early-stage disease and treated by hysterectomy and postoperative radiotherapy. However, hysterectomy remains an important part of the curative treatment. Chan et al. [144] analyzed 34 patients with cervical small cell carcinoma and the only long-term survivors were those with small tumors (<2.0 cm) amenable to radical surgery. Definitive radiation is also an alternative to surgery. Viswanathan et al. [145] reported 21 patients with small cell carcinoma of the cervix treated locally with either with hysterectomy or radiotherapy, and systemically with a platinum-based regimen. The overall survival was 29% at 5 years and adjuvant chemotherapy did not result in a significant increase in relapse-free survival.

In fact, the role of chemotherapy in the treatment of cervical small cell carcinoma still remains unclear. Due to the aggressive course of the disease and pattern of recurrence, adjuvant chemotherapy is currently given to amenable patients even without strong evidences of benefit. One recent retrospective study could demonstrate benefits of chemotherapy in the treatment of cervical small cell carcinoma. Cohen et al. [146] collected 136 from case-series reported in the literature and 52 patients from tumor registry databases at four north-American hospitals. Of 188 patients, 135 had stage

I–IIA, 45 had IIB–IVA, and 8 had stage IVB disease. Overall survival at 5 years based on stage was 36.8% for stage I-IIA and 8.9% for stage IIB-IVA. Furthermore, adjuvant chemotherapy or chemoradiation was associated with improved survival in stage IIB–IVA disease versus surgical resection alone (3-year survival: 17.8 vs. 12.0%, $P=0.043$). In conclusion, radical hysterectomy followed by platinum-based chemotherapy with or without external radiation should be considered for all early-stage patients. Upfront platinum-based chemotherapy followed by chemoradiotherapy, or surgery in selected cases, should be offered for amenable high-stage patients.

Conclusion

Extra-pulmonary PDNET comprise a heterogeneous and complex group of diseases. They are associated with a poor outcome, with median survival seldom achieving 1 year among patients with advanced disease. The treatment of PDNET follows the same principles of those for small cell carcinoma of the lung, with platinum-based chemotherapy reserved for metastatic disease and chemoradiation delivered to localized tumors. Because of its low frequency, the management of PDNET has relied on retrospective series. Multicenter, randomized clinical trials, preferably with collaborative groups, are warranted to help us determine the best therapeutic approach to this aggressive cancers.

References

1. Remick SC, Ruckdeschel JC. Extrapulmonary and pulmonary small-cell carcinoma: tumor biology, therapy, and outcome. Med Pediatr Oncol. 1992;20(2):89–99.
2. Walenkamp AM, Sonke GS, Sleijfer DT. Clinical and therapeutic aspects of extrapulmonary small cell carcinoma. Cancer Treat Rev. 2009;35(3):228–36.
3. Remick SC, Hafez GR, Carbone PP. Extrapulmonary small-cell carcinoma. A review of the literature with emphasis on therapy and outcome. Medicine (Baltimore). 1987;66(6):457–71.
4. Watson KJ, Shulkes A, Smallwood RA, et al. Watery diarrhea-hypokalemia-achlorhydria syndrome and carcinoma of the esophagus. Gastroenterology. 1985;88(3):798–803.
5. O'Byrne KJ, Cherukuri AK, Khan MI, et al. Extrapulmonary small cell gastric carcinoma. A case report and review of the literature. Acta Oncol. 1997;36(1):78–80.
6. Tateishi R, Taniguchi K, Horai T, Iwanaga T, Taniguchi H. Argyrophil cell carcinoma (apudoma) of the esophagus. A histopathologic entity. Virchows Arch A Pathol Anat Histol. 1976;371(4):283–94.
7. Doherty MA, McIntyre M, Arnott SJ. Oat cell carcinoma of esophagus: a report of six British patients with a review of the literature. Int J Radiat Oncol Biol Phys. 1984;10(1):147–52.
8. Rindi G, de Herder WW, O'Toole D, Wiedenmann B. Consensus guidelines for the management of patients with digestive neuroendocrine tumors: why such guidelines and how we went about it. Neuroendocrinology. 2006;84(3):155–7.
9. Rindi G, Kloppel G, Couvelard A, et al. TNM staging of midgut and hindgut (neuro) endocrine tumors: a consensus proposal including a grading system. Virchows Arch. 2007;451(4):757–62.

10. Sobin L, Gospodarowicz M, Wittekind C, editors. UICC: TNM classification of malignant tumours. 7th ed. Oxford: Wiley-Blackwell; 2009.
11. Van Der Gaast A, Verwey J, Prins E, Splinter TA. Chemotherapy as treatment of choice in extrapulmonary undifferentiated small cell carcinomas. Cancer. 1990;65(3):422–4.
12. Jass J, Sobin LH. Histological typing of intestinal tumors. WHO International Histological Classification of Tumors. Berlin: Springer; 1989.
13. Wick MR, Weatherby RP, Weiland LH. Small cell neuroendocrine carcinoma of the colon and rectum: clinical, histologic, and ultrastructural study and immunohistochemical comparison with cloacogenic carcinoma. Hum Pathol. 1987;18(1):9–21.
14. Burke AB, Shekitka KM, Sobin LH. Small cell carcinomas of the large intestine. Am J Clin Pathol. 1991;95(3):315–21.
15. Ho KJ, Herrera GA, Jones JM, Alexander CB. Small cell carcinoma of the esophagus: evidence for a unified histogenesis. Hum Pathol. 1984;15(5):460–8.
16. Takubo K, Nakamura K, Sawabe M, et al. Primary undifferentiated small cell carcinoma of the esophagus. Hum Pathol. 1999;30(2):216–21.
17. Maitra A, Tascilar M, Hruban RH, Offerhaus GJ, Albores-Saavedra J. Small cell carcinoma of the gallbladder: a clinicopathologic, immunohistochemical, and molecular pathology study of 12 cases. Am J Surg Pathol. 2001;25(5):595–601.
18. Sarsfield P, Anthony PP. Small cell undifferentiated ('neuroendocrine') carcinoma of the colon. Histopathology. 1990;16(4):357–63.
19. WHO. The World Health Organization histological typing of lung tumours. Second edition. Am J Clin Pathol. 1982;77(2):123–36.
20. Gaffey MJ, Mills SE, Lack EE. Neuroendocrine carcinoma of the colon and rectum. A clinicopathologic, ultrastructural, and immunohistochemical study of 24 cases. Am J Surg Pathol. 1990;14(11):1010–23.
21. Yaziji H, Broghamer Jr WL. Primary small cell undifferentiated carcinoma of the rectum associated with ulcerative colitis. South Med J. 1996;89(9):921–4.
22. Sarker AB, Hoshida Y, Akagi S, et al. An immunohistochemical and ultrastructural study of case of small-cell neuroendocrine carcinoma in the ampullary region of the duodenum. Acta Pathol Jpn. 1992;42(7):529–35.
23. Bunn Jr PA, Linnoila I, Minna JD, Carney D, Gazdar AF. Small cell lung cancer, endocrine cells of the fetal bronchus, and other neuroendocrine cells express the Leu-7 antigenic determinant present on natural killer cells. Blood. 1985;65(3):764–8.
24. Lloyd RV, Cano M, Rosa P, Hille A, Huttner WB. Distribution of chromogranin A and secretogranin I (chromogranin B) in neuroendocrine cells and tumors. Am J Pathol. 1988;130(2):296–304.
25. Tapia FJ, Polak JM, Barbosa AJ, et al. Neuron-specific enolase is produced by neuroendocrine tumours. Lancet. 1981;1(8224):808–11.
26. Ordonez NG. Value of thyroid transcription factor-1 immunostaining in distinguishing small cell lung carcinomas from other small cell carcinomas. Am J Surg Pathol. 2000;24(9):1217–23.
27. Agoff SN, Lamps LW, Philip AT, et al. Thyroid transcription factor-1 is expressed in extrapulmonary small cell carcinomas but not in other extrapulmonary neuroendocrine tumors. Mod Pathol. 2000;13(3):238–42.
28. Cheuk W, Chan JK. Thyroid transcription factor-1 is of limited value in practical distinction between pulmonary and extrapulmonary small cell carcinomas. Am J Surg Pathol. 2001;25(4):545–6.
29. Jones TD, Kernek KM, Yang XJ, et al. Thyroid transcription factor 1 expression in small cell carcinoma of the urinary bladder: an immunohistochemical profile of 44 cases. Hum Pathol. 2005;36(7):718–23.
30. Lyda MH, Weiss LM. Immunoreactivity for epithelial and neuroendocrine antibodies are useful in the differential diagnosis of lung carcinomas. Hum Pathol. 2000;31(8):980–7.
31. Kalhor N, Zander DS, Liu J. TTF-1 and p63 for distinguishing pulmonary small-cell carcinoma from poorly differentiated squamous cell carcinoma in previously pap-stained cytologic material. Mod Pathol. 2006;19(8):1117–23.

32. Rindi G, Kloppel G, Alhman H, et al. TNM staging of foregut (neuro)endocrine tumors: a consensus proposal including a grading system. Virchows Arch. 2006;449(4):395–401.
33. Kloppel G, Perren A, Heitz PU. The gastroenteropancreatic neuroendocrine cell system and its tumors: the WHO classification. Ann NY Acad Sci. 2004;1014:13–27.
34. Ibrahim NB, Briggs JC, Corbishley CM. Extrapulmonary oat cell carcinoma. Cancer. 1984;54(8):1645–61.
35. Bensch KG, Corrin B, Pariente R, Spencer H. Oat-cell carcinoma of the lung. Its origin and relationship to bronchial carcinoid. Cancer. 1968;22(6):1163–72.
36. Gould VE, Memoli V, Chejfec G, Johannessen JV. The APUD cell system and its neoplasms: observations on the significance and limitations of the concept. Surg Clin North Am. 1979;59(1):93–108.
37. Skrabanek P, Powell D. Unifying concept of non-pituitary ACTH-secreting tumors: evidence of common origin of neural-crest tumors, carcinoids, and oat-cell carcinomas. Cancer. 1978;42(3):1263–9.
38. Pearse AG. Common cytochemical and ultrastructural characteristics of cells producing polypeptide hormones (the APUD series) and their relevance to thyroid and ultimobranchial C cells and calcitonin. Proc R Soc Lond B Biol Sci. 1968;170(18):71–80.
39. Pearse AG, Takor TT. Neuroendocrine embryology and the APUD concept. Clin Endocrinol (Oxf). 1976;5(Suppl):229S–44.
40. Sidhu GS. The endodermal origin of digestive and respiratory tract APUD cells. Histopathologic evidence and a review of the literature. Am J Pathol. 1979;96(1):5–20.
41. Bensch KG. The problem of classifying peripheral endocrine tumors. Hum Pathol. 1983;14(5):383–5.
42. Arai K, Matsuda M. Gastric small-cell carcinoma in Japan: a case report and review of the literature. Am J Clin Oncol. 1998;21(5):458–61.
43. Onuki N, Wistuba II, Travis WD, et al. Genetic changes in the spectrum of neuroendocrine lung tumors. Cancer. 1999;85(3):600–7.
44. Ledermann JA. Extrapulmonary small cell carcinoma. Postgrad Med J. 1992;68(796):79–81.
45. Carney D, McCann A, Corbally N. Molecular genetics of lung cancer. Chichester: John Wiley and Sons; 1990.
46. Lam KY, Law S, Tung PH, Wong J. Esophageal small cell carcinomas: clinicopathologic parameters, p53 overexpression, proliferation marker, and their impact on pathogenesis. Arch Pathol Lab Med. 2000;124(2):228–33.
47. Parwani AV, Geradts J, Caspers E, et al. Immunohistochemical and genetic analysis of non-small cell and small cell gallbladder carcinoma and their precursor lesions. Mod Pathol. 2003;16(4):299–308.
48. Kitamura H, Yazawa T, Sato H, Okudela K, Shimoyamada H. Small cell lung cancer: significance of RB alterations and TTF-1 expression in its carcinogenesis, phenotype, and biology. Endocr Pathol. 2009 Summer;20(2):101–7.
49. Nilsson O, Nilsson O, Delle Fave G, et al. Poorly differentiated carcinomas of the foregut (gastric, duodenal and pancreatic). Neuroendocrinology. 2006;84(3):212–5.
50. Kelsen DP, Weston E, Kurtz R, Cvitkovic E, Lieberman P, Golbey RB. Small-cell carcinoma of the esophagus: treatment by chemotherapy alone. Cancer. 1980;45(7):1558–61.
51. Einhorn LH. Initial therapy with cisplatin plus VP-16 in small-cell lung cancer. Semin Oncol. 1986;13(3 Suppl 3):5–9.
52. Batist G, Carney DN, Cowan KH, et al. Etoposide (VP-16) and cisplatin in previously treated small-cell lung cancer: clinical trial and in vitro correlates. J Clin Oncol. 1986;4(6):982–6.
53. Feld R, Evans WK, Coy P, et al. Canadian multicenter randomized trial comparing sequential and alternating administration of two non-cross-resistant chemotherapy combinations in patients with limited small-cell carcinoma of the lung. J Clin Oncol. 1987;5(9):1401–9.
54. Wolf M, Havemann K, Holle R, et al. Cisplatin/etoposide versus ifosfamide/etoposide combination chemotherapy in small-cell lung cancer: a multicenter German randomized trial. J Clin Oncol. 1987;5(12):1880–9.

55. Bunn PA Jr, Carney DN. Overview of chemotherapy for small cell lung cancer. Semin Oncol. 1997;24(2 Suppl 7):S7–69–S67–74.
56. Figoli F, Veronesi A, Ardizzoni A, et al. Cisplatin and etoposide as second-line chemotherapy in patients with small cell lung cancer. Cancer Invest. 1988;6(1):1–5.
57. Mascaux C, Paesmans M, Berghmans T, et al. A systematic review of the role of etoposide and cisplatin in the chemotherapy of small cell lung cancer with methodology assessment and meta-analysis. Lung Cancer. 2000;30(1):23–36.
58. Maksymiuk AW, Jett JR, Earle JD, et al. Sequencing and schedule effects of cisplatin plus etoposide in small-cell lung cancer: results of a North Central Cancer Treatment Group randomized clinical trial. J Clin Oncol. 1994;12(1):70–6.
59. Morant R, Bruckner HW. Complete remission of refractory small cell carcinoma of the pancreas with cisplatin and etoposide. Cancer. 1989;64(10):2007–9.
60. Fjallskog ML, Granberg DP, Welin SL, et al. Treatment with cisplatin and etoposide in patients with neuroendocrine tumors. Cancer. 2001;92(5):1101–7.
61. O'Connor J, Sade J, Pairola A, et al. Poorly differentiated neuroendocrine carcinoma – small cell of the gastrointestinal tract. Institutional experience. J Clin Oncol. 2006 ASCO Annual Meeting Proceedings Part I. 2006;24(18S):14142.
62. Jackson Jr DV, Case LD, Zekan PJ, et al. Improvement of long-term survival in extensive small-cell lung cancer. J Clin Oncol. 1988;6(7):1161–9.
63. Miranda FT, Spigel DR, Hainsworth JD, et al. Paclitaxel/carboplatin/etoposide (PCE) therapy for advanced poorly differentiated neuroendocrine (PDNE) carcinoma: a Minnie Pearl Cancer Research Network phase II trial. J Clin Oncol. 2005 ASCO Annual Meeting Proceedings. 2005:(abstr 4058).
64. Hou Z, Elasmar S, Lozano R, et al. A pilot study of irinotecan plus cisplatin in patients with metastatic high-grade neuroendocrine carcinoma. Proc Am Soc Clin Oncology. 2003;22:(abstr 1508):375.
65. Mani M, Shroff R, Jacobs C, et al. A phase II study of irinotecan and cisplatin for metastatic or unresectable high grade neuroendocrine carcinoma. J Clin Oncol. 2008;26S:15550.
66. Puglisi M, Dolly S, Faria A, Myerson JS, Popat S, O'Brien ME. Treatment options for small cell lung cancer – do we have more choice? Br J Cancer. 2010;102(4):629–38.
67. Olofsson J, Van Nostrand AW. Anaplastic small cell carcinoma of larynx. Case report. Ann Otol Rhinol Laryngol. 1972;81(2):284–7.
68. Ferlito A. Diagnosis and treatment of small cell carcinoma of the larynx: a critical review. Ann Otol Rhinol Laryngol. 1986;95(6 Pt 1):590–600.
69. Mills SE, Cooper PH, Garland TA, Johns ME. Small cell undifferentiated carcinoma of the larynx. Report of two patients and review of 13 additional cases. Cancer. 1983;51(1): 116–20.
70. Ferlito A, Polidoro F. Simultaneous primary oat cell carcinoma (apudoma) and squamous cell carcinoma of the hypopharynx. ORL J Otorhinolaryngol Relat Spec. 1980;42(3):146–57.
71. Aguilar 3rd EA, Robbins KT, Stephens J, Dimery IW, Batsakis JG. Primary oat cell carcinoma of the larynx. Am J Clin Oncol. 1987;10(1):26–32.
72. Baugh RF, Wolf GT, Beals TF, Krause CJ, Forastiere A. Small cell carcinoma of the larynx: results of therapy. Laryngoscope. 1986;96(11):1283–90.
73. Gnepp DR, Ferlito A, Hyams V. Primary anaplastic small cell (oat cell) carcinoma of the larynx. Review of the literature and report of 18 cases. Cancer. 1983;51(9):1731–45.
74. Barker Jr JL, Glisson BS, Garden AS, et al. Management of nonsinonasal neuroendocrine carcinomas of the head and neck. Cancer. 2003;98(11):2322–8.
75. Nagao K, Matsuzaki O, Saiga H, et al. Histopathologic studies of undifferentiated carcinoma of the parotid gland. Cancer. 1982;50(8):1572–9.
76. Rosenthal DI, Barker Jr JL, El-Naggar AK, et al. Sinonasal malignancies with neuroendocrine differentiation: patterns of failure according to histologic phenotype. Cancer. 2004;101(11): 2567–73.
77. Galanis E, Frytak S, Lloyd RV. Extrapulmonary small cell carcinoma. Cancer. 1997; 79(9):1729–36.

78. Turnbull AD, Rosen P, Goodner JT, Beattie EJ. Primary malignant tumors of the esophagus other than typical epidermoid carcinoma. Ann Thorac Surg. 1973;15(5):463–73.
79. Horai T, Kobayshi A, Tateishi R, et al. A cytologic study on small cell carcinoma of the esophagus. Cancer. 1978;41(5):1890–6.
80. Huncharek M, Muscat J. Small cell carcinoma of the esophagus. The Massachusetts General Hospital experience, 1978 to 1993. Chest. 1995;107(1):179–81.
81. Vrouvas J, Ash DV. Extrapulmonary small cell cancer. Clin Oncol (R Coll Radiol). 1995;7(6):377–81.
82. Sabanathan S, Graham GP, Salama FD. Primary oat cell carcinoma of the oesophagus. Thorax. 1986;41(4):318–21.
83. McFadden DW, Rudnicki M, Talamini MA. Primary small cell carcinoma of the esophagus. Ann Thorac Surg. 1989;47(3):477–80.
84. Ohmura Y, Takiyama W, Mandai K, Doi T, Nishikawa Y. Small cell carcinoma of the esophagus: a case report. Jpn J Clin Oncol. 1997;27(2):95–100.
85. Nichols GL, Kelsen DP. Small cell carcinoma of the esophagus. The Memorial Hospital experience 1970 to 1987. Cancer. 1989;64(7):1531–3.
86. Rosenthal SN, Lemkin JA. Multiple small cell carcinomas of the esophagus. Cancer. 1983;51(10):1944–6.
87. Craig SR, Carey FA, Walker WS, Cameron EW. Primary small-cell cancer of the esophagus. J Thorac Cardiovasc Surg. 1995;109(2):284–8.
88. Medgyesy CD, Wolff RA, Putnam Jr JB, Ajani JA. Small cell carcinoma of the esophagus: the University of Texas M. D. Anderson Cancer Center experience and literature review. Cancer. 2000;88(2):262–7.
89. Madroszyk A, Egreteau J, Martin L, Queneau PE, Bosset JF, Merrouche Y. Small-cell carcinoma of the esophagus: report of three cases and review of the literature with emphasis on therapy. Ann Oncol. 2001;12(9):1321–5.
90. Yachida S, Matsushita K, Usuki H, Wanibuchi H, Maeba T, Maeta H. Long-term survival after resection for small cell carcinoma of the esophagus. Ann Thorac Surg. 2001;72(2):596–7.
91. Matsusaka T, Watanabe H, Enjoji M. Oat-cell carcinoma of the stomach. Fukuoka Igaku Zasshi. 1976;67(2):65–73.
92. Matsui K, Kitagawa M, Miwa A, Kuroda Y, Tsuji M. Small cell carcinoma of the stomach: a clinicopathologic study of 17 cases. Am J Gastroenterol. 1991;86(9):1167–75.
93. Bernatz P. Small cell neoplasm of the stomach: a clinicoplathologic study. Minnesota: Graduate School, University of Minnesota; 1950.
94. Richardson RL, Weiland LH. Undifferentiated small cell carcinomas in extrapulmonary sites. Semin Oncol. 1982;9(4):484–96.
95. Clery AP, Dockerty MB, Waugh JM. Small-cell carcinoma of the colon and rectum. A clinicopathologic study. Arch Surg. 1961;83:164–72.
96. Hussein AM, Feun LG, Sridhar KS, Otrakji CL, Garcia-Moore M, Benedetto P. Small cell carcinoma of the large intestine presenting as central nervous systems signs and symptoms. Two case reports with literature review. J Neurooncol. 1990;8(3):269–74.
97. Pazdur R, Bonomi P, Gould VE, et al. Neuroendocrine small cell carcinomas in miscellaneous primary sites: implications for staging and therapy. Anticancer Res. 1981;1(6):335–40.
98. Redman BG, Pazdur R. Colonic small cell undifferentiated carcinoma: a distinct pathological diagnosis with therapeutic implications. Am J Gastroenterol. 1987;82(4):382–5.
99. Mills SE, Cohen AR, Allen Jr MS. Small-cell undifferentiated carcinoma of the colon. A clinicopathological study of five cases and their association with colonic adenomas. Am J Surg Pathol. 1983;7(7):643–51.
100. Balachandra B, Marcus V, Jass JR. Poorly differentiated tumours of the anal canal: a diagnostic strategy for the surgical pathologist. Histopathology. 2007;50(1):163–74.
101. Miller JR, Baggenstoss AH, Comfort MW. Carcinoma of the pancreas; effect of histological types and grade of malignancy on its behavior. Cancer. 1951;4(2):233–41.

102. Cubilla AL, Fitzgerald PJ. Cancer of the pancreas (nonendocrine): a suggested morphologic classification. Semin Oncol. 1979;6(3):285–97.
103. Wahid NA, Neugut AI, Hibshoosh H, Brunetti JC, Fountain KS, Rubin M. Response of small cell carcinoma of pancreas to a small cell lung cancer regimen: a case report. Cancer Invest. 1996;14(4):335–9.
104. Toker C. Oat cell tumor of the small bowel. Am J Gastroenterol. 1974;61(6):481–3.
105. Fer MF, Greco FA, Oldham RK. Poorly differentiated neoplasms and tumors of unknown origin: introduction. Semin Oncol. 1982;9(4):393–5.
106. Swanson PE, Dykoski D, Wick MR, Snover DC. Primary duodenal small-cell neuroendocrine carcinoma with production of vasoactive intestinal polypeptide. Arch Pathol Lab Med. 1986;110(4):317–20.
107. Lee CS, Machet D, Rode J. Small cell carcinoma of the ampulla of vater. Cancer. 1992;70(6):1502–4.
108. Yao JL, Madeb R, Bourne P, et al. Small cell carcinoma of the prostate: an immunohistochemical study. Am J Surg Pathol. 2006;30(6):705–12.
109. Wenk RE, Bhagavan BS, Levy R, Miller D, Weisburger W. Ectopic ACTH, prostatic oat cell carcinoma, and marked hypernatremia. Cancer. 1977;40(2):773–8.
110. Miyoshi Y, Uemura H, Kitami K, Satomi Y, Kubota Y, Hosaka M. Neuroendocrine differentiated small cell carcinoma presenting as recurrent prostate cancer after androgen deprivation therapy. BJU Int. 2001;88(9):982–3.
111. Sella A, Konichezky M, Flex D, Sulkes A, Baniel J. Low PSA metastatic androgen- independent prostate cancer. Eur Urol. 2000;38(3):250–4.
112. Turbat-Herrera EA, Herrera GA, Gore I, Lott RL, Grizzle WE, Bonnin JM. Neuroendocrine differentiation in prostatic carcinomas. A retrospective autopsy study. Arch Pathol Lab Med. 1988;112(11):1100–5.
113. Tanaka M, Suzuki Y, Takaoka K, et al. Progression of prostate cancer to neuroendocrine cell tumor. Int J Urol. 2001;8(8):431–6. discussion 437.
114. Yu DS, Hsieh DS, Chen HI, Chang SY. The expression of neuropeptides in hyperplastic and malignant prostate tissue and its possible clinical implications. J Urol. 2001;166(3):871–5.
115. di Sant'Agnese PA. Neuroendocrine differentiation in carcinoma of the prostate. Diagnostic, prognostic, and therapeutic implications. Cancer. 1992;70(1 Suppl):254 68.
116. Wang W, Epstein JI. Small cell carcinoma of the prostate. A morphologic and immunohistochemical study of 95 cases. Am J Surg Pathol. 2008;32(1):65–71.
117. Abbas F, Civantos F, Benedetto P, Soloway MS. Small cell carcinoma of the bladder and prostate. Urology. 1995;46(5):617–30.
118. Delahunt B, Abernethy DA, Johnson CA, Nacey JN. Prostate carcinoma and the Lambert-Eaton myasthenic syndrome. J Urol. 2003;169(1):278–9.
119. Smith DC, Tucker JA, Trump DL. Hypercalcemia and neuroendocrine carcinoma of the prostate: a report of three cases and a review of the literature. J Clin Oncol. 1992; 10(3):499–505.
120. Okada H, Gotoh A, Ogawa T, Arakawa S, Ohbayashi C, Kamidono S. Two cases of small cell carcinoma of the prostate. Scand J Urol Nephrol. 1996;30(6):503–8.
121. Kinebuchi Y, Noguchi W, Irie K, Nakayama T, Kato H, Nishizawa O. Relapsed prostate cancer with neuroendocrine differentiation and high serum levels of carcinoembryonic antigen without elevation of prostrate-specific antigen: a case report. Int J Urol. 2007; 14(2):147–9.
122. Spiess PE, Pettaway CA, Vakar-Lopez F, et al. Treatment outcomes of small cell carcinoma of the prostate: a single-center study. Cancer. 2007;110(8):1729–37.
123. Deorah S, Gaitonde K, Raman R, Rao MB, Donovan JF. Survival of patients with small cell carcinoma of the prostate during 1973–2003: a population based study. J Urol. 2009;181(4):63.
124. Rubenstein JH, Katin MJ, Mangano MM, et al. Small cell anaplastic carcinoma of the prostate: seven new cases, review of the literature, and discussion of a therapeutic strategy. Am J Clin Oncol. 1997;20(4):376–80.

125. Tremont-Lukats IW, Bobustuc G, Lagos GK, Lolas K, Kyritsis AP, Puduvalli VK. Brain metastasis from prostate carcinoma: The M. D. Anderson Cancer Center experience. Cancer. 2003;98(2):363–8.
126. Erasmus CE, Verhagen WI, Wauters CA, van Lindert EJ. Brain metastasis from prostate small cell carcinoma: not to be neglected. Can J Neurol Sci. 2002;29(4):375–7.
127. Mackey JR, Au HJ, Hugh J, Venner P. Genitourinary small cell carcinoma: determination of clinical and therapeutic factors associated with survival. J Urol. 1998;159(5):1624–9.
128. Asmis TR, Reaume MN, Dahrouge S, Malone S. Genitourinary small cell carcinoma: a retrospective review of treatment and survival patterns at The Ottawa Hospital Regional Cancer Center. BJU Int. 2006;97(4):711–5.
129. Cramer SF, Aikawa M, Cebelin M. Neurosecretory granules in small cell invasive carcinoma of the urinary bladder. Cancer. 1981;47(4):724–30.
130. Cheng L, Pan CX, Yang XJ, et al. Small cell carcinoma of the urinary bladder: a clinicopathologic analysis of 64 patients. Cancer. 2004;101(5):957–62.
131. Cheng L, Jones TD, McCarthy RP, et al. Molecular genetic evidence for a common clonal origin of urinary bladder small cell carcinoma and coexisting urothelial carcinoma. Am J Pathol. 2005;166(5):1533–9.
132. Choong NW, Quevedo JF, Kaur JS. Small cell carcinoma of the urinary bladder. The Mayo Clinic experience. Cancer. 2005;103(6):1172–8.
133. Abrahams NA, Moran C, Reyes AO, Siefker-Radtke A, Ayala AG. Small cell carcinoma of the bladder: a contemporary clinicopathological study of 51 cases. Histopathology. 2005;46(1):57–63.
134. Siefker-Radtke AO, Dinney CP, Abrahams NA, et al. Evidence supporting preoperative chemotherapy for small cell carcinoma of the bladder: a retrospective review of the M. D. Anderson cancer experience. J Urol. 2004;172(2):481–4.
135. Bex A, de Vries R, Pos F, Kerst M, Horenblas S. Long-term survival after sequential chemoradiation for limited disease small cell carcinoma of the bladder. World J Urol. 2009;27(1):101–6.
136. Lohrisch C, Murray N, Pickles T, Sullivan L. Small cell carcinoma of the bladder: long term outcome with integrated chemoradiation. Cancer. 1999;86(11):2346–52.
137. Davis MP, Murthy MS, Simon J, Wise H, Minton JP. Successful management of small cell carcinoma of the bladder with cisplatin and etoposide. J Urol. 1989;142(3):817.
138. Mukesh M, Cook N, Hollingdale AE, Ainsworth NL, Russell SG. Small cell carcinoma of the urinary bladder: a 15-year retrospective review of treatment and survival in the Anglian Cancer Network. BJU Int. 2009;103(6):747–52.
139. Bex A, Nieuwenhuijzen JA, Kerst M, et al. Small cell carcinoma of bladder: a single-center prospective study of 25 cases treated in analogy to small cell lung cancer. Urology. 2005;65(2):295–9.
140. Lester JF, Hudson E, Barber JB. Bladder preservation in small cell carcinoma of the urinary bladder: an institutional experience and review of the literature. Clin Oncol (R Coll Radiol). 2006;18(8):608–11.
141. Crowder S, Tuller E. Small cell carcinoma of the female genital tract. Semin Oncol. 2007;34(1):57–63.
142. Lee SW, Nam JH, Kim DY, et al. Unfavorable prognosis of small cell neuroendocrine carcinoma of the uterine cervix: a retrospective matched case-control study. Int J Gynecol Cancer. 2010;20(3):411–6.
143. Sheets EE, Berman ML, Hrountas CK, Liao SY, DiSaia PJ. Surgically treated, early-stage neuroendocrine small-cell cervical carcinoma. Obstet Gynecol. 1988;71(1):10–4.
144. Chan JK, Loizzi V, Burger RA, Rutgers J, Monk BJ. Prognostic factors in neuroendocrine small cell cervical carcinoma: a multivariate analysis. Cancer. 2003;97(3):568–74.
145. Viswanathan AN, Deavers MT, Jhingran A, Ramirez PT, Levenback C, Eifel PJ. Small cell neuroendocrine carcinoma of the cervix: outcome and patterns of recurrence. Gynecol Oncol. 2004;93(1):27–33.
146. Cohen JG, Kapp DS, Shin JY, et al. Small cell carcinoma of the cervix: treatment and survival outcomes of 188 patients. Am J Obstet Gynecol. 2010;203:347.e1–6.

Chapter 11
Hereditary and Sporadic Medullary Thyroid Carcinoma

Ana O. Hoff, Cleber Camacho, and Rui M.B. Maciel

Abstract Medullary thyroid carcinoma (MTC) is an uncommon neuroendocrine tumor that arises from the parafollicular cells of the thyroid gland. These cells produce calcitonin, a peptide that is a useful marker of disease. MTC accounts for approximately 5% of all thyroid carcinomas. Most of the cases are sporadic; 25–30% is hereditary and associated with the multiple endocrine neoplasia type 2 syndrome (MEN2). In 1961, 2 years after the initial description of MTC by Hazard and colleagues, Sipple described the association of MTC with pheochromocytoma, a syndrome that was later denominated multiple endocrine neoplasia type 2 (MEN2). For the past 5 decades, an extensive amount of knowledge has been acquired. Before the discovery of the genetic abnormality associated with the syndrome, the diagnosis and management of patients with hereditary MTC and their family members were based on basal and stimulated levels of calcitonin. In this context, families with MEN2 were characterized, variants of MEN2 were identified, and carriers identified by biochemical screening were treated with thyroidectomy. With the discovery of the gene associated with MEN2 (*RET* gene) in 1993, management was further refined and genetic analysis became the most sensitive and specific modality to distinguish normal individuals from carriers of MEN2, and the risk of performing a prophylactic thyroidectomy in a normal individual was not a concern anymore. In these past 15 years, new knowledge continues to emerge. We can now correlate fine differences in phenotype with different types of *RET* mutations and have questioned the significance of different genetic backgrounds, specifically *RET* polymorphisms, in time of onset and aggressiveness of disease. Furthermore, the discovery of how the RET receptor functions and which signaling pathways are activated has permitted the development of small molecules that target these pathways, inhibiting cell proliferation and tumor growth.

A.O. Hoff (✉)
Department of Endocrinology, Fleury Group, São Paulo, Brazil

Endocrine Neoplasia Unit, Instituto do Cancer do Estado de São Paulo, Faculdade de Medicina da Universidade de São Paulo, São Paulo, Brazil
e-mail: ana.hoff@fleury.com

J.C. Yao et al. (eds.), *Neuroendocrine Tumors*, Current Clinical Oncology,
DOI 10.1007/978-1-60327-997-0_11,

Keywords Parafollicular cells of the thyroid • Calcitonin • MEN2 • Pheochromocytoma • Thyroidectomy • RET polymorphisms • Hypoparathyroidism

Introduction

Medullary thyroid carcinoma (MTC) is an uncommon neuroendocrine tumor that arises from the parafollicular cells of the thyroid gland. These cells produce calcitonin, a peptide that is a useful marker of disease. MTC accounts for approximately 5% of all thyroid carcinomas. Most of the cases are sporadic; 25–30% is hereditary and associated with the multiple endocrine neoplasia type 2 syndrome (MEN2). In 1961, 2 years after the initial description of MTC by Hazard and colleagues, Sipple described the association of MTC with pheochromocytoma, a syndrome that was later denominated multiple endocrine neoplasia type 2 (MEN2) [1, 2]. For the past 5 decades, an extensive amount of knowledge has been acquired. Before the discovery of the genetic abnormality associated with the syndrome, the diagnosis and management of patients with hereditary MTC and their family members were based on basal and stimulated levels of calcitonin [3, 4]. In this context, families with MEN2 were characterized, variants of MEN2 were identified, and carriers identified by biochemical screening were treated with thyroidectomy. With the discovery of the gene associated with MEN2 (*RET* gene) in 1993 [5, 6], management was further refined and genetic analysis became the most sensitive and specific modality to distinguish normal individuals from carriers of MEN2, and the risk of performing a prophylactic thyroidectomy in a normal individual was not a concern anymore. In these past 15 years new knowledge continues to emerge. We can now correlate fine differences in phenotype with different types of *RET* mutations and have questioned the significance of different genetic backgrounds, specifically *RET* polymorphisms, in time of onset and aggressiveness of disease. Furthermore, the discovery of how the RET receptor functions and which signaling pathways are activated has permitted the development of small molecules that target these pathways inhibiting cell proliferation and tumor growth.

This chapter provides an overview of sporadic and hereditary MTC. The importance of the discovery of the *RET* gene and the current management of MTC is discussed.

Clinical Presentation

Most cases of MTC (65–70%) are sporadic, not associated with a germline mutation of the *RET* gene. Patients with sporadic disease present with a thyroid nodule identified by palpation or by an ultrasound examination commonly after the fourth decade of life. Sporadic MTC tends to be unicentric and not associated with C-cell hyperplasia. In contrast, hereditary MTC is multifocal, bilateral and is associated with C-cell hyperplasia, a precursor lesion [7–9].

Hereditary MTC is caused by a germline mutation of the *RET* gene and is associated with the multiple endocrine neoplasia type 2 syndrome (MEN2) [5, 6]. MEN2 is an autosomal dominant syndrome characterized by MTC, pheochromocytoma, and primary hyperparathyroidism. There are three different subtypes: multiple endocrine neoplasia type 2A (MEN2A), multiple endocrine neoplasia type 2B (MEN2B), and familial medullary thyroid carcinoma (FMTC). In all these subtypes, MTC is the cardinal manifestation occurring in more than 90% of affected individuals. Pheochromocytoma manifests in 50% of individuals with MEN2A and MEN2B, and primary hyperparathyroidism occurs in approximately 10–20% of patients with MEN2A. In FMTC, the only manifestation is MTC [10]. In addition to MTC and the risk for pheochromocytoma, individuals with MEN2B have a typical phenotype that includes a marphanoid habitus, thickened lips, and the presence of ganglioneuromas in the oral mucosa and gastrointestinal tract [11–13].

Hereditary MTC manifests earlier, usually before the third decade of life [10, 14]. The onset of disease is associated with the aggressiveness of the *RET* mutation; development of MTC occurs in the first year of life in MEN2B, in the first decade in MEN2A, and in the second or third decade of life in individuals harboring *RET* mutations associated with FMTC [10, 14]. Since genetic analysis became an integral part of the evaluation of any patient diagnosed with MTC, the identification of an individual with a germline *RET* mutation leads to earlier recognition of affected asymptomatic family members and earlier treatment [14, 15]. Therefore, a greater number of patients with hereditary MTC are diagnosed with localized disease to the thyroid, making cure an outcome much more frequent than 2 decades ago.

In summary, most patients with sporadic MTC presents with clinically apparent disease detected by ultrasound or by physical examination. When MEN2 is known to a family, the diagnosis of hereditary MTC is usually early and based on the genetic analysis of the *RET* gene. In most of these individuals, minimal or no disease is present at diagnosis. A handful of patients with hereditary MTC may present similarly to patients with sporadic disease; in general, these individuals do not have family history of MTC, either because they are the first ones to develop the syndrome due to a *de novo* *RET* mutation or, they are part of a kindred harboring an indolent mutation associated with lower penetrance and later onset of disease. This latter situation occurs mostly with mutations associated with familial MTC and less frequently with MEN2A [16].

When the disease is outside the thyroid gland, the chance of cure reduces and the chance of recurrence rises significantly. Both in sporadic and hereditary MTC, it is known that two thirds of patients who present with palpable thyroid disease or a tumor greater than 1 cm will also have cervical lymphadenopathy and, approximately 5% will present with distant metastatic disease [8, 9].

Lymph node metastases occur more frequently in the central compartment (level VI) followed by involvement of the ipsilateral nodes (levels II–V). Involvement of contra-lateral nodes may also occur in up to 40% of patients presenting with a palpable primary tumor [17, 18]. Patients with MTC can also present with mediastinal and hilar lymphadenopathy. Mediastinum and hilar disease are more difficult to treat and to control and it may be associated with increased morbidity from the growth and infiltration of adjacent tissues [8].

In addition to regional involvement, patients who have more advanced disease can present with metastatic involvement of the lungs, liver, and bone. Metastasis to abdominal lymph nodes and brain can also be observed in few patients.

The metastatic process is hematogenous and the involvement of lungs and liver is commonly diffuse and multifocal. Bone metastases are essentially lytic, involving not only long bones but also the spine. MRI is the best study to evaluate for spinal metastasis [19]. These patients should be carefully followed because of the potential for spinal cord involvement. Progression of metastatic disease is slow in most cases, allowing patients who have extensive disease to have prolonged survival. Patients with extensive MTC may also develop flushing and/or diarrhea; symptoms that are a result of the release of vasoactive peptides by the tumor cells. In few cases, ectopic production of ACTH can result in Cushing's syndrome [20].

The *RET* Gene and Receptor

The *RET* gene is located on chromosome 10q11.2, contains 21 exons and is expressed by neuroendocrine and neural cells including thyroid C-cells, adrenal medullary cells, parasympathetic, sympathetic and colonic ganglia, cells of the urogenital tract, and parathyroid cells [21, 22]. The *RET* gene encodes a tyrosine kinase receptor denominated RET that consists of two extracellular domains (a cadherin-like and a cysteine-rich domain), a transmembrane domain, and two intracellular tyrosine kinase domains (Fig. 11.1). The RET receptor is a functional receptor for neurotrophic ligands of the glial cell line-derived neurotrophic factor (GDNF) family [23, 24]. The GDNF family is composed by GDNF, neurturin, artemin, and persephin. These ligands cannot bind the RET receptor directly; they require a high-affinity ligand-binding coreceptor called GFRα-1 [alpha] for full activation and signal transduction (Fig. 11.1).

The RET receptor system is important for normal differentiation of the gastrointestinal neuronal system, parts of the sympathetic nervous and neuroendocrine systems, and renal development [25]. In mice, deletion of one of the genes that encodes part of this system results in kidney agenesis and in lack of the enteric nervous system [26]. In humans, loss of function of RET is associated with congenital megacolon or Hirschsprung's disease, whereas germline activating *RET* mutations causes MEN2 syndrome [5, 6, 27].

RET Mutations in MEN 2 Syndrome

MEN2A, familial MTC, and MEN2B are caused by activating mutations of the *RET* gene (Table 11.1). The most common mutations in MEN2A are located in exons 10 and 11 of the *RET* gene, encoding the highly conserved cysteine-rich domain (see Table 11.1, Fig. 11.1) [10]. Codon 634 mutations are the most common and are

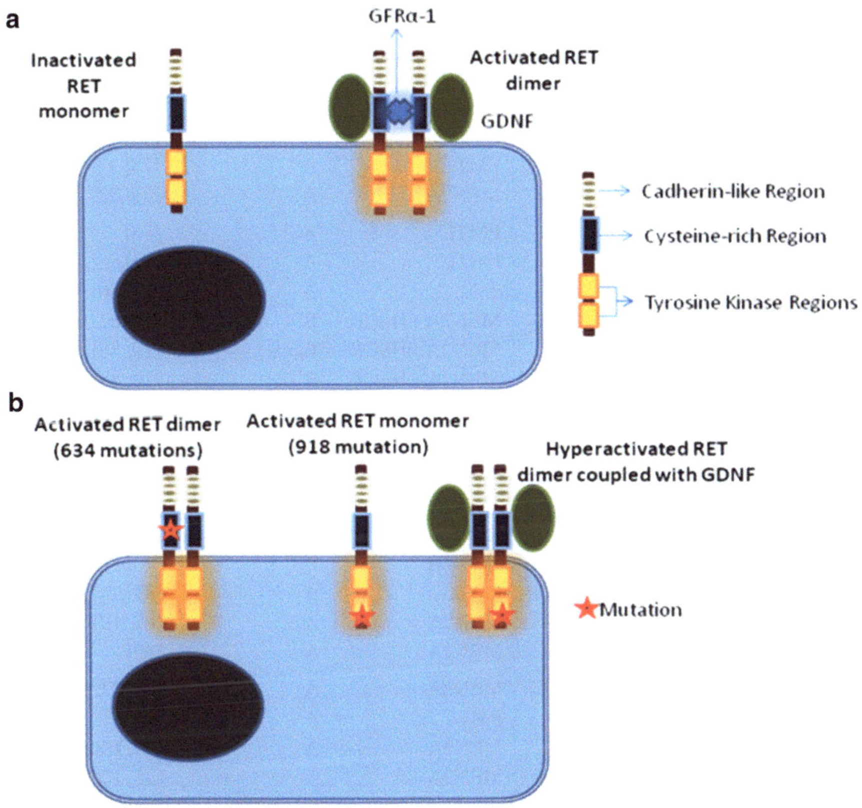

Fig. 11.1 Schematic representation of the RET receptor system. (**a**) RET is a tyrosine kinase receptor with an extracellular domain containing a cysteine-rich region important for dimerization and two tyrosine kinase intracellular domains important for phosphorylation. (**b**) Cysteine-rich domain mutations (codon 634) cause ligand-independent dimerization and autophosphorylation of the RET receptor while tyrosine kinase domain mutations (codon 918) can result in activation of the receptor with or without dimerization or ligand-binding. GFRα-1 [alpha](glial cell line-derived neurotrophic factor receptor); GDNF (glial cell line-derived factor)

found in 85% of MEN2A patients [10]. A single coding change (cys634arg) accounts for 52% of all 634 mutations [10]. Intracellular tyrosine kinase domain mutations (codons 768, 790, 791, 804, 891) have also been reported in MEN2A kindreds but are less common (see Table 11.1) [10]. There are two variants of MEN2A; MEN2A associated with cutaneous lichen amyloidosis (CLA) and MEN2A associated with Hirschsprung's disease [8, 28, 29]. CLA is a pruritic skin lesion that involves the upper back; this lesion is specifically associated with mutations involving codon 634 of exon 11. MEN2A associated with Hirschsprung's disease is associated with mutations involving codons 609, 611, 618, and 620 (Table 11.1).

In FMTC, most of the mutations occur at the extracellular, cysteine-rich domain but mutations involving the intracellular tyrosine kinase domain are not

Table 11.1 Mutations associated with hereditary medullary thyroid carcinoma

EXON	Mutation	Phenotype	ATA risk level	References
5	G321R	FMTC	A	[75]
8	531/9 base pair duplication	FMTC[a]	A	[76]
	532 duplication	?	A	[77]
	C515S	FMTC	A	[78]
	G533C	MEN2A	A	[79–82]
10	R600Q	FMTC	A	[83]
	K603E	FMTC	A	[84]
	Y606C	?	A	[85, 86]
	C609F/R/G/S/Y	MEN2A+HSCR	B	[10, 87–91]
	C611R/G/F/S/W/Y	MEN2A+HSCR	B	[10, 88]
	C618R/G/F/S/Y	MEN2A+HSCR	B	[10, 88]
	C620R/G/F/S/W/Y	MEN2A+HSCR	B	[10, 88, 90]
11	C630R/F/S/Y	MEN2A	B	[92–94]
	D631Y	?	B	[95]
	633/9 base pair duplication	MEN2A	B	[96]
	C634R/G/F/S/W/Y	MEN2A+CLA	C	[10, 88, 97–99]
	634/12 base pair duplication	MEN2A	B	[100]
	635/insertion ELCR; T636P	FMTC	A	[85]
	S649L	MEN2A	A	[87, 101–103]
	K666E	MEN2A	A	[85]
13	E768D	MEN2A	A	[10, 92, 95, 104]
	N777S	FMTC	A	[105]
	L790F	MEN2A	A	[95, 106]
	Y791F	MEN2A	A	[95, 106, 107]
14	V804L	MEN2A	A	[10, 73]
	V804M	MEN2A+CLA	A	[10, 73, 108, 109]
	G819K	?	A	[86]
	R833C	?	A	[110]
	R844Q	?	A	[86, 95]
15	R866W	FMTC	A	[111]
	A883F	MEN2B	D	[34, 112]
	A883T	FMTC	Not classified	[113, 114]
	S891A	MEN2A	A	[115–117]
16	R912P	FMTC	A	[30, 90]
	M918T	MEN2B	D	[10]
RET mutation associations				
13/14	V804M+V778I	FMTC	B	[118]
14	V804M+E805K	MEN2B	D	[119]
14	V804M+Y806C	MEN2B	D	[92, 120, 121]
14/15	V804M+S904C	MEN2B	D	[122]

RET mutations and ATA risk classification

Adapted from ATA Medullary Thyroid Cancer Guideline [15]

[a]Association with Hirschsprung's disease (HSCR) not confirmed

infrequent (see Table 11.1) [10, 30, 31]. At least 95% of individuals who have MEN2B have a germline met918thr mutation [32, 33]. The other mutation identified in patients who have MEN2B involves codon 883 [34].

Germline *RET* mutations are also found in a few apparent sporadic MTC cases [35, 36]. Investigation of patients with MTC and no family history of thyroid carcinoma has identified germline *RET* gene mutations in 6–7% of these patients [35, 36]. For this reason, genetic analysis is recommended to all patients with MTC [15].

A *RET* mutation is the most frequent and most important molecular abnormality observed in MTC. *RET* mutations are not only seen in patients with hereditary MTC, approximately 40–50% of sporadic MTCs have a somatic *RET* mutation [37, 38]. The most common somatic mutation is the met918thr, the same one that when germline causes MEN2B [37 39]. Tumors harboring this mutation are believed to have a more aggressive course [39].

Diagnosis and Management of Medullary Thyroid Carcinoma

Clinically Apparent Sporadic or Hereditary Medullary Thyroid Carcinoma

The diagnosis of MTC in an individual with clinically apparent disease is based on cytological analysis of the thyroid nodule or of cervical lymph nodes. When the fine needle aspiration biopsy (FNAB) is suspicious or diagnostic for MTC, patients should undergo a preoperative evaluation that includes: basal serum calcitonin and CEA level, genetic analysis of the *RET* gene, calcium and PTH level to exclude primary hyperparathyroidism, and urinary and/or plasma metanephrines to exclude pheochromocytoma [15]. In case a pheochromocytoma is diagnosed, patients should undergo adrenalectomy prior to thyroidectomy. In addition, an evaluation assessing the extent of disease is paramount to plan the surgical intervention [15]. A detailed ultrasound (US) of the cervical area is essential in all patients to exclude lymph node involvement of the superior mediastinum, central compartment, and bilateral lateral cervical areas [15, 40].

Patients with extensive LN involvement by US and/or basal calcitonin level greater than 400 pg/mL should undergo evaluation to exclude distant metastatic disease [15, 41]. In these cases, in addition to a cervical US, the current guidelines of the American Thyroid Association recommend a computed tomography (CT) of the neck, chest, and abdomen. It is important to note that the detection of liver metastases from MTC can be challenging and for this reason, it is recommended the use of a three-phase contrast-enhanced multidetector liver CT (liver protocol) or contrast-enhanced magnetic resonance imaging (MRI) of the liver. A bone scintigraphy is also useful to exclude bone metastases.

Surgery is the mainstay treatment of MTC, and cure from a surgical procedure depends on the extent of disease. Patients with tumor <1 cm and no LN involvement have the greatest chance of cure; while patients with distant metastatic disease cure is very unlikely [42].

Total thyroidectomy (TT) is indicated for most patients and the extent of lymph node resection depends on the extent of disease at presentation. Patients with disease localized to the thyroid gland should undergo TT with bilateral central compartment (level VI) dissection. In patients with LN involvement, the recommended surgical intervention includes dissection of the lateral compartment in which disease was detected [15]. In patients with extensive distant metastatic disease, the extent of surgery should be tailored to achieve local control; extensive resections with risk of morbidity should be avoided. Patients with unresectable disease should be directed to systemic therapy and participation in clinical trials considered [15].

Postoperative Monitoring and Management of Residual or Recurrent Disease

Calcitonin is a highly sensitive marker of disease and is used to assess cure after the initial surgical treatment [43]. CEA is another marker of disease; it is less sensitive and less specific than calcitonin but the levels are more stable making it useful to follow patients with more extensive disease [44]. In addition, it is useful in the follow up of patients with poorly differentiated MTC that lost the ability to produce calcitonin.

It is recommended to analyze calcitonin and CEA levels 3 months after surgery; an undetectable level of calcitonin (basal or after stimulation with calcium and/or pentagastrin) indicates biochemical remission [45]. These patients should be followed with calcitonin measurements every 6–12 months and a neck US could be done as baseline and repeated once a year or in case the calcitonin level rises. However, persistence of residual disease after initial treatment is extremely common. Retrospective studies indicate that 35–90% of patients with MTC remain with detectable levels of calcitonin after initial surgery [41, 46]. Machens and co-authors evaluated 224 patients treated surgically for MTC, calcitonin was undetectable in 65% of patients with disease confined to the thyroid gland and in only 10% of patients with LN metastases [41]. A calcitonin level ≤150 pg/mL is usually associated with Loco-regional disease that in most cases is occult in imaging studies [47]. In these cases, long-term surveillance with periodic measurements of calcitonin and CEA allows an assessment of the biologic behavior of the disease. In most cases, the disease is indolent and remains stable for a prolonged period of time. An increase in calcitonin or CEA level of at least 20% should prompt an US examination of the neck; a calcitonin level greater than 150 pg/mL should prompt another metastatic assessment to exclude distant metastases.

Patients with no identifiable disease should be observed. If suspicious disease is identified in the neck, an FNAB should be performed for cytological analysis and measurement of calcitonin in the washout fluid [48]. The latter improves the sensitivity and specificity of the diagnosis. Upon diagnosis of residual/recurrent disease, surgical resection of the biopsy proven compartment may be considered. In patients not submitted to an LN dissection in the initial surgery, a second surgery provides a chance for cure. However, the decision to reoperate patients submitted to adequate LN dissection in initial surgery should be carefully balanced between the risk of hypoparathyroidism with the small chance of calcitonin normalization (6–20% of the cases) [49, 50] and a favorable long-term outcome of patients with low-volume residual MTC (86%, 10-year survival rate) [51].

Patients with advanced loco-regional disease may benefit from external-beam radiotherapy (EBRT) for local tumor control. EBRT can be used with an adjuvant or palliative intent. Adjuvant EBRT can be indicated for patients with extensive regional LN involvement with high risk of recurrence such as gross or microscopic residual disease after an extensive and final surgical procedure, extra-thyroidal disease, and disease outside lymph nodes. In these cases, EBRT may reduce the risk of recurrent disease and may provide long-term loco-regional control [52–55].

The indolence of metastatic MTC and the lack of an effective systemic treatment make observation the best approach for these patients. Only patients with an extensive tumor burden or with evidence of progressive disease should be considered for systemic treatment. Progression of disease can be determined by imaging studies and/or by a progressive rise of tumor markers. The concept of the doubling time (DT) of calcitonin and CEA has gained acceptance in the last few years [56, 57]. Barbet and colleagues have successfully shown that a short DT was associated with lower survival; a calcitonin DT <6 months was associated with a 5- and 10-year survival of 25 and 8%, respectively; while a CT DT between 6 and 24 months was associated with a 5- and 10-year survival of 92 and 37% and a calcitonin DT longer than 2 years was associated with 100% survival at the end of the study [56]. Calculation of CEA DTs is also recommended, especially in those patients with poorly differentiated disease that loses ability to produce calcitonin [15]. Calculation of DTs can be done through a calculator available at http://www.thyroid.org.

Patients with a DT <2 years or rapidly progressive disease by imaging studies should be considered for systemic treatment [15]. Systemic chemotherapy is historically not very effective in MTC. Dacarbazine and doxorubicin are the most effective agents. Dacarbazine in combination with doxorubicin or other agents have resulted in control of tumor growth in approximately 20–30% of patients; however, in these studies, it has not resulted in any complete remissions [58–63]. The lack of effective treatment and the recent development of tyrosine kinase inhibitors (TKI) capable of disrupting RET signaling, and signaling of other tyrosine kinase pathways activated in MTC cells, such as the VEGF receptor, have resulted in the development of several clinical trials [64]. Schlumberger and colleagues have investigated the role of motesanib, inhibitor of RET, VEGFR and PDGFR, in patients with advanced metastatic MTC who were either symptomatic or who had progressive disease by RECIST criteria [65]. Most patients achieved stable disease (81%), partial response was observed in only 2% of patients and 8% had progressive disease. No patients achieved complete response [66]. Other TKIs that have been investigated include sorafenib, axitinib, sunitinib, and imatinib [66–70]. Two very promising TKIs include vandetanib and XL 184 which are under investigation.

Asymptomatic Hereditary Medullary Thyroid Carcinoma

Genetic analysis of the *RET* gene is recommended for all patients diagnosed with MTC. Upon detection of a germline *RET* mutation, all first-degree relatives should undergo DNA analysis to detect or exclude a *RET* mutation [14, 15]. Genetic analysis of family members should occur as early as possible. In kindreds with MEN2B, the recommended age of *RET* testing is within the first year of life or as soon as MEN2B is suspected and in kindreds with MEN2A or FMTC between 3 and 5 years of age [14, 15]. Individuals without a *RET* mutation are not at risk to develop MTC, pheochromocytoma or hyperparathyroidism and therefore are excluded from long-term surveillance. When a mutation is identified, preoperative evaluation and management will depend on the type of mutation detected, on the age in which the mutation was detected, and on the presence or absence of disease [15]. Carriers identified with apparent disease should undergo the same evaluation and treatment outlined in the earlier section.

When the identification of a carrier status occurs at a preclinical stage, the work-up and management will depend on the aggressiveness/type (risk level) of the *RET* mutation. All carriers of a MEN2B mutation should undergo a cervical US examination and if older than 6 months a measurement of serum calcitonin. Carriers of a MEN2A or a FMTC mutation older than 3–5 years of age should be evaluated with a neck US, serum calcitonin, and calcium level. Screening for pheochromocytoma should start at age 8 in carriers of MEN2B mutations and carriers of mutations involving exons 634 and 630 of the *RET* gene. In all other mutations, pheochromocytoma screening can start at 20 years of age.

Prophylactic thyroidectomy is the procedure of choice for all asymptomatic carriers with a *RET* mutation. The experience collected over the past 15 years has demonstrated that *RET* testing has excellent sensitivity, and prophylactic thyroidectomy is safe and results in a high rate of surgical cure. Despite not having a very prolonged follow-up period, several studies have demonstrated that when performed early, prophylactic thyroidectomy is associated with no evidence of post-operatively persistent or recurrent disease [71–74]. Based on information acquired through genotype–phenotype correlation, mutations have been classified according to their risk of aggressiveness (Table 11.1). Phenotypic features taken into account were the age of earliest development of MTC, age of earliest development of lymph node metastases, penetrance of MTC, and lifelong behavior of MTC associated with each mutation. The recommended age for prophylactic thyroidectomy is based on each risk category. Highest risk mutations (ATA level D) are associated with MEN2B and the recommended age for prophylactic thyroidectomy is as soon as possible or within the first year of life [15]. Mutations that involve codon 634 (ATA level C), associated with MEN2A, TT should be performed before age 5 years [15]. ATA level B mutations include other cysteine-rich domain mutations (exons 609, 611, 618, 620, and 630) with a lower risk of aggressive MTC; in these cases prophylactic thyroidectomy should also be considered before age 5 but could be delayed to a later age if the following criteria are met; normal detailed cervical US, normal basal or stimulated calcitonin level, and indolent biologic behavior of MTC in the specific kindred [15]. Level-A mutations are associated with the least aggressive phenotype and include mutations at codons 768, 790, 791, 804, and 891. In this group, surgery may be delayed beyond age 5 if above criteria are met [15].

As prophylactic level VI (central) compartment LN dissection increases the risk of surgical hypoparathyroidism and/or vocal cord paralysis, its recommendation is restricted to MEN2B carriers when older than 1 year of age. MEN2B carriers that undergo surgery prior to 1 year, level VI LN dissection should be performed only when LN involvement is detected by US or intraoperatively [15].

Summary and Conclusions

MTC is a rare neuroendocrine tumor originated from the parafollicular C-cells of the thyroid gland. In approximately 30% of the cases, it is hereditary and associated with the multiple endocrine neoplasia type 2 syndrome. The most important molecular abnormality associated with MTC is an activating mutation of the *RET* gene; germline mutations of this gene are present in generally all of the hereditary cases, and somatic mutations in approximately 40% of sporadic tumors. The knowledge acquired since the discovery of the *RET* gene has been of utmost importance for a better understanding and treatment of this disease. Further research will not only solidify current knowledge but will also provide further insights on how to better treat patients with metastatic disease.

References

1. Hazard JB, Hawk WA, Crile Jr G. Medullary (solid) carcinoma of the thyroid; a clinicopathologic entity. J Clin Endocrinol Metab. 1959;19(1):152–61.
2. Sipple JH. The association of pheochromocytoma with carcinoma of the thyroid gland. Am J Med. 1961;31:163–6.
3. Gagel RF, Tashjian Jr AH. Cummings T, et al. The clinical outcome of prospective screening for multiple endocrine neoplasia type 2a. An 18-year experience. N Engl J Med. 1988; 318(8):478–84.
4. Lips CJ, Landsvater RM, Hoppener JW, et al. Clinical screening as compared with DNA analysis in families with multiple endocrine neoplasia type 2A. N Engl J Med. 1994;331(13):828–35.
5. Donis-Keller H, Dou S, Chi D, et al. Mutations in the RET proto-oncogene are associated with MEN 2A and FMTC. Hum Mol Genet. 1993;2(7):851–6.

6. Mulligan LM, Kwok JB, Healey CS, et al. Germ-line mutations of the RET proto-oncogene in multiple endocrine neoplasia type 2A. Nature. 1993;363(6428):458–60.
7. Wolfe HJ, Melvin KE, Cervi-Skinner SJ, et al. C-cell hyperplasia preceding medullary thyroid carcinoma. N Engl J Med. 1973;289(9):437–41.
8. Gagel RF, Marx SJ. Multiple endocrine neoplasia. In: Kronenberg HM, Melmed S, Polonsky KS, Larsen PR, editors. William textbook of endocrinology. 11th ed. Philadelphia: Saunders Elsevier; 2008. p. 1705–46.
9. Hoff AO, Gagel RF. Multiple endocrine neoplasia type 2. In: DeGroot LJ, Jameson JL, editors. Endocrinology. 5th ed. Elsevier Saunders: Philadelphia; 2005.
10. Eng C, Clayton D, Schuffenecker I, et al. The relationship between specific RET proto-oncogene mutations and disease phenotype in multiple endocrine neoplasia type 2. International RET mutation consortium analysis. JAMA. 1996;276(19):1575–9.
11. Skinner MA, DeBenedetti MK, Moley JF, Norton JA, Wells SA, Jr. Medullary thyroid carcinoma in children with multiple endocrine neoplasia types 2A and 2B. J Pediatr Surg. 1996;31(1):177–81; discussion 181–72.
12. Camacho CP, Hoff AO, Lindsey SC, et al. Early diagnosis of multiple endocrine neoplasia type 2B: a challenge for physicians. Arq Bras Endocrinol Metabol. 2008;52(8): 1393–8.
13. Santarpia L, Gagel RF, Sherman SI, Sarlis NJ, Evans DB, Hoff AO. Diabetes insipidus and panhypopituitarism due to intrasellar metastasis from medullary thyroid cancer. Head Neck. 2009;31(3):419–23.
14. Brandi ML, Gagel RF, Angeli A, et al. Guidelines for diagnosis and therapy of MEN type 1 and type 2. J Clin Endocrinol Metab. 2001;86(12):5658–71.
15. Kloos RT, Eng C, Evans DB, et al. Medullary thyroid cancer: management guidelines of the American Thyroid Association. Thyroid. 2009;19(6):565–612.
16. Eng C, Smith DP, Mulligan LM, et al. A novel point mutation in the tyrosine kinase domain of the RET proto-oncogene in sporadic medullary thyroid carcinoma and in a family with FMTC. Oncogene. 1995;10(3):509–13.
17. Moley JF, DeBenedetti MK. Patterns of nodal metastases in palpable medullary thyroid carcinoma: recommendations for extent of node dissection. Ann Surg. 1999;229(6):880–7; discussion 887–8.
18. Scollo C, Baudin E, Travagli JP, et al. Rationale for central and bilateral lymph node dissection in sporadic and hereditary medullary thyroid cancer. J Clin Endocrinol Metab. 2003;88(5):2070–5.
19. Mirallie E, Vuillez JP, Bardet S, et al. High frequency of bone/bone marrow involvement in advanced medullary thyroid cancer. J Clin Endocrinol Metab. 2005;90(2):779–88.
20. Keusch G, Binswanger U, Dambacher MA, Fischer JA. Ectopic ACTH syndrome and medullary thyroid carcinoma. Acta Endocrinol Copenh. 1977;86(2):306–16.
21. Pachnis V, Mankoo B, Costantini F. Expression of the c-ret proto-oncogene during mouse embryogenesis. Development. 1993;119(4):1005–17.
22. Tsuzuki T, Takahashi M, Asai N, Iwashita T, Matsuyama M, Asai J. Spatial and temporal expression of the ret proto-oncogene product in embryonic, infant and adult rat tissues. Oncogene. 1995;10(1):191–8.
23. Takahashi M. The GDNF/RET signaling pathway and human diseases. Cytokine Growth Factor Rev. 2001;12(4):361–73.
24. Santoro M, Carlomagno F, Melillo RM, Fusco A. Dysfunction of the RET receptor in human cancer. Cell Mol Life Sci. 2004;61(23):2954–64.
25. Skinner MA, Safford SD, Reeves JG, Jackson ME, Freemerman AJ. Renal aplasia in humans is associated with RET mutations. Am J Hum Genet. 2008;82(2):344–51.
26. Schuchardt A, D'Agati V, Larsson-Blomberg L, Costantini F, Pachnis V. RET-deficient mice: an animal model for Hirschsprung's disease and renal agenesis. J Intern Med. 1995;238(4):327–32.
27. Edery P, Lyonnet S, Mulligan LM, et al. Mutations of the RET proto-oncogene in Hirschsprung's disease. Nature. 1994;367(6461):378–80.

28. Gagel RF, Levy ML, Donovan DT, Alford BR, Wheeler T, Tschen JA. Multiple endocrine neoplasia type 2a associated with cutaneous lichen amyloidosis. Ann Intern Med. 1989; 111(10):802–6.
29. Decker RA, Peacock ML, Watson P. Hirschsprung disease in MEN 2A: increased spectrum of RET exon 10 genotypes and strong genotype-phenotype correlation. Hum Mol Genet. 1998;7(1):129–34.
30. Jimenez C, Dang GT, Schultz PN, et al. A novel point mutation of the RET protooncogene involving the second intracellular tyrosine kinase domain in a family with medullary thyroid carcinoma. J Clin Endocrinol Metab. 2004;89(7):3521–6.
31. Bolino A, Schuffenecker I, Luo Y, et al. RET mutations in exons 13 and 14 of FMTC patients. Oncogene. 1995;10(12):2415–9.
32. Carlson KM, Dou S, Chi D, et al. Single missense mutation in the tyrosine kinase catalytic domain of the RET protooncogene is associated with multiple endocrine neoplasia type 2B. Proc Natl Acad Sci USA. 1994;91(4):1579–83.
33. Rossel M, Schuffenecker I, Schlumberger M, et al. Detection of a germline mutation at codon 918 of the RET proto-oncogene in French MEN 2B families. Hum Genet. 1995;95(4):403–6.
34. Gimm O, Marsh DJ, Andrew SD, et al. Germline dinucleotide mutation in codon 883 of the RET proto-oncogene in multiple endocrine neoplasia type 2B without codon 918 mutation. J Clin Endocrinol Metab. 1997;82(11):3902–4.
35. Wohllk N, Cote GJ, Bugalho MM, et al. Relevance of RET proto-oncogene mutations in sporadic medullary thyroid carcinoma. J Clin Endocrinol Metab. 1996;81(10):3740–5.
36. Scurini C, Quadro L, Fattoruso O, et al. Germline and somatic mutations of the RET proto-oncogene in apparently sporadic medullary thyroid carcinomas. Mol Cell Endocrinol. 1998;137(1):51–7.
37. Zedenius J, Wallin G, Hamberger B, Nordenskjold M, Weber G, Larsson C. Somatic and MEN 2A de novo mutations identified in the RET proto-oncogene by screening of sporadic MTCs. Hum Mol Genet. 1994;3(8):1259–62.
38. Marsh DJ, Learoyd DL, Andrew SD, et al. Somatic mutations in the RET proto-oncogene in sporadic medullary thyroid carcinoma. Clin Endocrinol (Oxf). 1996;44(3):249–57.
39. Eng C, Mulligan LM, Smith DP, et al. Mutation of the RET protooncogene in sporadic medullary thyroid carcinoma. Genes Chromosom Cancer. 1995;12(3):209–12.
40. Kouvaraki MA, Shapiro SE, Fornage BD, et al. Role of preoperative ultrasonography in the surgical management of patients with thyroid cancer. Surgery. 2003;134(6):946–54; discussion 954–45.
41. Machens A, Schneyer U, Holzhausen HJ, Dralle H. Prospects of remission in medullary thyroid carcinoma according to basal calcitonin level. J Clin Endocrinol Metab. 2005;90(4):2029–34.
42. Modigliani E, Cohen R, Campos JM, et al. Prognostic factors for survival and for biochemical cure in medullary thyroid carcinoma: results in 899 patients. The GETC Study Group. Groupe d'etude des tumeurs a calcitonine. Clin Endocrinol (Oxf). 1998;48(3):265–73.
43. DeLellis RA, Rule AH, Spiler I, Nathanson L, Tashjian Jr AH, Wolfe HJ. Calcitonin and carcinoembryonic antigen as tumor markers in medullary thyroid carcinoma. Am J Clin Pathol. 1978;70(4):587–94.
44. Saad MF, Fritsche Jr HA, Samaan NA. Diagnostic and prognostic values of carcinoembryonic antigen in medullary carcinoma of the thyroid. J Clin Endocrinol Metab. 1984;58(5):889–94.
45. Franc S, Niccoli-Sire P, Cohen R, et al. Complete surgical lymph node resection does not prevent authentic recurrences of medullary thyroid carcinoma. Clin Endocrinol (Oxf). 2001;55(3):403–9.
46. Weber T, Schilling T, Frank-Raue K, et al. Impact of modified radical neck dissection on biochemical cure in medullary thyroid carcinomas. Surgery. 2001;130(6):1044–9.
47. Yen TW, Shapiro SE, Gagel RF, Sherman SI, Lee JE, Evans DB. Medullary thyroid carcinoma: results of a standardized surgical approach in a contemporary series of 80 consecutive patients. Surgery. 2003;134(6):890–9; discussion 899–901.

48. Boi F, Maurelli I, Pinna G, et al. Calcitonin measurement in wash-out fluid from fine needle aspiration of neck masses in patients with primary and metastatic medullary thyroid carcinoma. J Clin Endocrinol Metab. 2007;92(6):2115–8.
49. Kebebew E, Ituarte PH, Siperstein AE, Duh QY, Clark OH. Medullary thyroid carcinoma: clinical characteristics, treatment, prognostic factors, and a comparison of staging systems. Cancer. 2000;88(5):1139–48.
50. Tisell LE, Hansson G, Jansson S, Salander H. Reoperation in the treatment of asymptomatic metastasizing medullary thyroid carcinoma. Surgery. 1986;99(1):60–6.
51. van Heerden JA, Grant CS, Gharib H, Hay ID, Ilstrup DM. Long-term course of patients with persistent hypercalcitoninemia after apparent curative primary surgery for medullary thyroid carcinoma. Ann Surg. 1990;212(4):395–400; discussion 400–1.
52. Brierley J, Tsang R, Simpson WJ, Gospodarowicz M, Sutcliffe S, Panzarella T. Medullary thyroid cancer: analyses of survival and prognostic factors and the role of radiation therapy in local control. Thyroid. 1996;6(4):305–10.
53. Fersht N, Vini L, A'Hern R, Harmer C. The role of radiotherapy in the management of elevated calcitonin after surgery for medullary thyroid cancer. Thyroid. 2001;11(12):1161–8.
54. Nguyen TD, Chassard JL, Lagarde P, et al. Results of postoperative radiation therapy in medullary carcinoma of the thyroid: a retrospective study by the French Federation of Cancer Institutes – the Radiotherapy Cooperative Group. Radiother Oncol. 1992; 23(1):1–5.
55. Schwartz DL, Rana V, Shaw S, et al. Postoperative radiotherapy for advanced medullary thyroid cancer – local disease control in the modern era. Head Neck. 2008;30(7):883–8.
56. Barbet J, Campion L, Kraeber-Bodere F, Chatal JF. Prognostic impact of serum calcitonin and carcinoembryonic antigen doubling-times in patients with medullary thyroid carcinoma. J Clin Endocrinol Metab. 2005;90(11):6077–84.
57. Laure Giraudet A, Al Ghulzan A, Auperin A, et al. Progression of medullary thyroid carcinoma: assessment with calcitonin and carcinoembryonic antigen doubling times. Eur J Endocrinol. 2008;158(2):239–46.
58. Scherubl H, Raue F, Ziegler R. Combination chemotherapy of advanced medullary and differentiated thyroid cancer. Phase II study. J Cancer Res Clin Oncol. 1990;116(1):21–3.
59. Orlandi F, Caraci P, Berruti A, et al. Chemotherapy with dacarbazine and 5-fluorouracil in advanced medullary thyroid cancer. Ann Oncol. 1994;5(8):763–5.
60. Wu LT, Averbuch SD, Ball DW, de Bustros A, Baylin SB, McGuire 3rd WP. Treatment of advanced medullary thyroid carcinoma with a combination of cyclophosphamide, vincristine, and dacarbazine. Cancer. 1994;73(2):432–6.
61. Schlumberger M, Abdelmoumene N, Delisle MJ, Couette JE. Treatment of advanced medullary thyroid cancer with an alternating combination of 5 FU-streptozocin and 5 FU-dacarbazine. The Groupe d'Etude des Tumeurs a Calcitonine (GETC). Br J Cancer. 1995;71(2):363–5.
62. Di Bartolomeo M, Bajetta E, Bochicchio AM, et al. A phase II trial of dacarbazine, fluorouracil and epirubicin in patients with neuroendocrine tumours. A study by the Italian Trials in Medical Oncology (I.T.M.O.) Group. Ann Oncol. 1995;6(1):77–9.
63. Bajetta E, Rimassa L, Carnaghi C, et al. 5-Fluorouracil, dacarbazine, and epirubicin in the treatment of patients with neuroendocrine tumors. Cancer. 1998;83(2):372–8.
64. Sherman SI. Advances in chemotherapy of differentiated epithelial and medullary thyroid cancers. J Clin Endocrinol Metab. 2009;94(5):1493–9.
65. Schlumberger MJ, Elisei R, Bastholt L, et al. Phase II study of safety and efficacy of motesanib in patients with progressive or symptomatic, advanced or metastatic medullary thyroid cancer. J Clin Oncol. 2009;27(23):3794–801.
66. Gupta-Abramson V, Troxel AB, Nellore A, et al. Phase II trial of sorafenib in advanced thyroid cancer. J Clin Oncol. 2008;26(29):4714–9.
67. Frank-Raue K, Fabel M, Delorme S, Haberkorn U, Raue F. Efficacy of imatinib mesylate in advanced medullary thyroid carcinoma. Eur J Endocrinol. 2007;157(2):215–20.

68. de Groot JW, Zonnenberg BA, van Ufford-Mannesse PQ, et al. A phase II trial of imatinib therapy for metastatic medullary thyroid carcinoma. J Clin Endocrinol Metab. 2007;92(9): 3466–9.
69. Cohen EE, Rosen LS, Vokes EE, et al. Axitinib is an active treatment for all histologic subtypes of advanced thyroid cancer: results from a phase II study. J Clin Oncol. 2008;26(29): 4708–13.
70. Kelleher FC, McDermott R. Response to sunitinib in medullary thyroid cancer. Ann Intern Med. 2008;148(7):567.
71. Frank-Raue K, Buhr H, Dralle H, et al. Long-term outcome in 46 gene carriers of hereditary medullary thyroid carcinoma after prophylactic thyroidectomy: impact of individual RET genotype. Eur J Endocrinol. 2006;155(2):229–36.
72. Skinner MA, Moley JA, Dilley WG, Owzar K, Debenedetti MK, Wells Jr SA. Prophylactic thyroidectomy in multiple endocrine neoplasia type 2A. N Engl J Med. 2005;353(11): 1105–13.
73. Learoyd DL, Gosnell J, Elston MS, et al. Experience of prophylactic thyroidectomy in multiple endocrine neoplasia type 2A kindreds with RET codon 804 mutations. Clin Endocrinol (Oxf). 2005;63(6):636–41.
74. Gimm O, Ukkat J, Niederle BE, et al. Timing and extent of surgery in patients with familial medullary thyroid carcinoma/multiple endocrine neoplasia 2A-related RET mutations not affecting codon 634. World J Surg. 2004;28(12):1312–6.
75. Dvorakova S, Vaclavikova E, Duskova J, Vlcek P, Ryska A, Bendlova B. Exon 5 of the RET proto-oncogene: a newly detected risk exon for familial medullary thyroid carcinoma, a novel germ-line mutation Gly321Arg. J Endocrinol Invest. 2005;28(10):905–9.
76. Pigny P, Bauters C, Wemeau JL, et al. A novel 9-base pair duplication in RET exon 8 in familial medullary thyroid carcinoma. J Clin Endocrinol Metab. 1999;84(5):1700–4.
77. Niccoli-Sire P, Murat A, Rohmer V, et al. When should thyroidectomy be performed in familial medullary thyroid carcinoma gene carriers with non-cysteine RET mutations? Surgery. 2003;134(6):1029–36; discussion 1036–27.
78. Fazioli F, Piccinini G, Appolloni G, et al. A new germline point mutation in Ret exon 8 (cys515ser) in a family with medullary thyroid carcinoma. Thyroid. 2008;18(7): 775–82.
79. Da Silva AM, Maciel RM, Da Silva MR, Toledo SR, De Carvalho MB, Cerutti JM. A novel germ-line point mutation in RET exon 8 (Gly(533)Cys) in a large kindred with familial medullary thyroid carcinoma. J Clin Endocrinol Metab. 2003;88(11):5438–43.
80. Kaldrymides P, Mytakidis N, Anagnostopoulos T, et al. A rare RET gene exon 8 mutation is found in two Greek kindreds with familial medullary thyroid carcinoma: implications for screening. Clin Endocrinol (Oxf). 2006;64(5):561–6.
81. Bethanis S, Koutsodontis G, Palouka T, et al. A newly detected mutation of the RET protooncogene in exon 8 as a cause of multiple endocrine neoplasia type 2A. Hormones (Athens). 2007;6(2):152–6.
82. Peppa M, Boutati E, Kamakari S, et al. Multiple endocrine neoplasia type 2A in two families with the familial medullary thyroid carcinoma associated G533C mutation of the RET proto-oncogene. Eur J Endocrinol. 2008;159(6):767–71.
83. Saez ME, Ruiz A, Cebrian A, et al. A new germline mutation, R600Q, within the coding region of RET proto-oncogene: a rare polymorphism or a MEN 2 causing mutation? Hum Mutat. 2000;15(1):122.
84. Rey JM, Brouillet JP, Fonteneau-Allaire J, et al. Novel germline RET mutation segregating with papillary thyroid carcinomas. Genes Chromosom Cancer. 2001;32(4):390–1.
85. Ahmed SA, Snow-Bailey K, Highsmith WE, Sun W, Fenwick RG, Mao R. Nine novel germline gene variants in the RET proto-oncogene identified in twelve unrelated cases. J Mol Diagn. 2005;7(2):283–8.
86. Ercolino T, Lombardi A, Becherini L, et al. The Y606C RET mutation causes a receptor gain of function. Clin Endocrinol (Oxf). 2008;69(2):253–8.

87. Paszko Z, Sromek M, Czetwertynska M, et al. The occurrence and the type of germline mutations in the RET gene in patients with medullary thyroid carcinoma and their unaffected kindred's from Central Poland. Cancer Invest. 2007;25(8):742–9.
88. Quayle FJ, Fialkowski EA, Benveniste R, Moley JF. Pheochromocytoma penetrance varies by RET mutation in MEN 2A. Surgery. 2007;142(6):800–5; discussion 805, e801.
89. Igaz P, Patocs A, Racz K, Klein I, Varadi A, Esik O. Occurrence of pheochromocytoma in a MEN2A family with codon 609 mutation of the RET proto-oncogene. J Clin Endocrinol Metab. 2002;87(6):2994.
90. Fialkowski EA, DeBenedetti MK, Moley JF, Bachrach B. RET proto-oncogene testing in infants presenting with Hirschsprung disease identifies 2 new multiple endocrine neoplasia 2A kindreds. J Pediatr Surg. 2008;43(1):188–90.
91. Kinlaw WB, Scott SM, Maue RA, et al. Multiple endocrine neoplasia 2A due to a unique C609S RET mutation presents with pheochromocytoma and reduced penetrance of medullary thyroid carcinoma. Clin Endocrinol (Oxf). 2005;63(6):676–82.
92. Kameyama K, Okinaga H, Takami H. RET oncogene mutations in 75 cases of familial medullary thyroid carcinoma in Japan. Biomed Pharmacother. 2004;58(6–7):345–7.
93. Yonekawa H, Sugitani I, Fujimoto Y, Arai M, Yamamoto N. A family of multiple endocrine neoplasia type 2A (MEN 2A) with Cys630Tyr RET germline mutation: report of a case. Endocr J. 2007;54(4):531–5.
94. Raue F, Frank-Raue K. Multiple endocrine neoplasia type 2. Horm Res. 2007;68(5): 101–104.
95. Berndt I, Reuter M, Saller B, et al. A new hot spot for mutations in the ret protooncogene causing familial medullary thyroid carcinoma and multiple endocrine neoplasia type 2A. J Clin Endocrinol Metab. 1998;83(3):770–4.
96. Hoppner W, Dralle H, Brabant G. Duplication of 9 base pairs in the critical cysteine-rich domain of the RET proto-oncogene causes multiple endocrine neoplasia type 2A. Hum Mutat. 1998;Suppl 1:S128–30.
97. Punales MK, Graf H, Gross JL, Maia AL. RET codon 634 mutations in multiple endocrine neoplasia type 2: variable clinical features and clinical outcome. J Clin Endocrinol Metab. 2003;88(6):2644–9.
98. Zhou YL, Zhu SX, Li JJ, et al. The clinical patterns and RET proto-oncogene in fifteen multiple endocrine neoplasia type 2A pedigrees. Zhonghua Nei Ke Za Zhi. 2007;46(6):466–70.
99. Lemos MC, Carrilho F, Rodrigues FJ, et al. Early onset of medullary thyroid carcinoma in a kindred with multiple endocrine neoplasia type iia associated with cutaneous lichen amyloidosis. Endocr Pract. 2002;8(1):19–22.
100. Hoppner W, Ritter MM. A duplication of 12 bp in the critical cysteine rich domain of the RET proto-oncogene results in a distinct phenotype of multiple endocrine neoplasia type 2A. Hum Mol Genet. 1997;6(4):587–90.
101. Colombo-Benkmann M, Li Z, Riemann B, et al. Characterization of the RET protooncogene transmembrane domain mutation S649L associated with nonaggressive medullary thyroid carcinoma. Eur J Endocrinol. 2008;158(6):811–6.
102. Wiench M, Wygoda Z, Gubala E, et al. Estimation of risk of inherited medullary thyroid carcinoma in apparent sporadic patients. J Clin Oncol. 2001;19(5):1374–80.
103. Vierhapper H, Bieglmayer C, Heinze G, Baumgartner-Parzer S. Frequency of RET proto-oncogene mutations in patients with normal and with moderately elevated pentagastrin-stimulated serum concentrations of calcitonin. Thyroid. 2004;14(8):580–3.
104. Dabir T, Hunter SJ, Russell CF, McCall D, Morrison PJ. The RET mutation E768D confers a late-onset familial medullary thyroid carcinoma – only phenotype with incomplete penetrance: implications for screening and management of carrier status. Fam Cancer. 2006; 5(2):201–4.
105. D'Aloiso L, Carlomagno F, Bisceglia M, et al. Clinical case seminar: in vivo and in vitro characterization of a novel germline RET mutation associated with low-penetrant nonaggressive familial medullary thyroid carcinoma. J Clin Endocrinol Metab. 2006;91(3): 754–9.

106. Frank-Raue K, Machens A, Scheuba C, Niederle B, Dralle H, Raue F. Difference in development of medullary thyroid carcinoma among carriers of RET mutations in codons 790 and 791. Clin Endocrinol (Oxf). 2008;69(2):259–63.
107. Vestergaard P, Vestergaard EM, Brockstedt H, Christiansen P. Codon Y791F mutations in a large kindred: is prophylactic thyroidectomy always indicated? World J Surg. 2007;31(5): 996–1001; discussion 1002–4.
108. Recasens M, Oriola J, Fernandez-Real JM, et al. Asymptomatic bilateral adrenal pheochromocytoma in a patient with a germline V804M mutation in the RET proto-oncogene. Clin Endocrinol (Oxf). 2007;67(1):29–33.
109. Rothberg AE, Raymond VM, Gruber SB, Sisson J. Familial medullary thyroid carcinoma associated with cutaneous lichen amyloidosis. Thyroid. 2009;19(6):651–5.
110. Cranston A, Carniti C, Martin S, et al. A novel activating mutation in the RET tyrosine kinase domain mediates neoplastic transformation. Mol Endocrinol. 2006;20(7):1633–43.
111. Prazeres HJ, Rodrigues F, Figueiredo P, et al. Occurrence of the Cys611Tyr mutation and a novel Arg886Trp substitution in the RET proto-oncogene in multiple endocrine neoplasia type 2 families and sporadic medullary thyroid carcinoma cases originating from the central region of Portugal. Clin Endocrinol (Oxf). 2006;64(6):659–66.
112. Smith DP, Houghton C, Ponder BA. Germline mutation of RET codon 883 in two cases of de novo MEN 2B. Oncogene. 1997;15(10):1213–7.
113. Elisei R, Cosci B, Romei C, et al. Identification of a novel point mutation in the RET gene (Ala883Thr), which is associated with medullary thyroid carcinoma phenotype only in homozygous condition. J Clin Endocrinol Metab. 2004;89(11):5823–7.
114. Elisei R, Romei C, Cosci B, et al. RET genetic screening in patients with medullary thyroid cancer and their relatives: experience with 807 individuals at one center. J Clin Endocrinol Metab. 2007;92(12):4725–9.
115. Hofstra RM, Fattoruso O, Quadro L, et al. A novel point mutation in the intracellular domain of the ret protooncogene in a family with medullary thyroid carcinoma. J Clin Endocrinol Metab. 1997;82(12):4176–8.
116. Dang GT, Cote GJ, Schultz PN, Khorana S, Decker RA, Gagel RF. A codon 891 exon 15 RET proto-oncogene mutation in familial medullary thyroid carcinoma: a detection strategy. Mol Cell Probes. 1999;13(1):77–9.
117. Jimenez C, Habra MA, Huang SC, et al. Pheochromocytoma and medullary thyroid carcinoma: a new genotype-phenotype correlation of the RET protooncogene 891 germline mutation. J Clin Endocrinol Metab. 2004;89(8):4142–5.
118. Kasprzak L, Nolet S, Gaboury L, et al. Familial medullary thyroid carcinoma and prominent corneal nerves associated with the germline V804M and V778I mutations on the same allele of RET. J Med Genet. 2001;38(11):784–7.
119. Cranston AN, Carniti C, Oakhill K, et al. RET is constitutively activated by novel tandem mutations that alter the active site resulting in multiple endocrine neoplasia type 2B. Cancer Res. 2006;66(20):10179–87.
120. Iwashita T, Murakami H, Kurokawa K, et al. A two-hit model for development of multiple endocrine neoplasia type 2B by RET mutations. Biochem Biophys Res Commun. 2000; 268(3):804–8.
121. Miyauchi A, Futami H, Hai N, et al. Two germline missense mutations at codons 804 and 806 of the RET proto-oncogene in the same allele in a patient with multiple endocrine neoplasia type 2B without codon 918 mutation. Jpn J Cancer Res. 1999;90(1):1–5.
122. Menko FH, van der Luijt RB, de Valk IA, et al. Atypical MEN type 2B associated with two germline RET mutations on the same allele not involving codon 918. J Clin Endocrinol Metab. 2002;87(1):393–7.

Chapter 12
Adrenocortical Carcinoma

Alexandria T. Phan and Camilo Jimenez

Abstract Adrenal tumors can be adrenal incidentalomas, adenomas, adrenocortical carcinoma (ACC), or pheochromocytoma (malignant or benign). Making up the majority of adrenal tumors are benign, nonfunctioning (not producing hormones) adenomas that are discovered incidentally on abdominal imagining studies referred to as adrenal incidentalomas. Another large part of adrenal tumors are benign, functioning (secreting hormones) adenomas. From most frequent to least, these functioning adrenal adenomas can cause Cushing's syndrome, primary aldosteronism, and virilization. Adrenocortical carcinomas (ACCs) are the least common among adrenal tumors but are extremely heterogeneous and can be aggressive and fatal. Evaluation of adrenal incidentalomas and adrenocortical adenomas are discussed briefly here. This chapter will focus on adrenocortical carcinomas (ACCs), discussing all aspects of ACCs including management and treatment of this rarest disease.

Keywords Adrenal incidentalomas • Adrenocortical adenomas • Adrenocortical carcinoma • Pheochromocytoma • Cushing's syndrome • Primary aldosteronism • Virilization

Introduction

The adrenal cortex is an outer portion of the adrenal gland. Different layers in the adrenal cortex produce different hormones. Together, the adrenal cortex secretes corticosteroids and other hormones directly into the bloodstream. The hormones produced by the adrenal cortex include corticosteroid, aldosterone, and androgen

A.T. Phan (✉)
Department of Gastrointestinal Medical Oncology, The University of Texas
M.D. Anderson Cancer Center, Houston, TX, USA
e-mail: atphan@mdanderson.org

J.C. Yao et al. (eds.), *Neuroendocrine Tumors*, Current Clinical Oncology,
DOI 10.1007/978-1-60327-997-0_12,

hormones. Corticosteroid hormones include hydrocortisone hormone, also known as cortisol, which controls the body's use of fats, proteins, and carbohydrates; and corticosterone, which, together with hydrocortisone hormones, suppresses inflammatory reactions in the body and also affects the immune system. Aldosterone hormone inhibits the level of sodium excreted into the urine, maintaining blood volume and blood pressure. Androgen hormones have minimal effect on the development of male characteristics.

Adrenal tumors arising from the cortex can be incidentalomas, adenomas or adrenocortical carcinoma (ACC), while those arising from the medulla can be pheochromocytoma (malignant or benign). Making up the majority of adrenal tumors are benign, nonfunctioning (not producing hormones) adenomas that are discovered incidentally on abdominal imagining studies referred to as adrenal incidentalomas. Another large part of adrenal tumors are benign, functioning (secreting hormones) adenomas. From most frequent to least, these functioning adrenal adenomas can cause Cushing's syndrome, primary aldosteronism, and virilization. Adrenocortical carcinomas (ACCs) are the least common among adrenal tumors but are extremely heterogeneous and can be aggressive and fatal. Evaluation of adrenal incidentalomas and adrenocortical adenomas are discussed briefly here. This chapter will focus on adrenocortical carcinomas (ACCs), discussing all aspects of ACCs including management and treatment of this rarest disease.

Epidemiology

Primary malignancy from the adrenal cortex is referred to as ACC. The maximum diameter of the adrenal mass is predictive of malignancy. In a study of 887 patients with adrenal incidentalomas from the National Italian Study Group [1] ACC were significantly associated with mass size, with 90% being more than 4 cm in diameter when discovered. ACC accounts approximately for 0.02% [2] of all cancers reported. ACC has an estimated incidence of one to two cases per 1.7 million of the population, roughly 200–300 new cases being diagnosed in the United States annually [3, 4]. Because of its rarity and fatality, any epidemiologic figures for ACC are only estimated based on retrospective analysis of population-based or large case-series cohorts.

ACC has a bimodal age distribution, with an increased incidence in children less than 5 years old, and adults in their fourth and fifth decades of life. ACC has no specific racial predilection, although case series suggested a higher ACC prevalence among Caucasian- than African-Americans. The female-to-male ratio is approximately 2.5–3.1 [5]. At presentation, men tend to be older and have a worse overall prognosis than their female counterparts. Women are more likely to have an associated endocrine syndrome (functional ACC); functional ACC has shorter survival duration in comparison to that in nonfunctional disease. A major percentage of functional ACC will have corticosteroid-producing tumors, and is known to be associated with several comorbid conditions – diabetes, hypertension, steroid myopathy, and immunosuppression from dysfunctional macrophages. Generally, systemic cytotoxic chemotherapy has narrow therapeutic index in these patients with functional ACCs. Several case series had suggested that patients with functional ACCs would present with earlier cancer stages because of overt signs and symptoms of associated hormonal excess. Women develop functional ACCs more often than men [6, 7]. Adults with ACCs generally present with unresectable locally advanced or distant metastatic disease.

Complete surgical resection still remains the best chance of cure. However, even after complete curative surgery (R0 resection), the rate of recurrence is still high, estimated to be 70–80% [8]. The overall survival of patients with ACC has not changed significantly. There have not been any practice changing advancement over the past 2–3 decades; there are many more publications on molecular profiles of small cohorts of ACC than there are results of clinical studies. However, the hope remains that improved understanding of the molecular pathogenesis of this rare malignancy can lead to development of drugs effective in improving patient's survival.

Tumorigenesis

Approximately less than 15% of ACC cases are associated with hereditary conditions, while the majority of newly diagnosed ACC occur sporadically and not associated with inheritance. These hereditary syndromes contribute to small percentage of cases of ACC. Hereditary cases of ACC are frequently found in Li-Fraumeni, multiple endocrine neoplasia type 1 (MEN-1), Sarcoma, Breast, Lung and adrenal cancers (SBLA) syndrome, Carney syndrome, and Beckwith-Wiedemann syndrome (see Table 12.1) [9, 10].

Li-Fraumeni syndrome is an autosomal dominant hereditary syndrome due to a germline mutation of the tumor-suppressor gene p53 gene on 17p13 [11]. Patients within this family are at risk for ACC, breast cancer, soft tissue and bone sarcoma, as well as brain tumors. The TP53 gene is a tumor suppressor gene and is the most frequently mutated gene in human cancers [12]. The p53 protein controls the cell cycle at the G1/S interface and plays an important role in inducing programmed cell death in response to severe cellular DNA damage [13]. Loss of TP53 has at least three roles in progression: suppressing apoptosis, preventing cell cycle arrest and permitting genetic instability, which may be in favor of the generation of viable genetic variants [14]. MEN-1 is another autosomal dominant syndrome associated with adrenal tumors along with other tumors of the endocrine system. Patients with MEN-1 syndrome will frequently have adenomas of pituitary and parathyroid, pancreatic neuroendocrine carcinoma, and adenoma and carcinoma of the adrenal gland. Unilateral or bilateral adrenal tumors can be found in 20–40% of patients with MEN-1. The Majority of adrenal tumors associated with MEN-1 is benign adenomas, and rarely functional. MEN-1 syndrome is a result of the germline mutation

Table 12.1 Hereditary syndromes associated with adrenal neoplasms

	Syndromes	Genes	Clinical features	Peptides/ hormones secreted by tumors
Associated with adrenocortical carcinoma (ACC)	Li-Fraumeni	TP53 (17p13) Specifically for sporadic ACC TP53 somatic mutations 17p13 LOH	Soft tissue sarcoma Breast cancers Brain tumors Leukemia ACC	Variable[a]
	Beckwith-Wiedemann	11p15 mutation IGF-11 overexpression P57kip2 mutation KCNQ10T epigenetic defect H19 epigenetic defect Specifically for sporadic ACC LOH 11p15 Overexpression IGF-II	Omphalocele Macroglossia Macrosomia Hemi-hypertrophy Wilms' tumor ACC	Variable[a]
	Familial aenomatous polyposis	APC (5q12-22) Specifically for sporadic ACC β-Catenin somatic mutations	Colonic polyps/ colorectal cancers Peri-ampullary pancreatic cancer Thyroid tumors Hepatoblastoma Adrenal adenomas ACC	Variable[a]
	Multiple endocrine neoplasms 1	Menin (11q13) Specifically for sporadic ACC LOH 11q13	Parathyroid adenoma Pituitary adenoma Pancreatic tumors (pNET)/cysts Adrenal adenomas Adrenal hyperplasia ACC	Variable[a]

LOH loss of heterozygosity

[a]Hormonal secretions can be cortisol, sex steroids, and aldosterone, or combinations of all

of the MEN-1 gene on 11q13, which encodes for a protein called menin. The exact function of the menin is uncertain, but it has been suggested that it is likely involved in apoptosis. Because it interacts with many other proteins, including several transcription factors, menin is important in cellular growth and division [15, 16]. SBLA is a newer syndrome and thus has not been localized to any particular chromosomal loci [17]. Along with ACC, patients with SBLA syndrome will have increased risk for sarcoma, breast, and lung cancers.

Carney and Beckwith-Wiedemann syndromes are commonly diagnosed during childhood or adolescence because their characterized clinical features are usually discovered earlier than adulthood. Beckwith-Wiedemann is an autosomal dominant familial disease, where the chromosomal locus responsible for this syndrome was mapped to chromosome 11p15 [18], which includes the insulin-like growth factor II (IGF-II), H19, and cyclin-dependent kinase inhibitor C (p57/kip2). This locus is subject to parental imprinting with IGF-II solely expressed from the paternal allele, and H19 and p57/kip2 normally expressed from the maternal allele. The pathogenesis of the Beckwith-Wiedemann syndrome has been ascribed to genetic and epigenetic changes in the 11p15 locus resulting in overexpression of IGF-II and low expression of p57/kip2 and H19 [19]. IGF-II is predominantly expressed during embryonic development. In the actively growing fetal human adrenal gland, high levels of IGF-II are detected whereas in adult adrenal tissue, only low IGF-II levels are found. P57/kip2 is a cyclin-dependent kinase inhibitor and regulates cell cycle progression from the G1 to the S phase. H19 mRNA is not translated to protein and is hypothesized to regulate IGF-II expression [20]. Affected patients in this hereditary syndrome will be characterized by macroglosia, exomphalos, gigantism, and development of embryonic tumors such as Wilms' tumor, hepatoblastoma, rhabdomyosarcoma, and ACC [20, 21]. Cushing's syndrome due to primary pigmented nodular adrenocortical disease (PPNAD) has been observed in Carney complex patients. Carney syndrome is caused by inactivation of germline protein receptor kinase cAMP-dependent regulatory type I alpha (tissue specific extinguisher 1) or PRKAR1A. Mutation of PRKAR1A is mostly due to the LOH on 17q24. Protein receptor kinase A (PRKA) is involved in the regulation of lipid and glucose metabolism and is a component of the signal transduction mechanism of certain G-protein-coupled signal transduction. PRKA is composed of two regulatory subunits and two catalytic subunits. There are multiple isoforms of the regulatory subunit (RIalpha- and RIbeta-, RIIalpha- and RIIbeta-). Binding of cAMP to the regulatory subunit releases the catalytic subunits, which then phosphorylate a diverse set of proteins including the transcription factor CREB, ion channels, and metabolic enzymes. Pathology in patients with Carney complex syndrome includes skin pigmentation, paragangliomas, gastric or cardiac sarcoma, hereditary leiomyomatosis and renal cancer, along with endocrine tumors [22].

While the molecular mechanisms of hereditary ACC associated with hereditary syndromes are well characterized, the exact molecular tumorigenesis of sporadic ACC remained elusive. The identification of germline molecular defects in the hereditary syndrome responsible for adrenal tumors has facilitated improved understanding into the molecular pathogenesis associated with sporadic ACC. Indeed, similar molecular defects have since been identified as somatic alterations in sporadic adrenal tumors as well. For example, allelic losses at 17p13 (loci of TP53) and 11p15 (loci for IGF-II) have been demonstrated in sporadic ACC, and somatic mutations at 17q24 (loci for PRKAR1A) have been found in secreting adrenal adenomas. The frequent findings of mutations such as 17p13 and 11p15 give credence to the suggestion for their roles in tumorigenesis of sporadic ACC.

In the era of array analyses of DNA, RNA and proteins, additional molecular pathology has been identified from ACC cell lines and tumor tissues. Specifically, in situ mutations of tumor suppressor genes, TP53 and TP57, and increased production of IGF-II were observed from analyses of HR925 ACC cell lines [23]. Definite germ cell mutations of the TP53 gene have also been demonstrated in more than 90% of children with sporadic ACC from southern Brazil, which has the highest prevalence of sporadic ACC in the world [24, 25]. In addition to TP53, amplification of steroidogenic factor-1 (SF-1) expression has also been described in Brazilian children afflicted with ACCs [26]. Other studies demonstrate that some of ACC tumor cells express menin, the aberrant gene product in patients with type I [MEN-1] [23]. Overexpression of insulin-like growth factor (IGF-I and IGF-II) genes also related strongly to the tumorigenesis of sporadic ACC. Both IGF-I and IGF-II are involved in differentiation of the adrenal cortex. High levels of these factors may play a role in tumorigenesis and dedifferentiation [27–29]. Though commonly associated with IGF-I/IGF-II genes, LOH at 11p can result in amplifications of other growth factors not yet identified, which will likely have important involvement in ACC tumorigenesis.

In the review by Libe and Bertherat [23] and later further elucidated by Stratakis [22], tumor formation of ACC was represented by multistep model going from adrenal hyperplasia to adenoma and then to carcinoma, where each advancing step acquires additional genetic mutations. In this model, mutations of PRKAR1A and MEN-1 genes occur earlier in the process, while allelic losses in the TP53 and IGF-II genes occur later. In addition the mutation of genes which have important role in cell cycle and signal transduction, aberrant receptor expressions in the adrenocortical tissues have also be proposed as important contributor to stepwise transition from hyperplasia to adenoma, and subsequently carcinoma. For example, in cortisol-secreting adenoma, aberrant receptors that are independent of ACTH interaction with its receptor in the adrenocortical tissues include gastric inhibitory polypeptide (GIP), beta-adrenergic agonists, V1-vasopressin, serotonin (5-HT4 receptor), and luteinizing hormone (LH)/human chorionic gonadotropin (GnRH) [30]. In several small case series of patients with rennin-independent aldosterone-secreting adenomas, aberrant receptors found were GIP, 5-HT4, LH, GnRH, vasopressin, or thyroid-stimulating hormone (TSH) [31, 32].

Recently, genes belonging to the Wnt, Ras, and squamous cell carcinoma-related oncogene (SCCRO) family have been identified as three additional suspect involved in sporadic ACC tumorigenesis. Signaling by the Wnt family of secreted lipoproteins has central roles in embryogenesis and in adult tissue homeostatic processes.

The central event in the Wnt pathway is the stabilization of the transcription cofactor β-catenin in the cytoplasm and following its nuclear translocation and interaction with T-cell factor/lymphoid enhancer factor, β-catenin-dependent gene expression [33]. β-Catenin has also a function in cell–cell adhesion by interacting with E-cadherin and α-catenin. Activating mutations of the Wnt signaling pathway have been described in a large number of sporadic tumors [34]. Specifically activating mutations of exon 3 of the β-catenin gene (CTNNB1) were found with similar frequencies in adrenal adenomas and carcinomas, suggesting involvement of the β-catenin gene in the tumorigenesis of ACC [35].

The Ras gene family is composed of three genes (H-, K-, and N-Ras) and encodes low-molecular-weight GTPases which cycle between the GDP-bound (inactive) and GTP-bound (active) state at the plasma membrane. These molecular switches are involved in signaling pathways that modulate proliferation, differentiation, motility, and death [36]. Due to its pivotal roles, it is not surprising that Ras genes are the most frequently mutated oncogenes in human cancer [37]. However, evidence of the Ras genes being involved in adrenal tumorigenesis is still inconsistent. Activating N-Ras mutations were identified in 12.5% of adrenal carcinomas and adenomas tested, whereas no mutations were found in K- and H-Ras [38]. In a smaller number of adrenal tumors, Moul et al. [39] did not detect any point mutations in N-, H-, or K-Ras. Finally, Ocker et al. [40] also did not identify K-Ras mutations in 40 AAs. It is interesting to note that epidermal growth factor receptor (EGFR) is overexpressed in both adrenal adenomas and carcinomas [41, 42]. Moreover, as the signal transducing tyrosine kinase activity of the EGFR is mediated by Ras proteins among others, it is conceivable that chronically active wild-type Ras promotes tumorigenesis through activation of multiple Ras effectors that contribute to deregulated cell growth, dedifferentiation, and increased survival, migration and invasion. Epidermal growth factor (EGF) is not overexpressed in ACCs, but EGFR may be bound by TGFα, which is a natural ligand for EGFR and is often found in adrenal tumors [42].

SCCRO is a novel gene involved in the hedgehog-signaling pathway of mammalian development, including the adrenal cortex. SCCRO is one of the newly described "onco-developmental" genes, important in normal cellular function in the regulated state and carcinogenesis in the deregulated state. In a recent study of murine ACC [43] high levels of SCCRO were observed in 94% of benign adrenal adenomas, while loss of SCCRO was related to over 65% of ACC. Loss of expression was related to a worse outcome and may represent a marker of dedifferentiation.

Genetic mutation is an important player in the development of adrenal tumor. The other important players include proteins in the tumor microenvironment. Bleuschlein and colleagues described newly discovered roles of proteins and peptides in both the murine and human models of adrenal tumors [44]. Inhibin and activin are dimeric glycoproteins in the TGFβ (Βετα) family of ligands. Activin is a ubiquitous protein, while inhibin is expressed mostly in the gonads, adrenal cortex, and pituitary gland. They are known to play as important paracrine and autocrine effectors, regulating growth and differentiation. Archival ACC immunostaining has shown the presence of strong inhibin and activin receptor [45]. Activin has been shown to inhibit proliferation, induce apoptosis, and modulate ACTH-induced cortisol secretion. In vitro, activin treatment of ACC-cultured cells inhibits steroidogenesis in a dose-dependent manner.

Significant progress has been made through molecular studies of the pathogenesis of adrenal tumors, both adenoma and carcinomas. Since the 1990s, molecular understanding of adrenal tumorigenesis has significantly progressed beyond TP53. Other alterations have been described at the genomic, transcript, or protein levels [46–48]. These mutations or alterations can involve growth factors (IGF-II) [49], cell cycle regulation (TP53, CHEK2) [22], signal transduction (cAMP and Wnt) [50], and cellular receptor, resulting in deregulated cellular pathways in adrenal adenomas and ACCs. Synthesizing these observations, a proposed multistep model of tumorigenesis had been described, where progress from one step to another is associated with acquiring additional gene mutations [22]. Additionally, paracrine and autocrine factors, such as activin and inhibin, had been observed to be important in regulating growth and differentiation of adrenal tumors. The complex interplay of molecular genetic alterations and autocrine and paracrine signals in the microenvironment is just the simplest and most superficial understanding of the molecular pathogenesis of adrenal tumors. Expanding the molecular pathogenesis of adrenal tumor will improve the ability for further drug development to deliver personalized cancer care.

Clinical Presentations

Most commonly encountered in primary care medicine or endocrinology are adrenal incidentalomas or hormone-secreting ademonas. Incidentalomas are adrenal tumors most commonly discerned as an incidental finding, in up to 3% of abdominal imaging and 10% of autopsies [51]. These are mass lesions greater than 1 cm that are serendipitously discovered by radiologic examination. In the Mayo Clinic series of 61,054 abdominal CT scans performed from 1985 to 1990, adrenal masses were seen in 2,066 patients (3%) and adrenal incidentalomas were observed in 259 patients (1%) [51]. Bilateral adrenal masses are seen in about 10–15% of adrenal incidentalomas where 9% are caused by adrenal metastases and 10% had bilateral adrenal incidentalomas [52]. Although most incidentalomas are nonfunctional, functional tumors are observed in small subset of patients with incidentalomas. Based on large series of 1,004 adrenal incidentalomas, approximately 15% are functional, where most frequent is cortisol (9%) producing and causing subclinical Cushing's syndrome, and the remaining functional incidentalomas are pheochromocytomaS (4%) and aLdosteronomas (2%) [53]. Therefore, many experts and treatment guidelines had endorsed evaluation of adrenal incidentalomas suggesting that all of these patients should be screened for the possibility of malignancy and subclinical hormonal hyper-function. A homogeneous adrenal mass <4 cm in diameter, with a smooth border, and an attenuation value of <10 Housefield unit (HU) on unenhanced CT and a rapid contrast medium washout (>50% at 10 min) is very likely to be a benign adenoma of the adrenal cortex [1, 54]. Subclinical Cushing's syndrome and pheochromocytoma must be ruled out in all patients with newly discovered incidentalomas or adenomas; this step is especially important prior to any invasive or diagnostic tissue procurement. Measurement of 24-h urinary fractionated metanephrines and catecholamines as well as cortisol will help to exclude pheochromocytoma and Cushing's syndrome. However, subclinical Cushing's syndrome will require 1 mg overnight dexamethasone suppression test (DST), where the postovernight DST 8 AM serum cortisol concentration cutoff is >5 μg/dL (>138 nmol/L).

Less frequent than adrenal incidentalomas and adenomas are ACCs. As a result, ACC are not commonly considered as a differential diagnosis of abdominal pain or hormonal syndromes. Typically ACC will appear as unilateral and large adrenal mass. Imaging characteristics suggestive of malignancy (ACC or metastases from elsewhere) include: diameter >4 cm, irregular contour, heterogeneous density, greater than 20 HU, and delayed contrast medium washout (<50% at 10 min) [55]. Symptoms of ACC depend on whether the tumor is a nonsecretor of hormones (nonfunctional) or producer of hormones (functional). Different from adrenal incidentalomas, and adenomas with subclinical hormonal syndromes, patients with functional ACC will manifest overt, characterized manifestation of end-organ effects of the hormones being overproduced, while patients with nonfunctional ACCs will present with vague signs and symptoms relating to the location, bulky, and burden of the cancerous mass.

Approximately 60% of ACC are functional [56–58]. Overproduction of corticosteroids, sex steroids, and least common minerocorticosteroids will cause Cushing's syndrome, virilization and Conn's syndrome, respectively. Adults with hormone-secreting ACCs usually present with Cushing's syndrome alone (45%), mixed Cushing's and virilization syndrome, with overproduction of both glucocorticoids and androgens (25%) [56–58]. Less than 5% with virilization alone, but the presence of virilization in a patient with an adrenal neoplasm suggests an ACC rather than an adenoma. In fact, most ACCs may secrete multiple hormones and may change profile of hormone secretion according to size, growth rate, and histologic differentiation.

Cushing's syndrome results from functional tumors overproducing cortisol. Symptoms vary, but most patients have upper body or truncal obesity, rounded face, and thinning arms and legs. Skin becomes fragile and thin, with frequent ecchymoses. Cutaneous straie may appear on the abdomen, thighs, buttocks, arms, and breasts. Many patients have severe fatigue, proximal muscle weakness, and osteoporosis, hypertension, and glucose intolerance. Neuropsychological manifestations of irritability, anxiety, and depression can be frequent. Women usually have hirsutism, dysmenorrhea or amenorrhea and rarely clitomegaly. Men have decreased fertility with diminished or absent libido. There tends to be more marked virilization in Cushing's syndrome caused by ACC than adrenal adenomas, given a higher rate of cosecretion of 17-ketosteroids and dihydroepiandosterone (DHEA) in malignant tumors [59]. Virilization in women with ACC may be rarely due to free testosterone secretion, while feminization in men with ACC, such as gynecomastia, testicular atrophy and low sperm count, has been observed in patients with tumors secreting aldostenedione, which is peripherally converted to estrogen [3]. Because the incidence of ACC is so rare, a broad differential diagnoses list inclusive of ACC should be considered when evaluating patients with Cushing's or virilizing syndrome.

Patients with nonfunctioning ACC usually present with symptoms relating to the mass-effect of the tumor on its nearby organs, i.e. General or diffuse abdominal discomfort, fullness or early satiety. On radiologic imaging nonfunctioning ACC typically will be large and unilateral.

Regardless of hormonal production or not, most patients with ACC typically will present with advanced disease. Eighty percent of patients, at diagnosis, will have advanced disease, and of those with locally advanced disease, less than 20% will have resectable disease. It remains controversial if patients with functional ACC would be diagnosed at earlier stages of cancer because of symptoms relating to overproduction of hormones.

Pathology

Pathological diagnosis should be done by an experienced pathologist. Differentiation between benign vs. malignant adrenal tumors is still based on macroscopic and microscopic features. Macroscopic features worrisome for malignant process include tumor weight, hemorrhage, tumor capsule invasion, and/or gross vascular invasion. Weiss score is most widely used for grading microscopic features suggestive of a malignant tumor [60, 61]. This classification lists nine histologic criteria associated with adrenal tumors that metastasized or recurred locally. These features include (1) high nuclear grade using the criteria of Fuhrman et al. [62]; (2) mitotic rate >5 per 50 high-power fields; (3) atypical mitotic figures; (4) eosinophilic tumor cell cytoplasm (+75% of tumor cells); (5) diffuse architecture present in >33% of the tumor; (6) necrosis; (7) invasion of venous structures; (8) invasion of sinusoidal structures; and (9) capsular invasion. Using this system of scoring, Weiss found originally and later updated that clinically malignant tumors exhibited >3 of the nine features [61].

Important additional information is gained from immunohistochemistry. Ki67 expression has been suggested to have prognostic implication, as its expression is often the measurement of tumor proliferation index. The Melan-A (MART-1) gene encodes an antigen recognized by cytotoxic T cells. It has been said to be restricted in its expression to melanocytes. However, investigators from Memorial Sloan Kettering Cancer Center have reported that MART-1 has potential diagnostic application in ACC. Once melanoma is excluded, the presence of immunoreactivity for A103 (an antibody to MART-1) excludes any other carcinoma that may enter into differential diagnosis of ACC [63]. Several new markers (LOH at 17p13, IGF-2 overexpression, Cyclin E) have been proposed to separate benign from malignant adrenal lesions [64–66].

Even when diagnostic material is available, the distinction between benign and malignant adrenal tumors may be difficult. Unfortunately, the only definitive diagnostic criteria for a malignant adrenal tumor are presence of distant metastasis or local vascular invasion. In the absence of these findings, even using the Weiss scoring system will only provide the likelihood of malignant behavior.

Diagnostic Evaluation and Cancer Staging

Careful endocrine assessment is crucial prior to adrenal surgery. Because subclinical Cushing's adenomas are common and because pheochromocytomas have serious implications in perioperative management, these two diagnoses need to be part of the differential diagnoses of any workup of adrenal mass, and exclude before invasive intervention. The pattern of hormonal secretion may point to malignant potential of the lesion and may affect surgical strategy. Autonomous cortisol secretion by the tumor is associated with the risk of postoperative adrenal insufficiency. Additionally, endocrine evaluation at baseline will establish tumor markers for monitoring in tumor progression or recurrence. Lastly because medical and surgical management of ACC is different from pheochromomocytoma, it is important to differentiate the two disease processes by hormonal profile.

Both size and appearance of adrenal mass on computerized tomography (CT), magnetic resonance imagining (MRI), and more recently 18F-fluorodeoxyglucose positron emission tomography (FDG-PET) have been used to distinguish between benign and malignant lesions. None of these imaging tests are specific for malignancy but each modality serves as complementary to each other. The size of the adrenal mass, as measured by CT or MRI, remains one of the best indicators of malignant potential. According to National Institute of Health (NIH) consensus conference, adrenal mass larger than 6 cm is highly suspicious for malignancy, requiring surgically removal [67]. On the other hand, adrenal mass smaller than 3 cm is less likely to be malignant and can be monitored. Adrenal masses between 3 and 6 cm represent the main diagnostic challenge. Though no single diagnostic method or approach will resolve this challenge, clinical suspicion, imaging quality, and rate or quality adrenal mass change, together will contribute to improve the diagnostic accuracy to differentiate malignant from benign adrenal tumors.

Malignant adrenal tumor or ACC will appear on CT scans as inhomogeneous with irregular margins and irregular enhancement of solid components after IV contrast administration. Local invasion or tumor extension into the inferior vena cava along with spread to nonregional lymph nodes are common in advanced ACCs. Measurement of HU in unenhanced CT is useful for differentiating malignant from benign adrenal lesions. Using a threshold value of 10 HU sensitivity and specificity for characterization, an adrenal lesion as a benign adenoma in unenhanced CT was 71 and 98% in a meta-analysis of ten studies [68, 69]. Adrenal lesions with an attenuation value of >10 HU in unenhanced CT or an enhancement washout of less than 50% and a delayed attenuation of greater than 35 HU (on 10–15 min delayed enhanced CT) are suspicious for malignancy [69]. There is no clear evidence that MRI is any more effective as CT in distinguishing malignant from benign lesions. Sensitivity of MRI from differentiating benign and malignant adrenal masses ranged between 81 and 89% with specificity between 92 and 99% (Fig. 12.1) [70]. One useful characteristic of MRI is the fact that it can identify tumor invasion into the inferior vena cava, allowing for better surgical planning. In few published case series, suggestions were made that FDG-PET could be better for differentiating malignant from benign

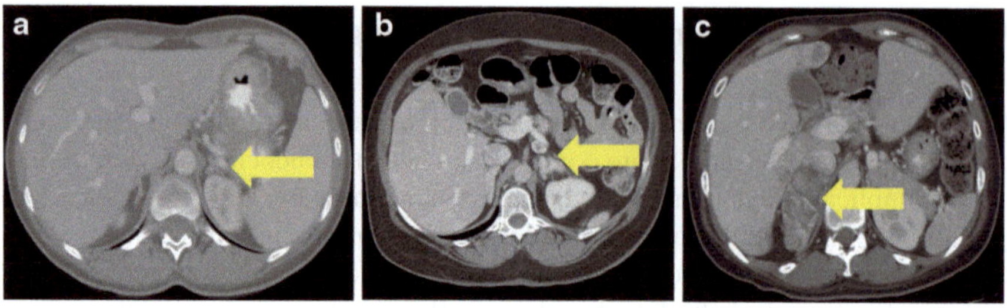

Fig. 12.1 Patient with (**a**) normal adrenal gland, (**b**) adrenal hyperplasia, and (**c**) adrenocortical carcinoma

adrenal tumors. However, without prospective or consistent data, no conclusion can be made about the applicability of FDG-PET for diagnosing and staging of ACCs. Depending on which discipline of medicine is caring for patients with adrenal tumors, tissue diagnosis may or may not be required. In traditional oncology, tissue diagnosis is necessary especially since the risks to the patients with already advanced and unresectable disease are outweighed by the benefits of certainty of diagnosis. in non-oncology disciplines, common belief that fine needle aspiration may result in tract metastases and is of limited diagnostic value, and should be reserved for adrenal tumor that is unresectable or metastatic. However, there is no real concrete evidence to validate this belief. In fact, because of the narrow therapeutic index of systemic therapy for ACCs, little evidence of seeding of cancer cells with a fine needle aspiration, and benefit of accurate and consistent diagnosis for communication between different research disciplines as well as for clinical extrapolation of data into treatment practice, tissue diagnosis is encouraged and recommended when working up patients with adrenal tumors. Once a diagnosis of ACC is made, cancer staging is performed to assess spread of disease and its hormonal functionality.

Hormonal evaluation in apparently asymptomatic patients has been debated. Most suggest that even in asymptomatic patients, the following tests should be performed to determine the secretory capacity of the tumor: fasting blood glucose, serum potassium, 24-h urinary free cortisol, fasting serum cortisol at 8 AM following a 1-mg DST at bedtime, serum estradiol, estrone, and adrenal androgens. Because of the significant adverse clinical outcomes with undiagnosed pheochromocytoma, most experts advocated that plasma metanephrines or urinary metanephrines and catecholamines be obtained in all patients to exclude pheochromocytoma, regardless of clinical suspicion. Additionally because of the infrequency of aldosterone over-secreting tumor in malignant adrenal tumors, plasma aldosterone and renin should be at baseline and with clinical suspicion for hyperaldosteronism.

Cancer treatment is dependent on stage of disease. Diagnostic imaging with CT, MRI, and FDG-PET scans formulate the foundation for staging. Bones scan or bone survey is indicated if there are relevant clinical signs and symptoms of bony involvement. In recent years, FDG-PET scan has been used by clinicians to distinguish benign and malignant lesions as well as staging of asymptomatic or occult metastatic sites [71]. However, the use of FDG-PET scan to diagnosis and stage patients with

ACC has yet to be validated. Integrated PET-CT imaging improves the performance of PET because adrenal adenomas can be better differentiated from nonadenomas using a combination of CT attenuation measurements plus the intensity of FDG update, as described by the standardized uptake value (SUV) for the adrenal lesion [71]. Using PET alone (with an SUV cutoff of 3.1), the sensitivity, specificity, positive predictive value, and negative predictive values for malignant lesions vs. adenomas were 99, 92, 89, and 99%, respectively. The corresponding values for PET-CT were 100, 98, 97, and 100%, respectively [71]. A new method of adrenal imagining is ^{11}C-methodmidate-PET. Metomidate binds to adrenal 11-β-hydroxylase and is, therefore, an excellent tool to distinguish lesions of adrenal origin from other lesions [72]. This is still mostly available in research centers in Europe.

For practical reasons, most experts and investigators in the field of adrenal tumors use surgical staging systems, based upon tumor size, nodal involvement and the presence or absence of metastases that was developed initially by MacFarlane et al. in 1958, and subsequently modified by Sullivan et al. in 1978. The variability in the staging systems used in individual studies complicates any comparison of reported results. Using data from most of other publications, particularly the staging system proposed in Lee et al. [73], the latest proposal for unification and revision of TNM staging system was suggested in 2009 by the European Network for the Study of Adrenal Tumors Classification (ENSAT 2008) [74], which was recently validated [75]. Five-year disease-specific survival rates were 82% (stage I), 61% (stage II), 50% (stage III), and 13% (stage IV) [74]. The American Joint Cancer Committee (AJCC) introduced their first TNM staging system for ACC in version 7 [76]. Table 12.2 summarized the AJCC staging system for ACC.

Natural History and Prognosis

The Majority of patients will present with advanced stage disease. Almost 70% of ACC has spread beyond the adrenal gland at the time of diagnosis. At diagnosis, patients with stages I and II will comprise about 32% of the population and 68% will present with stages III and IV. Stage by stage, the more advanced stage of disease correlates with less durable survival rate. Complete resection is the chance for cure among patients who present with locally advanced and resectable disease. Eighty percent of ACC patients will have local recurrence or metastatic disease, after radical resection and/or curative resection. Published data on cohorts with adult ACCs have suggested that risk of recurrence is increased among patients with large primary tumor size (>10 cm), capsular extension, vascular invasion, incomplete resection, and possibly even type of surgical approaches (laparatomy vs. laparoscope) [77]. Other case series also reported that the overall survival time was higher in patients with recurrent cancer, having prior radiologic and/or clinical responses to mitotane than in patients who had disease progression while on mitotane [78]. Observations from moderate-sized case–control series had suggested that patients with functional ACCs will typical have poorer survival than those without hormonal overproduction. In practice, these

Table 12.2 Adrenocortical carcinoma TNM staging modified from AJCC version 7

Definitions of T, N, and M	
Primary tumor (T)	
TX	Primary tumor cannot be assessed
T0	No evidence of primary tumor
T1	Tumor ≤5 cm in greatest diameter, no extra-adrenal invasion
T2	Tumor >5 cm in greatest diameter, no extra-adrenal invasion
T3	Tumor of any size with local invasion, but not invading adjacent organs (kidney, diaphragm, great vessels, pancreas, spleen, and liver)
T4	Tumor of any size with invasion of adjacent organs (kidney, diaphragm, great vessels, pancreas, spleen, and liver)
Regional lymph nodes (N)	
NX	Regional lymph nodes (aortic, para- or peri-aortic, retroperitoneal) cannot be assessed
N0	No regional lymph node metastasis
N1	Metastasis in regional lymph node(s)
Distant metastasis (M)	
M0	No distant metastasis
M1	Distant metastasis

Clinical cancer stage grouping	Five years survival rate[a] (%)	T	N	M
Stage I	65	T1	N0	M0
Stage II	65	T2	N0	M0
Stage III	40	T1	N1	M0
		T2	N1	M0
		T3	N0	M0
Stage IV	<10	T3	N1	M0
		T4	N0	M0
		T4	N1	M0
		Any T	Any N	M1

[a]http://www.cancer.org/cancer/adrenalcorticalcancer/overviewguide/adrenal-cortical-cancer-overview-survival-rates (accessed on 8/23/2010)

observations make sense, since most patients with Cushing's syndrome would be already immunosuppressed even prior to any systemic cytotoxic therapy [79]. However, validation of any potential predictive or prognostic factors will be very difficult since the incidence and prevalence of ACC are extremely rare. The most frequently reported pattern of spread in patients with ACC included distant metastases to the liver, lung, lymph nodes, and bone [56].

The most consistent and reliable clinical factors for predicting prognosis of ACC are stage of disease and quality of surgical resection [56, 58]. Morphologic characteristics of highly proliferative or very aggressive cancer had been included in factors of poor prognosis for patients with ACCs. These include tumor necrosis, high atypical mitotic figures, and Ki67 [25]. Additional factors, not commonly recognized, but been associated with poor prognosis are nuclear grade, clear cell component, diffuse architecture, vascular, or tumor capsule invasions [60]. In recent years, with the advances of the human genome, tissue microarray has enabled multimolecular profiling. Investigators from Memorial Sloan-Kettering Cancer Center analyzed molecular profile of 124 patients with ACC or adrenal adenomas, correlating with disease outcome, particularly the disease-specific survival. These investigators discovered that there was a significant variation in cell cycle regulatory protein expression among ACCs and between tumor and normal tissue. Furthermore, the presence of distant metastases, older age (>45 years), and incomplete resection (R1) were determinants of poor survival [25]. Molecular alterations reported to have poor prognostic implication in ACCs including amplification of 6q, 7p, 12q and 19p, losses of 3, 8, 10p, 16q, 17q and 19q [80]. Other investigators had suggested that *PINK1* and *BUB1B* are predicative of survival [81]. Investigators from the University of Michigan reported that poor prognosis is being associated with mutations at 1q, 22p, 10p, and 6p [82], whereas good prognosis is being correlated with mutations at 16p and 5q. Predictive of survival was consistently found to be associated with aberrant expressions of genes involved in cell-cycle function and chromosomal instability.

Despite or perhaps because of being a rare malignancy, natural history of disease in patients with ACC is variable especially among patients with advanced disease. At the time of diagnosis, 40–70% of the patients would have advanced unresectable or metastatic ACCs [73]. Prognosis for patients with ACC is very poor, with 13% 5-year survival rate for stage IV. Recurrence would be frequent after surgery, and most common site of recurrence would be the resected bed. Most common site of distant metastasis included liver, lung, lymph nodes, and bone. Many had been reported, but the most commonly recognized predictive histologic characteristics include number of atypical mitotic figures, level of Ki67 staining, presence of tumor necrosis, lymphovascular, and/or tumor capsule invasion. Significant progress had been gained to better understand the molecular tumorigenesis of ACCs. Molecular alterations of genes involved in cell-cycle and chromosomal instability may be prognostic, and differential expressions of these genes may explain the clinical heterogeneity in advanced ACC. However, current molecular signatures are inadequate evidence for practice changing. The most reliable survival factors are stage of disease at the time of diagnosis and completeness of initial curative surgery.

Treatment and Management

Accurate diagnosis and complete staging of patients presenting with newly diagnosed ACC will provide health providers with an opportunity for optimize treatment planning. Surgery still has the best chance for cure. Simply, the size of ACC at the time of diagnosis plays an important role in determining if curative surgery is even possible. Despite curability with complete surgical resection, rate of recurrence is unacceptably high. On the other hand, for metastatic or recurrent diseases that are not resectable, treatment options are limited to chemotherapy with or without mitotane. However, options for systemic treatment are associated with significant therapy-related toxicities without clear survival improvement. At most centers of excellence, specialized in the management of adrenal tumors, multidisciplinary approach to patients with ACC usually produced the best clinical outcomes.

Localized Resectable Disease

Surgery: Complete surgical resection is the only potentially curative treatment for ACC. Curative surgery would be possible only in the minority of patients with locally advanced disease. Median survival of patients with completely resected tumors is 46 months, compared with only 8.5 months if the tumor were incompletely resected [83]. Laparoscopic adrenalectomy should be reserved for presumed benign cortical tumors (<3 cm), aldosteromas, and pheochromomocytomas and for the rare patient who requires palliative adrenalectomy for metastatic disease. Consensus from experts recommend for a trans-abdominal approach through a subcostal incision for any suspected or proven adrenal malignancy, facilitating maximal exposure for complete surgical resection and minimizing tumor spillage. In a retrospective review of 88 patients (71 laparatomy, 17 laparoscope) who underwent curative surgery, Miller et al. [77] observed no statistical difference in rates of local (20 vs. 25%, $p=0.23$) and peritoneal (11 vs. 18%, $p=0.22$). However, the type of surgery has a significant adverse impact on clearing margins of resection/intraoperative tumor spillage (18 vs. 50%, $p=0.01$) and time to local recurrence (19 vs. 10 months, $p<0.005$). Definitive interpretation of this finding can be made, since the study was underpowered. The presence of IVC invasion should not be considered as metastatic disease, but rather, as tumor extension. The indication of total tumor excision in patients with stage III and IV disease remains controversial.

Recurrence rate remains unacceptably high even after curative surgery. Consistent with findings for other complex surgeries [84], outcomes appear to favor patients who had their primary curative surgeries at academic institutions or centers of excellence [8]. In the analysis of 218 cases of ACC patients who had underwent curative surgeries, Grubbs et al. from University of Texas at M D Anderson Cancer Center [8] reported 82% recurrence rate, where the rate of cancer recurrence was negatively correlated with where surgery was performed; recurrence occurred in 50% of patients who had surgeries at M D Anderson (index group), while occurred in 86% of those who had surgeries at outside institutions/communities (outside group). When survival outcomes were compared between index and outside groups, the quality of surgery also significantly impact survival outcomes; median overall survival (OS: not reach vs. 44 months, $p=0.02$) and disease-free survival (DFS: 25 vs. 12 months, $p=0.003$).

Postoperative (Adjuvant) Therapy

Looking to improve poor survival and high recurrence rates after curative surgery, adjuvant therapy had been used. By definition, adjuvant therapy is additional therapy given after curative surgery, and appropriate design to evaluate the role of adjuvant therapy is a randomized study comparing therapy vs. observation after curative surgery. Anecdotal reports suggest that there are benefits but definitive evidence in favor of adjuvant therapy is lacking. At best the existing evidence came from retrospective analyses of case–control series, as there are no randomized controlled clinical studies. Different modalities had been used to reduce the rate of ACC recurrence, including adjuvant radiotherapy, chemotherapy, and mitotane.

The use of radiotherapy had been limited to palliation of symptoms in cases of unresectable or metastatic ACC. Adjuvant radiotherapy is less clearly defined as very little information about its efficacy has been reported. Fassnacht et al. [85] reported on a retrospective analysis of matching case–control comparison between 28 patients (Control: 14 received no adjuvant radiotherapy, Treatment: 14 received adjuvant radiotherapy) with resected ACC who were treated with or without adjuvant radiotherapy. This exercise was able to demonstrate that adjuvant radiotherapy to the resected tumor bed is effective in reducing the local recurrence, where the probability of local recurrence significantly decreased compared to surgery alone (79 vs. 12%, $p<0.01$). Recurrence frequently developed at the inter-aortocaval region [86]. No significant DFS and OS improvement was seen with adjuvant radiotherapy [85]. Review of published data on adjuvant radiotherapy after curative surgery further justify the need for large well-designed clinical study to better define the role of radiotherapy [86]. Based on current evidence, adjuvant radiotherapy should be considered for selected patients with high risk features such as lymphovascular or capsular invasion, high proliferative indices such as Ki-67 or atypical mitotic figures, large and bulky tumor (stage III), after incomplete resection (R1), and lymph node involvement to regional location (N1 station).

Currently, there are no reports of preoperative or perioperative chemotherapy for patients with resectable ACC going for curative intent. Chemotherapy had been used adjuvantly to improve local and systemic recurrence. Similarly, results from clinical studies are lacking, and so practice of adjuvant chemotherapy remains unknown. Streptozocin is an old cytotoxic chemotherapy, and its mechanism of action is mainly to cause DNA damage by forming cross-links with the guanine nucleotide bases in the DNA. ACC patients who had curative surgery were enrolled into a phase II parallel study of combination of streptozocin plus mitotane (treatment arm = 17 patients) and observation alone (control arm = 11 patients). DFS being the primary endpoint of the study was found to be superior with combination chemotherapy [87]. However, the result did not allow for robust confidence in effectiveness of adjuvant streptozocin because the study was underpowered, nonrandomized, and lacked appropriate control. Furthermore, because there was no adjuvant mitotane alone arm, the role of streptozocin plus mitotane compared to mitotane alone will remain unanswered.

Mitotane (o,p′-DDT) is a derivative of the insecticide dichlorodiphenyltrichloroethane (DDT). Acting as an adrenocorticolytic agent, mitotane is used to control symptoms of hormonal overproduction. Though antitumor activity with mitotane is well-recognized, the exact mechanism for its cytotoxic activity remains poorly understood. While several uncontrolled reports suggest that adjuvant mitotane may delay or prevent recurrence in patients undergoing curative surgery [88–90], others fail to support any benefit in terms of DFS or OS [91, 92]. Reasons for this disparity in results include lack of well-designed clinical trials and inconsistency in dose and duration of mitotane administered. The best available evidence for meaningful benefit with adjuvant mitotane came from a retrospective analysis of 177 combined patients with ACC after undergoing R0 (complete) or R1 (microscopically incomplete) from Italy and Germany. Specifically, adjuvant low dose (2–3 g daily) mitotane for median duration of 2–3 years can favorably modify median recurrence-free survival (42 vs. 10–25 months), death (25 vs. 41–51%), and overall survival (110 vs. 52–67 months) [93]. Despite the study results, adjuvant mitotane remains controversial until randomized controlled study powered to detect meaningful improvement of survival outcomes. It is necessary to weigh risks and benefits of mitotane and decision to recommend for adjuvant therapy should be made case-by-case.

Locally Advanced Unresectable and Metastatic Disease

Medical therapy: The Majority of ACC patients will present with unresectable disease or metastatic disease, requiring medical therapy with either hormonal control if disease is functional and/or cytotoxic therapy with combination chemotherapy or mitotane alone.

Hormonal management: Hyper-secretion of hormonal steroids in ACC frequently contributes to the disease burden and can severely affect quality of life. Therapy for endocrine syndromes of ACC can be either with surgical removal of hormonogenic tissues, or with medical treatment. Medical treatment can be either blockade of hormonal secretion, anti-tumor therapy or both hormonal suppression and anti-tumor like mitotane. Due to its slow-to-reach therapeutic level and its dose-limiting toxicity, mitotane alone is frequently insufficient to rapidly control hyper-secretion of all patients. The Majority of medical treatments use for hormonal control does not translate into tumor response, as the objective of therapy in medical hormonal control is to improve quality of life and is not associated with therapeutic tumor response. Agents used for hormonal control include ketoconazole (weakly and nonselectively inhibits several p450 enzymes involved in adrenal steroid synthesis), metyrapone (inhibits adrenal 11β-hydroxylase), aminoglutethimide (inhibits enzymatic conversion of cholesterol to pregnenolone), mifepristone (blocks progesterone and glucocorticoid receptors), etomidate (inhibits adrenal 11β-hydroxylase), and mitotane. Single agent or combination of different agents is used to control hormonal overproduction.

Cytotoxic chemotherapy: Experience with cytotoxic chemotherapy in ACC is limited, probably due to the rarity of disease leading to very few well-designed studies to assess the efficacy of therapy. Several combinations of cytotoxic agents have been used and the available evidence suggests that cisplatin-based chemotherapy has activity in ACC. Various chemotherapy regimens have been combined with mitotane, which theoretically added to the efficacy of the cytotoxic agent by blocking cellular efflux via MDR suppression. Berruti et al. reported an objective response rate with mitotane–etoposide–adriamycin–cisplatin (M-EAP) combination chemotherapy of 49% among 28 patients with advanced ACC [94]. This success comes at the cost of significant toxicity. Since then other studies have not been able to reproduce the same tumor efficacy, and response rate with cisplatin-based chemotherapy is approximately 20–30% [95]. Another regimen proposed because of less side effects profile is a combination of mitotane–streptozotocin (M-S), where Khan et al. reported an objective response rate of 36% among eight patients with advanced ACC [87]. Review of selected published data using combination chemotherapy in advanced ACC resulted in tumor response rate of about 32%. Without randomized control trial via large international efforts, the optimal frontline chemotherapy regimen cannot be determined. The same large cooperative effort will also be required to assess whether or not the addition of mitotane to chemotherapy regimen will increase tumor response rate. Currently international cooperation has lead to the ongoing trial, FIRM-ACT, where patients with advanced ACC are randomized between the M-EAP and M-S as frontline therapy [96]. Though no results had been released, the study was reported to be near completion.

Mitotane: Mitotane (Lysodren, HRA Pharma Paris, Bristol Meyer Squibb New York, o,p′-DDD) is the only FDA-approved drug for the treatment of ACC. It is developed in 1960 as an insecticide (DDT) and is taken up by adrenal cortex, causing necrosis of the adrenal cortex. Uniquely, mitotane is used for both blockage of hormonal production in functional ACC as well as anti-tumor for metastatic or unresectable ACC. Mechanism of action remains unclear, but mitotane is thought to exert specific cytotoxic effect on adrenocortical cells producing focal degeneration of the fasicular and particularly the reticular zone whereas changes of the zona glomerulosa are relatively slight. Impairment of adrenal steroidogenesis is due to a direct inhibitory effect of the enzymes, particularly 11β-hydroxylase and cholesterol side chain cleavage [97].

Mitotane is a difficult drug to manage as it has a narrow therapeutic index, where antitumor activity occurred at level >14 mg/L but toxic side effects occurred at level >22 mg/L. Only a few patients reach target levels within 4–6 weeks, whereas in the majority of patients it takes several weeks to months [98]. Aside from adrenal suppression/insufficiency, side effects of mitotane are many but frequently gastrointestinal or involve the central nervous system [99]. In general, adverse effects are reversible after cessation of mitotane. However since mitotane accumulate in adipose tissue, half-life is long, blood levels and adverse effects usually increase over time even if the dose remains unchanged. Patients on mitotane should be monitored for side effects and have close surveillance of blood level of mitotane, adrenal function, and clinical evidence of side effects. Due to its adrenolytic activity and increased metabolic clearance of glucocorticoids, adrenal replacement with long-acting glucocorticoids such as decadron and prednisone are necessary. Because the clinical manifestations of mitotane side effects and those of mitotane-induced adrenal insufficiency are the same, high awareness of the both will allow for better compliance. We recommend that patients start with low dose (1.5–2 g/day) of mitotane and titrate 0.5 g weekly, to reach therapeutic serologic level. Concurrent administration of glucocorticoids is also recommended. Blood level of mitotane can be evaluated after 2 weeks of starting therapy, and serum ACTH, renin, 24-h urine free cortisol (UFC) or 17-OH cortisol (17OHCS) are used to monitor adequate adrenal function. Patients on mitotane are also recommended to discontinue the drug in case of trauma, surgery, shock or other medical insult (e.g., sepsis) and institute aggressive adrenal replacement therapy.

Mitotane is given in several clinical usages including recurrent, metastatic or unresectable disease alone or in combination with other cytotoxic agents. Though still considered controversial, mitotane has been used in the setting of adjuvant therapy after curative or complete surgical resection. It controls endocrine hypersecretion of patients with functional ACC as originally described more than 50 years ago by Bergenstal et al. [100]. As a single agent, the average objective tumor response rate of mitotane is seen in up to 20–30% of patients [97, 101]. Hormonal amelioration is usually – but not always – correlated with tumor response. Mitotane control of endocrine hyper-secretion usually occurs with serum mitotane concentrations >7 mg/L, and objective antitumor response and long-term survival benefits are observed only when serum mitotane concentrations are consistently >14 mg/L [101, 102].

For those patients lucky enough to present with resectable disease, approximately 70–80% will have recurrent or metastatic disease, after curative resection. Unfortunately, there is no curative therapy for recurrent ACCs. Management of patients with recurrent disease will also depend on the type of recurrence – locoregional or distant. The goal of therapy for distant recurrence of ACC is palliative and the foundation of therapy is systemic treatment with or without medical therapy for hormonal control. Patients with recurrent locoregional ACC should be assessed for completed surgical removal of disease. If complete removal of the recurrent ACC can be achieved, surgery would be recommended [103, 104]. However, if recurrent disease is not amenable to complete resection surgery is not feasible because of medical condition.

Summary and Future Direction

ACC is a rare malignancy. The Majority of patients will present with advanced disease, and thus majority of patients with ACC do not qualify for curative resection. Despite curative resection, approximately 80% of patients will recur, both at the resected bed or metastatic disease. Treatment options for advanced disease are often limited to either mitotane alone or combination chemotherapy with or without mitotane. Multidisciplinary approach has the best chance for optimized management of this lethal orphan disease. Improved understanding of the molecular pathogenesis had already initiated several large clinical trials. Improved understanding of the molecular tumorigenesis of this rare malignancy and collaborative effort will lead to advancement in the effective and tolerable therapies that may improve this disease outcome.

References

1. Angeli A, Osella G, Ali A, Terzolo M. Adrenal incidentaloma: an overview of clinical and epidemiological data from the National Italian Study Group. Horm Res. 1997; 47(4–6):279–83.
2. Wajchenberg BL, Albergaria Pereira MA, Medonca BB, et al. Adrenocortical carcinoma: clinical and laboratory observations. Cancer. 2000;88(4):711–36.
3. Luton JP, Cerdas S, Billaud L, et al. Clinical features of adrenocortical carcinoma, prognostic factors, and the effect of mitotane therapy. N Engl J Med. 1990;322(17): 1195–201.
4. Dackiw AP, Lee JE, Gagel RF, Evans DB. Adrenal cortical carcinoma. World J Surg. 2001;25(7):914–26.
5. Wooten MD, King DK. Adrenal cortical carcinoma. Epidemiology and treatment with mitotane and a review of the literature. Cancer. 1993;72(11):3145–55.
6. Crucitti F, Bellantone R, Ferrante A, Boscherini M, Crucitti P. The Italian Registry for Adrenal Cortical Carcinoma: analysis of a multiinstitutional series of 129 patients. The ACC Italian Registry Study Group. Surgery. 1996;119(2):161–70.
7. Xiao XR, Ye LY, Shi LX, Cheng GF, Li YT, Zhou BM. Diagnosis and treatment of adrenal tumours: a review of 35 years' experience. Br J Urol. 1998;82(2):199–205.
8. Grubbs EG, Callender GG, Xing Y, et al. Recurrence of adrenal cortical carcinoma following resection: surgery alone can achieve results equal to surgery plus mitotane. Ann Surg Oncol. 2010;17(1):263–70.
9. Koch CA, Pacak K, Chrousos GP. The molecular pathogenesis of hereditary and sporadic adrenocortical and adrenomedullary tumors. J Clin Endocrinol Metab. 2002;87(12): 5367–84.
10. Sidhu S, Sywak M, Robinson B, Delbridge L. Adrenocortical cancer: recent clinical and molecular advances. Curr Opin Oncol. 2004;16(1):13–8.
11. Lynch HT, Harris RE, Guirgis HA, Maloney K, Carmody LL, Lynch JF. Familial association of breast/ovarian carcinoma. Cancer. 1978;41(4):1543–9.
12. Hollstein M, Sidransky D, Vogelstein B, Harris CC. p53 mutations in human cancers. Science. 1991;253(5015):49–53.
13. Vogelstein B, Lane D, Levine AJ. Surfing the p53 network. Nature. 2000; 408(6810): 307–10.
14. Shao J, Fujiwara T, Kadowaki Y, et al. Overexpression of the wild-type p53 gene inhibits NF-kappaB activity and synergizes with aspirin to induce apoptosis in human colon cancer cells. Oncogene. 2000;19(6):726–36.
15. Lemos MC, Thakker RV. Multiple endocrine neoplasia type 1 (MEN1): analysis of 1336 mutations reported in the first decade following identification of the gene. Hum Mutat. 2008;29(1):22–32.
16. Balogh K, Racz K, Patocs A, Hunyady L. Menin and its interacting proteins: elucidation of menin function. Trends Endocrinol Metab. 2006;17(9):357–64.

17. Lynch HT, Radford B, Lynch JF. SBLA syndrome revisited. Oncology. 1990;47(1):75–9.
18. Henry I, Jeanpierre M, Couillin P, et al. Molecular definition of the 11p15.5 region involved in Beckwith-Wiedemann syndrome and probably in predisposition to adrenocortical carcinoma. Hum Genet. 1989;81(3):273–7.
19. Lam WW, Hatada I, Ohishi S, et al. Analysis of germline CDKN1C (p57KIP2) mutations in familial and sporadic Beckwith-Wiedemann syndrome (BWS) provides a novel genotype-phenotype correlation. J Med Genet. 1999;36(7):518–23.
20. Catchpoole D, Smallwood AV, Joyce JA, et al. Mutation analysis of H19 and NAP1L4 (hNAP2) candidate genes and IGF2 DMR2 in Beckwith-Wiedemann syndrome. J Med Genet. 2000;37(3):212–5.
21. Hertel NT, Carlsen N, Kerndrup G, et al. Late relapse of adrenocortical carcinoma in Beckwith-Wiedemann syndrome. Clinical, endocrinological and genetic aspects. Acta Paediatr. 2003;92(4):439–43.
22. Stratakis CA. New genes and/or molecular pathways associated with adrenal hyperplasias and related adrenocortical tumors. Mol Cell Endocrinol. 2009;300(1–2):152–7.
23. Libe R, Bertherat J. Molecular genetics of adrenocortical tumours, from familial to sporadic diseases. Eur J Endocrinol. 2005;153(4):477–87.
24. Latronico AC, Pinto EM, Domenice S, et al. An inherited mutation outside the highly conserved DNA-binding domain of the p53 tumor suppressor protein in children and adults with sporadic adrenocortical tumors. J Clin Endocrinol Metab. 2001;86(10):4970–3.
25. Stojadinovic A, Ghossein RA, Hoos A, et al. Adrenocortical carcinoma: clinical, morphologic, and molecular characterization. J Clin Oncol. 2002;20(4):941–50.
26. Figueiredo BC, Cavalli LR, Pianovski MA, et al. Amplification of the steroidogenic factor 1 gene in childhood adrenocortical tumors. J Clin Endocrinol Metab. 2005;90(2):615–9.
27. Gicquel C, Raffin-Sanson ML, Gaston V, et al. Structural and functional abnormalities at 11p15 are associated with the malignant phenotype in sporadic adrenocortical tumors: study on a series of 82 tumors. J Clin Endocrinol Metab. 1997;82(8):2559–65.
28. Gicquel C, Bertagna X, Schneid H, et al. Rearrangements at the 11p15 locus and overexpression of insulin-like growth factor-II gene in sporadic adrenocortical tumors. J Clin Endocrinol Metab. 1994;78(6):1444–53.
29. Gicquel C, Bertagna X, Gaston V, et al. Molecular markers and long-term recurrences in a large cohort of patients with sporadic adrenocortical tumors. Cancer Res. 2001;61(18):6762–7.
30. Libe R, Coste J, Guignat L, et al. Aberrant cortisol regulations in bilateral macronodular adrenal hyperplasia: a frequent finding in a prospective study of 32 patients with overt or subclinical Cushing's syndrome. Eur J Endocrinol. 2010;163(1):129–38.
31. Lampron A, Bourdeau I, Oble S, et al. Regulation of aldosterone secretion by several aberrant receptors including for glucose-dependent insulinotropic peptide in a patient with an aldosteronoma. J Clin Endocrinol Metab. 2009;94(3):750–6.
32. Zwermann O, Suttmann Y, Bidlingmaier M, Beuschlein F, Reincke M. Screening for membrane hormone receptor expression in primary aldosteronism. Eur J Endocrinol. 2009; 160(3):443–51.
33. Clevers H. Wnt/beta-catenin signaling in development and disease. Cell. 2006;127(3):469–80.
34. Giles RH, van Es JH, Clevers H. Caught up in a Wnt storm: Wnt signaling in cancer. Biochim Biophys Acta. 2003;1653(1):1–24.
35. Tissier F, Cavard C, Groussin L, et al. Mutations of beta-catenin in adrenocortical tumors: activation of the Wnt signaling pathway is a frequent event in both benign and malignant adrenocortical tumors. Cancer Res. 2005;65(17):7622–7.
36. Shields JM, Pruitt K, McFall A, Shaub A, Der CJ. Understanding Ras: 'it ain't over 'til it's over'. Trends Cell Biol. 2000;10(4):147–54.
37. Bos JL. ras oncogenes in human cancer: a review. Cancer Res. 1989;49(17):4682–9.
38. Yashiro T, Hara H, Fulton NC, Obara T, Kaplan EL. Point mutations of ras genes in human adrenal cortical tumors: absence in adrenocortical hyperplasia. World J Surg. 1994;18(4): 455–60; discussion 60–1.

39. Moul JW, Bishoff JT, Theune SM, Chang EH. Absent ras gene mutations in human adrenal cortical neoplasms and pheochromocytomas. J Urol. 1993;149(6):1389–94.
40. Ocker M, Sachse R, Rico A, Hensen J. PCR-SSCP analysis of human adrenocortical adenomas: absence of K-ras gene mutations. Exp Clin Endocrinol Diabetes. 2000; 108(8):513–4.
41. Kamio T, Shigematsu K, Sou H, Kawai K, Tsuchiyama H. Immunohistochemical expression of epidermal growth factor receptors in human adrenocortical carcinoma. Hum Pathol. 1990;21(3):277–82.
42. Sasano H, Suzuki T, Shizawa S, Kato K, Nagura H. Transforming growth factor alpha, epidermal growth factor, and epidermal growth factor receptor expression in normal and diseased human adrenal cortex by immunohistochemistry and in situ hybridization. Mod Pathol. 1994;7(7):741–6.
43. Sarkaria IS, Stojadinovic A, Talbot SG, et al. Squamous cell carcinoma-related oncogene is highly expressed in developing, normal, and adenomatous adrenal tissue but not in aggressive adrenocortical carcinomas. Surgery. 2004;136(6):1122–8.
44. Beuschlein F, Looyenga BD, Bleasdale SE, et al. Activin induces x-zone apoptosis that inhibits luteinizing hormone-dependent adrenocortical tumor formation in inhibin-deficient mice. Mol Cell Biol. 2003;23(11):3951–64.
45. Beuschlein F, Looyenga BD, Reincke M, Hammer GD. Role of the inhibin/activin system and luteinizing hormone in adrenocortical tumorigenesis. Horm Metab Res. 2004; 36(6):392–6.
46. Bourdeau I, Antonini SR, Lacroix A, et al. Gene array analysis of macronodular adrenal hyperplasia confirms clinical heterogeneity and identifies several candidate genes as molecular mediators. Oncogene. 2004;23(8):1575–85.
47. Horvath A, Boikos S, Giatzakis C, et al. A genome-wide scan identifies mutations in the gene encoding phosphodiesterase 11A4 (PDE11A) in individuals with adrenocortical hyperplasia. Nat Genet. 2006;38(7):794–800.
48. Bornstein SR, Hornsby PJ. What can we learn from gene expression profiling for adrenal tumor management? J Clin Endocrinol Metab. 2005;90(3):1900–2.
49. de Fraipont F, El Atifi M, Cherradi N, et al. Gene expression profiling of human adrenocortical tumors using complementary deoxyribonucleic Acid microarrays identifies several candidate genes as markers of malignancy. J Clin Endocrinol Metab. 2005;90(3):1819–29.
50. Gaujoux S, Tissier F, Groussin L, et al. Wnt/beta-catenin and 3',5'-cyclic adenosine 5' monophosphate/protein kinase A signaling pathways alterations and somatic beta-catenin gene mutations in the progression of adrenocortical tumors. J Clin Endocrinol Metab. 2008;93(10):4135–40.
51. Herrera MF, Grant CS, van Heerden JA, Sheedy PF, Ilstrup DM. Incidentally discovered adrenal tumors: an institutional perspective. Surgery. 1991;110(6):1014–21.
52. Kasperlik-Zaluska A, Walecki J, Brzezinski J, et al. MRI versus CT in the diagnosis of Nelson's syndrome. Eur Radiol. 1997;7(1):106–9.
53. Mantero F, Terzolo M, Arnaldi G, et al. A survey on adrenal incidentaloma in Italy. Study Group on Adrenal Tumors of the Italian Society of Endocrinology. J Clin Endocrinol Metab. 2000;85(2):637–44.
54. Young Jr WF. Clinical practice. The incidentally discovered adrenal mass. N Engl J Med. 2007;356(6):601–10.
55. Bovio S, Cataldi A, Reimondo G, et al. Prevalence of adrenal incidentaloma in a contemporary computerized tomography series. J Endocrinol Invest. 2006;29(4):298–302.
56. Ng L, Libertino JM. Adrenocortical carcinoma: diagnosis, evaluation and treatment. J Urol. 2003;169(1):5–11.
57. Allolio B, Fassnacht M. Clinical review: adrenocortical carcinoma: clinical update. J Clin Endocrinol Metab. 2006;91(6):2027–37.
58. Icard P, Goudet P, Charpenay C, et al. Adrenocortical carcinomas: surgical trends and results of a 253-patient series from the French Association of Endocrine Surgeons study group. World J Surg. 2001;25(7):891–7.

59. Michalkiewicz E, Sandrini R, Figueiredo B, et al. Clinical and outcome characteristics of children with adrenocortical tumors: a report from the International Pediatric Adrenocortical Tumor Registry. J Clin Oncol. 2004;22(5):838–45.
60. Weiss LM, Medeiros LJ, Vickery Jr AL. Pathologic features of prognostic significance in adrenocortical carcinoma. Am J Surg Pathol. 1989;13(3):202–6.
61. Medeiros LJ, Weiss LM. New developments in the pathologic diagnosis of adrenal cortical neoplasms. A review. Am J Clin Pathol. 1992;97(1):73–83.
62. Fuhrman SA, Lasky LC, Limas C. Prognostic significance of morphologic parameters in renal cell carcinoma. Am J Surg Pathol. 1982;6(7):655–63.
63. Busam KJ, Chen YT, Old LJ, et al. Expression of melan-A (MART1) in benign melanocytic nevi and primary cutaneous malignant melanoma. Am J Surg Pathol. 1998;22(8): 976–82.
64. Soon PS, Libe R, Benn DE, et al. Loss of heterozygosity of 17p13, with possible involvement of ACADVL and ALOX15B, in the pathogenesis of adrenocortical tumors. Ann Surg. 2008;247(1):157–64.
65. Schmitt A, Saremaslani P, Schmid S, et al. IGFII and MIB1 immunohistochemistry is helpful for the differentiation of benign from malignant adrenocortical tumours. Histopathology. 2006;49(3):298–307.
66. Tissier F, Louvel A, Grabar S, et al. Cyclin E correlates with malignancy and adverse prognosis in adrenocortical tumors. Eur J Endocrinol. 2004;150(6):809–17.
67. Grumbach MM, Biller BM, Braunstein GD, et al. Management of the clinically inapparent adrenal mass ("incidentaloma"). Ann Intern Med. 2003;138(5):424–9.
68. Hamrahian AH, Ioachimescu AG, Remer EM, et al. Clinical utility of noncontrast computed tomography attenuation value (hounsfield units) to differentiate adrenal adenomas/hyperplasias from nonadenomas: Cleveland clinic experience. J Clin Endocrinol Metab. 2005;90(2):871–7.
69. Szolar DH, Korobkin M, Reittner P, et al. Adrenocortical carcinomas and adrenal pheochromocytomas: mass and enhancement loss evaluation at delayed contrast-enhanced CT. Radiology. 2005;234(2):479–85.
70. Israel GM, Korobkin M, Wang C, Hecht EN, Krinsky GA. Comparison of unenhanced CT and chemical shift MRI in evaluating lipid-rich adrenal adenomas. AJR Am J Roentgenol. 2004;183(1):215–9.
71. Groussin L, Bonardel G, Silvera S, et al. 18F-Fluorodeoxyglucose positron emission tomography for the diagnosis of adrenocortical tumors: a prospective study in 77 operated patients. J Clin Endocrinol Metab. 2009;94(5):1713–22.
72. Hennings J, Hellman P, Ahlstrom H, Sundin A. Computed tomography, magnetic resonance imaging and 11C-metomidate positron emission tomography for evaluation of adrenal incidentalomas. Eur J Radiol. 2009;69(2):314–23.
73. Lee JE, Berger DH, el-Naggar AK, et al. Surgical management, DNA content, and patient survival in adrenal cortical carcinoma. Surgery. 1995;118(6):1090–8.
74. Fassnacht M, Johanssen S, Quinkler M, et al. Limited prognostic value of the 2004 International Union Against Cancer staging classification for adrenocortical carcinoma: proposal for a Revised TNM Classification. Cancer. 2009;115(2):243–50.
75. Lughezzani G, Sun M, Perrotte P, et al. The European Network for the Study of Adrenal Tumors staging system is prognostically superior to the international union against cancer-staging system: a North American validation. Eur J Cancer. 2010;46(4):713–9.
76. Edge SB, Byrd DR, Compton CC, Fritz A, Greene FL, Trotti A. AJCC cancer staging handbook. 7th ed. New York: Springer; 2010.
77. Miller BS, Gauger PG, Hammer GD, Giordano TJ, Doherty GM. Proposal for modification of the ENSAT staging system for adrenocortical carcinoma using tumor grade. Langenbecks Arch Surg. 2010;395(7):955–61.
78. Vassilopoulou-Sellin R, Schultz PN. Adrenocortical carcinoma. Clinical outcome at the end of the 20th century. Cancer. 2001;92(5):1113–21.

79. Abiven G, Coste J, Groussin L, et al. Clinical and biological features in the prognosis of adrenocortical cancer: poor outcome of cortisol-secreting tumors in a series of 202 consecutive patients. J Clin Endocrinol Metab. 2006;91(7):2650–5.
80. Stephan EA, Chung TH, Grant CS, et al. Adrenocortical carcinoma survival rates correlated to genomic copy number variants. Mol Cancer Ther. 2008;7(2):425–31.
81. de Reynies A, Assie G, Rickman DS, et al. Gene expression profiling reveals a new classification of adrenocortical tumors and identifies molecular predictors of malignancy and survival. J Clin Oncol. 2009;27(7):1108–15.
82. Giordano TJ, Kuick R, Else T, et al. Molecular classification and prognostication of adrenocortical tumors by transcriptome profiling. Clin Cancer Res. 2009;15(2):668–76.
83. Didolkar MS, Bescher RA, Elias EG, Moore RH. Natural history of adrenal cortical carcinoma: a clinicopathologic study of 42 patients. Cancer. 1981;47(9):2153–61.
84. Reavis KM, Smith BR, Hinojosa MW, Nguyen NT. Outcomes of esophagectomy at academic centers: an association between volume and outcome. Am Surg. 2008;74(10):939–43.
85. Fassnacht M, Hahner S, Polat B, et al. Efficacy of adjuvant radiotherapy of the tumor bed on local recurrence of adrenocortical carcinoma. J Clin Endocrinol Metab. 2006; 91(11):4501–4.
86. Polat B, Fassnacht M, Pfreundner L, et al. Radiotherapy in adrenocortical carcinoma. Cancer. 2009;115(13):2816–23.
87. Khan TS, Imam H, Juhlin C, et al. Streptozocin and o, p'DDD in the treatment of adrenocortical cancer patients: long-term survival in its adjuvant use. Ann Oncol. 2000;11(10):1281–7.
88. Kendrick ML, Lloyd R, Erickson L, et al. Adrenocortical carcinoma: surgical progress or status quo? Arch Surg. 2001;136(5):543–9.
89. Dickstein G, Shechner C, Arad E, Best LA, Nativ O. Is there a role for low doses of mitotane (o, p'-DDD) as adjuvant therapy in adrenocortical carcinoma? J Clin Endocrinol Metab. 1998;83(9):3100–3.
90. Kasperlik-Zaluska AA. Clinical results of the use of mitotane for adrenocortical carcinoma. Braz J Med Biol Res. 2000;33(10):1191–6.
91. Lubitz JA, Freeman L, Okun R. Mitotane use in inoperable adrenal cortical carcinoma. JAMA. 1973;223(10):1109–12.
92. Vassilopoulou-Sellin R, Guinee VF, Klein MJ, et al. Impact of adjuvant mitotane on the clinical course of patients with adrenocortical cancer. Cancer. 1993;71(10):3119–23.
93. Terzolo M, Angeli A, Fassnacht M, et al. Adjuvant mitotane treatment for adrenocortical carcinoma. N Engl J Med. 2007;356(23):2372–80.
94. Berruti A, Terzolo M, Sperone P, et al. Etoposide, doxorubicin and cisplatin plus mitotane in the treatment of advanced adrenocortical carcinoma: a large prospective phase II trial. Endocr Relat Cancer. 2005;12(3):657–66.
95. Quinkler M, Hahner S, Wortmann S, et al. Treatment of advanced adrenocortical carcinoma with erlotinib plus gemcitabine. J Clin Endocrinol Metab. 2008;93(6):2057–62.
96. Koschker AC, Fassnacht M, Hahner S, Weismann D, Allolio B. Adrenocortical carcinoma – improving patient care by establishing new structures. Exp Clin Endocrinol Diabetes. 2006;114(2):45–51.
97. Hahner S, Fassnacht M. Mitotane for adrenocortical carcinoma treatment. Curr Opin Investig Drugs. 2005;6(4):386–94.
98. Terzolo M, Pia A, Berruti A, et al. Low-dose monitored mitotane treatment achieves the therapeutic range with manageable side effects in patients with adrenocortical cancer. J Clin Endocrinol Metab. 2000;85(6):2234–8.
99. Fassnacht M, Allolio B. Clinical management of adrenocortical carcinoma. Best Pract Res Clin Endocrinol Metab. 2009;23(2):273–89.
100. Lipsett MB, Bergenstal DM. The metabolic and corticotrophin-suppressing activity of certain C21-deoxysteroids. Acta Endocrinol (Copenh). 1959;31(1):33–9.
101. Haak HR, Hermans J, van de Velde CJ, et al. Optimal treatment of adrenocortical carcinoma with mitotane: results in a consecutive series of 96 patients. Br J Cancer. 1994;69(5): 947–51.

102. van Slooten H, Moolenaar AJ, van Seters AP, Smeenk D. The treatment of adrenocortical carcinoma with o, p'-DDD: prognostic implications of serum level monitoring. Eur J Cancer Clin Oncol. 1984;20(1):47–53.
103. Schulick RD, Brennan MF. Adrenocortical carcinoma. World J Urol. 1999;17(1):26–34.
104. Bellantone R, Ferrante A, Boscherini M, et al. Role of reoperation in recurrence of adrenal cortical carcinoma: results from 188 cases collected in the Italian National Registry for Adrenal Cortical Carcinoma. Surgery. 1997;122(6):1212–8.

Chapter 13
Pheochromocytoma

Glenda G. Callender, Thereasa Rich, Jeffrey E. Lee, Nancy D. Perrier, and Elizabeth G. Grubbs

Abstract Pheochromocytomas and extra-adrenal paragangliomas are rare tumors that arise from neural crest-derived tissue that exists throughout the body in collections known as paraganglia. Sympathetic paraganglia arise along the distribution of the peripheral sympathetic nervous system, in locations such as the adrenal medulla and the organ of Zuckerkandl near the aortic bifurcation. Parasympathetic paraganglia arise along the cervical and thoracic branches of the vagus and glossopharyngeal nerves, in locations such as the carotid body.

Keywords Pheochromocytoma • Paraganglia • Peripheral sympathetic nervous system • Adrenal medulla • Vagus nerve • Glossopharyngeal nerve • Catecholamines • Hypertension • Diaphoresis

Introduction

Pheochromocytomas and extra-adrenal paragangliomas are rare tumors that arise from neural crest-derived tissue that exists throughout the body in collections known as paraganglia. Sympathetic paraganglia arise along the distribution of the peripheral sympathetic nervous system, in locations such as the adrenal medulla and the organ of Zuckerkandl near the aortic bifurcation. Parasympathetic paraganglia arise along the cervical and thoracic branches of the vagus and glossopharyngeal nerves, in locations such as the carotid body. The most recent World Health Organization classification utilizes the term *pheochromocytoma* for intra-adrenal tumors only,

E.G. Grubbs (✉)
Department of Surgical Oncology,
The University of Texas M.D. Anderson Cancer Center,
1515 Holcombe Boulevard, Unit 444, Houston, TX 77030, USA
e-mail: eggrubbs@mdanderson.org

J.C. Yao et al. (eds.), *Neuroendocrine Tumors*, Current Clinical Oncology,
DOI 10.1007/978-1-60327-997-0_13, © Springer Science+Business Media, LLC 2011

and the term *extra-adrenal paraganglioma* to refer to similar tumors that occur in other locations [1].

Fränkel [2] is credited with the first description of pheochromocytoma in 1886 when he discovered bilateral adrenal masses at the autopsy of an 18-year-old girl who died after suffering intermittent attacks of palpitations, headache, pallor, and sweats. In 1905, Poll [3] coined the term *pheochrome* from *pheo-* (dusky, gray) and *chromo-* (color) which describes the cut surface of this type of tumor after staining with potassium dichromate. In 1912, Pick [4] proposed the name *pheochromocytoma* to refer to adrenal and extra-adrenal tumors of chromaffin cell origin. The first successful operations for pheochromocytoma were performed by César Roux in Lausanne, Switzerland in February 1926, and by Charles Mayo in Rochester, MN in October 1926 [5]. By 1951, 125 operations for pheochromocytoma had been performed, with 33 deaths (26.4%) [6]. Shortly thereafter, availability of the vasoactive agents phentolamine and noradrenaline allowed for far superior intraoperative management, and in 1956, Priestley and colleagues at the Mayo Clinic published a series of 61 pheochromocytomas removed from 51 patients without operative mortality [7]. However, even with the advances of present-day science, pheochromocytoma remains a challenging entity, and meticulous medical and surgical care is required for successful management.

Epidemiology and Risk Factors

The incidence of pheochromocytoma is 2–8 per million persons per year [8, 9]. Pheochromocytoma represents a reversible cause of hypertension in 0.1–1% of hypertensive patients [10–12], and is identified in approximately 5% of incidentally discovered adrenal masses [13]. The incidence is equal between males and females [14], and the average age at diagnosis is 24.9 years in hereditary cases and 43.9 years in sporadic cases [15].

There are no known environmental, dietary, or lifestyle risk factors that have been linked to the development of pheochromocytoma. However, recent data suggest that 12–24% of pheochromocytomas and extra-adrenal paragangliomas occur in the setting of a hereditary syndrome [14–16]. Eight major genetic syndromes have been identified that carry increased risk of pheochromocytoma: multiple endocrine neoplasia types 1 and 2 (MEN1 and MEN2), von Hippel–Lindau disease (VHL), neurofibromatosis type 1 (NF1), and the familial pheochromocytoma–paraganglioma (PGL) syndromes types 1, 2, 3, and 4. Table 13.1 delineates the clinical features and associated gene mutations of each of these syndromes.

Pheochromocytoma is extremely rare in the setting of MEN1. Although approximately 30% of patients with MEN1 develop adrenal tumors, these are usually adrenal cortical lesions, and pheochromocytoma has been described in less than 1% [17].

Pheochromocytoma is seen in 1–5% of patients with NF1. However, patients with NF1 who are also hypertensive have a 20–50% incidence of catecholamine-producing

Table 13.1 Major genetic syndromes associated with pheochromocytoma or paraganglioma.14–16, 87

Syndrome	Gene	Locus	Protein	Inheritance pattern	Clinical features	Risk of Pheo/PGL	Features of Pheo/PGL
NF1	*NF1*	17q11.2	Neurofibromin	Autosomal dominant (AD)	Neurofibromas Café-au-lait spots Lisch nodules (iris hamartomas) Skin-fold freckling Pheochromocytoma/sympathetic PGL	1–5% (20–50% if hypertensive)	10–40% bilateral 10% malignant 5% extra-adrenal
VHL	*VHL*	3p25-26	VHL	AD	Hemangioblastomas (CNS, retina) Renal cysts and clear cell carcinoma Pancreatic cysts and islet cell tumors Endolymphatic sac tumors Epididymal cysts Pheochromocytoma/sympathetic PGL	10–20%	50–70% bilateral <10% malignant 10–15% extra-adrenal
MEN1	*Men1*	11q13	Menin	AD	Primary hyperparathyroidism Pituitary adenomas Pancreatic islet cell tumors Pheochromocytoma	<1%	Unilateral Rarely malignant
MEN2A	*RET*	10q11.2	RET	AD	Medullary thyroid carcinoma Pheochromocytoma Primary hyperparathyroidism	50%	50–70% bilateral <5% malignant Not extra-adrenal
MEN2B	*RET*	10q11.2	RET	AD	Medullary thyroid carcinoma Pheochromocytoma Ganglioneuromas Marfanoid body habitus	50%	50–70% bilateral <5% malignant Not extra-adrenal

(continued)

Table 13.1 (continued)

Syndrome	Gene	Locus	Protein	Inheritance pattern	Clinical features	Risk of Pheo/PGL	Features of Pheo/PGL
PGL1	*SDHD*	11q23	SDH subunit D	AD+parent of origin effects	Usually head and neck parasympathetic paragangliomas Occasionally pheo/sympathetic PGL	Up to 80%	30–40% multifocal Usually benign 40–60% extra-adrenal
PGL2	*SDH5*	11q13.1	SDH5	AD+parent of origin effects	Head and neck parasympathetic paragangliomas	Up to 80%	Only extra-adrenal paragangliomas
PGL3	*SDHC*	1q21	SDH subunit C	AD	Head and neck parasympathetic paragangliomas	Up to 80%	Seldom multi-focal Benign
PGL4	*SDHB*	1p36.1–35	SDH subunit B	AD	Head and neck parasympathetic paragangliomas Pheochromocytoma/sympathetic PGL	Up to 80%	Not multifocal 50–70% malignant 50–80% extra-adrenal

tumors [18, 19]. Pheochromocytomas in the setting of NF1 are often bilateral, usually not extra-adrenal, and are benign in 90% of cases.

Pheochromocytoma is more common in association with MEN2, and develops in approximately 50% of MEN2 gene carriers. However, well-defined genotype–phenotype correlations exist in MEN2, and therefore the incidence varies considerably by mutation. Pheochromocytoma occurs most frequently with codon 634 (MEN2A) and codon 918 (MEN2B) *RET* mutations [20]. Tumors are bilateral in 50–70% of patients, almost always benign, and almost never extra-adrenal.

The overall incidence of pheochromocytoma in patients with VHL is 10–20%, but genotype–phenotype correlations are also important in this syndrome. Patients with partial or complete *VHL* deletions (VHL type 1) have a low (6–9%) risk of pheochromocytoma, whereas patients with missense *VHL* mutations (VHL type 2) have a high (40–59%) risk of pheochromocytoma [21]. In VHL, tumors are bilateral in 50–70% of patients and malignant in less than 10% of patients. Sympathetic extra-adrenal paragangliomas occur in 10–15% of patients.

The familial pheochromocytoma–paraganglioma syndromes (PGL1–4) are a group of recently described syndromes that carry an increased risk of pheochromocytoma and extra-adrenal sympathetic or parasympathetic paraganglioma. The causative genes for PGL1, PGL3, and PGL4 are members of the succinate dehydrogenase (SDH) gene family (subunits D, C, and B, respectively). Inactivation of any of these subunits leads to insufficient activity of the mitochondrial complex II, which participates in electron transfer and succinate catabolism. The gene for PGL2 was recently identified as *SDH5*, a gene required for the flavination and subsequent functionality of SDH [22]. The clinical features of the various PGL syndromes are still incompletely defined, but gene carriers appear to have approximately 80% risk of developing tumors, and patterns of disease are emerging [23]. PGL1 (*SDHD*) is usually associated with head and neck parasympathetic paragangliomas, but pheochromocytomas and extra-adrenal sympathetic paragangliomas can also be seen. These tumors are often multifocal, and usually benign. PGL2 (*SDH5*) and PGL3 (*SDHC*) are associated with head and neck parasympathetic paragangliomas only, and are almost always benign. PGL4 (*SDHB*) is associated with sympathetic paragangliomas and pheochromocytomas, as well as parasympathetic paragangliomas. These tumors tend to be solitary, extra-adrenal, and carry up to a 70% risk of malignancy [23]. *SDHB* mutations also appear to confer an increased risk for renal carcinoma; this has been reported in several patients as early as their 20s, although the risk is likely to be quite small [23–25].

Pheochromocytomas and/or extra-adrenal paragangliomas also occur as a component of two other very rare syndromes: the Carney triad of extra-adrenal paraganglioma, gastrointestinal stromal tumor (GIST) and pulmonary chondroma [26], and the Carney–Stratakis dyad of paraganglioma and GIST [27]. Patients considered to have the Carney–Stratakis dyad have recently been shown to have a high rate of underlying *SDHB*, *SDHD*, or *SDHC* mutations; therefore, GIST may simply be a low-penetrant component tumor of the familial PGL syndromes [28].

The "rule of 10" has traditionally been applied to pheochromocytoma: 10% bilateral, 10% extra-adrenal, 10% extra-abdominal, 10% malignant, 10% in children,

10% asymptomatic, and 10% hereditary. However, this axiom has been challenged as data has accumulated regarding this rare disease [29]. For example, as described earlier, recent evidence suggests that considerably more than 10% of patients with apparently sporadic disease may in fact harbor an underlying germline gene mutation [15]. In addition, extra-adrenal paragangliomas are now recognized in up to 20% of patients with pheochromocytoma. Increasing numbers of asymptomatic patients are also being identified as more pheochromocytomas are diagnosed early in incidentally discovered adrenal masses or in patients undergoing screening for a known hereditary syndrome. Finally, the risk of malignancy must be taken in context of the underlying genetic mutation.

Clinical Presentation

Pheochromocytomas and sympathetic extra-adrenal paragangliomas classically present with "the 5 P's": *p*ressure (hypertension), *p*ain (headache), *p*erspiration, *p*alpitations, and *p*allor – symptoms of excess catecholamine production. Parasympathetic extra-adrenal paragangliomas do not secrete catecholamines, and are usually discovered as incidental findings on cervical or thoracic imaging or present as a neck mass with symptoms related to compression, such as dysphagia, dysphonia, or cranial nerve palsy.

Symptoms of catecholamine excess are often paroxysmal, and can be spontaneous or induced by a variety of events, including strenuous physical exertion; trauma; labor and delivery; surgery or other invasive procedures, including direct instrumentation of the tumor (e.g., fine needle aspiration); eating foods high in tyramine (e.g., red wine, chocolate, and cheese), which can cause the release of catecholamines from secretory granules; and rarely urination (bladder wall tumor). Episodes of hypertension can be variable in frequency, severity, and duration, and are often extremely difficult to manage medically. Hypertensive crisis can lead to cardiac arrhythmias, myocardial infarction, or death. Sustained hypertension in between paroxysmal episodes occurs in 50–60% of patients with pheochromocytoma [30], and these patients are often diagnosed with essential hypertension. Impaired glucose tolerance can also be seen in at least a third of patients with pheochromocytoma [31]. This state results from increased glycogenolysis, lipolysis, and gluconeogenesis related to excess catecholamine secretion and resolves after tumor resection.

In order to understand the pathophysiology of pheochromocytomas and extra-adrenal paragangliomas, it is important to understand the biochemical pathways of catecholamine metabolism (Fig. 13.1). Tyrosine is metabolized to dopamine and then to norepinephrine. The enzyme phenylethanolamine-*N*-methyltransferase (PNMT) catalyzes the conversion of norepinephrine to epinephrine in the adrenal medulla. Extra-adrenal sympathetic tissue lacks PNMT; therefore, extra-adrenal sympathetic paragangliomas manifest elevated norepinephrine levels and metabolites, whereas epinephrine levels remain normal. In the adrenal medulla, the PNMT-mediated conversion of norepinephrine to epinephrine becomes inefficient as tumors

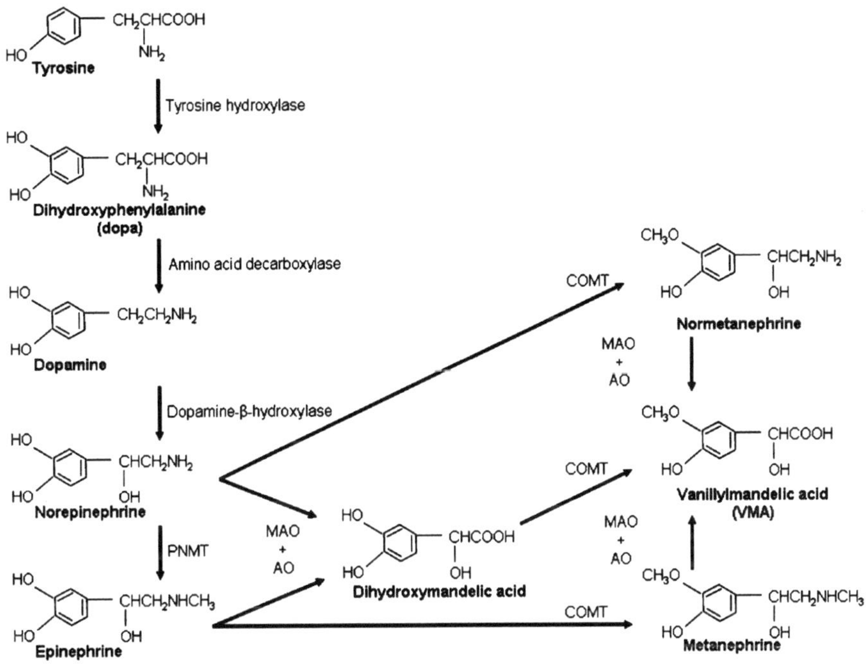

Fig. 13.1 Pathway of catecholamine metabolism [32]. *PNMT* Phenylethanolamine-*N*-methyltransferase; *MAO* monoamine oxidase; *AO* aldehyde oxidase; *COMT* catecholamine *O*-methyltransferase

Table 13.2 Actions of catecholamines [32]

Catecholamine receptor subtype	
α (norepinephrine-mediated)	β (epinephrine-mediated)
Arteriolar vasoconstriction (α1) (splanchnic, renal, cutaneous, genital)	Arteriolar vasodilation (β2) (muscle)
Sphincter contraction (α1) (gastrointestinal, urinary)	Muscle relaxation (β2) (gastrointestinal, urinary, bronchial)
Sweating	Increased cardiac contractility (β1)
Pupil dilation	Increased heart rate (β1)
Platelet aggregation (α2)	Increased cardiac conduction velocity (β1)
Increased gluconeogenesis (α)	Increased glycogenolysis
Decreased insulin secretion (α2)	Increased lipolysis and ketosis (β1)
	Increased insulin secretion (β2)
	Increased glucagon secretion (β2)
	Decreased glucose utilization
	Increased calorigenesis (β1)

increase in size. Thus, pheochromocytomas also often produce relatively more norepinephrine and its metabolites than epinephrine.

Norepinephrine and epinephrine have distinct end-organ effects (Table 13.2). Norepinephrine predominantly acts on α-receptors. It has limited β1 and very weak β2 activity. Conversely, epinephrine acts primarily on β1- and β2-receptors, and has less activity against α-receptors [32].

The pattern of catecholamine production in MEN2 differs from that seen in other inherited syndromes and sporadic cases. Expression of PNMT is preserved and thus epinephrine, instead of norepinephrine, is preferentially produced. Therefore, patients tend to present with attacks of paroxysmal hypertension, palpitations, anxiety, and headaches characteristic of β-adrenergic activity instead of the more common pattern of sustained hypertension characteristic of α-adrenergic activity [33].

Diagnostic Evaluation

History and Physical Exam

The diagnosis of pheochromocytoma begins with a careful history. Pheochromocytoma should be suspected in any patient with characteristic paroxysmal episodes; patients with labile, intermittent, or difficult-to-control hypertension; pregnant patients who develop hypertension without preeclampsia (i.e., without proteinuria); patients in whom hypertension develops at a young age; patients with anxiety attacks; patients with an asymptomatic incidentally discovered adrenal mass; and patients with a family history of pheochromocytoma or who are known to have an inherited condition that predisposes to pheochromocytoma. In apparently sporadic cases, a thorough family history is essential because it may influence a decision to obtain genetic testing. However, patients often do not know the details of their family members' medical problems, so it is important to ask about specific features suggestive of hereditary syndromes that a patient might recognize as the diagnosis of a family member. Table 13.3 provides a checklist of clinical features associated with each of the major hereditary syndromes that confer increased risk of pheochromocytoma.

Physical examination may reveal hypertension, tachycardia, a resting tremor, or diaphoresis. Unlike the clinical presentation of other neuroendocrine tumors such as carcinoid or medullary thyroid carcinoma, flushing is uncommon; α-adrenergic

Table 13.3 Clinical features suggestive of pheochromocytoma or paraganglioma [16]

Syndrome	Clinical features
Pheochromocytoma	Sudden death, hypertension, or stroke (especially at a young age or during pregnancy or anesthesia)
VHL	Cysts or cancer of the CNS, kidney, pancreas, or testes (especially in children) Early onset of deafness or blindness
MEN2	Kidney stones or high blood calcium Thyroid cancer or goiter Bumps on lips, tongue or eyelids
PGL1 or PGL4	Head and neck tumors, with symptoms from mass effect Abdominal tumors

vasoconstriction of skin arterioles results in the more typical pallor, especially during a hypertensive crisis. An effort should be made to identify physical manifestations of hereditary syndromes that may include pheochromocytoma or extra-adrenal paraganglioma. For example, cutaneous lichen amyloidosis, a plaque-like pruritic skin lesion, may be seen over the scapula and upper back in a subgroup of patients with MEN2A. Patients with MEN2B have very characteristic physical features, including neuromas of the lips, anterior tongue, and eyelids, and a marfanoid body habitus. The neurofibromas, café-au-lait spots, and skin-fold freckling of NF1 are often readily apparent.

Biochemical Testing

Biochemical testing to document excess catecholamine secretion is indicated in any patient in whom the diagnosis of pheochromocytoma is suspected. Controversy exists as to the optimal single test to make the diagnosis. Historically, a 24-h urine collection for catecholamines (epinephrine and norepinephrine) and their metabolites (metanephrine, normetanephrine, and vanillylmandelic acid [VMA]) was the test of choice. Recently, measurement of plasma free metanephrines (metanephrine and normetanephrine) has been hailed as the most accurate single test for the diagnosis of pheochromocytoma [34]. The sensitivity of plasma free metanephrines is 97–99%, compared to a sensitivity of 77–90% for urinary catecholamines and metanephrines. On the other hand, the specificity of plasma free metanephrines is relatively low at 85%, compared to a specificity of 98% for urinary measurements [35]. However, pretest probability is also important: the specificity of plasma free metanephrines is 82% in patients tested for sporadic pheochromocytoma vs. 96% in patients tested for hereditary pheochromocytoma [34]. Therefore, plasma free metanephrines appears to be an ideal screening test for patients at higher baseline risk of pheochromocytoma (such as patients with a family history or a known inherited predisposition, or patients with an incidentally discovered adrenal mass), but is associated with a relatively high false-positive rate in patients at lower baseline risk of pheochromocytoma. In general, it is reasonable to use plasma free metanephrines as an initial screening test, followed by 24-h measurement of urinary catecholamines and metabolites as a confirmatory test.

Regardless of the method used to measure excess catecholamines and/or their metabolites, it is often difficult to interpret test results because common foods and medications, physical or emotional stress, and even upright posture can interfere with measurement and can lead to a false-positive result [34]. For greatest accuracy, a blood sample for measurement of plasma free metanephrines should be drawn with the patient in the fasting state and supine, after lying unstimulated in a dark room for 30–45 min. Caffeine and nicotine, as well as medications such as tricyclic antidepressants, monoamine oxidase inhibitors, phenoxybenzamine, calcium-channel blockers, levodopa, α-methyldopa, amphetamines, and ephedrine, increase levels of catecholamines and/or metabolites in plasma and urine, and may cause false-positive results.

Coffee (including decaffeinated coffee), as well as medications such as labetalol, sotalol, buspirone, acetaminophen, levodopa, α-methyldopa, amphetamines, and ephedrine, interfere with the assays used for catecholamine and/or metabolite measurement and may lead to false-positive results [30].

In interpreting a positive test result, it is important to recognize that a mildly elevated catecholamine or metanephrine level is usually due to some type of interference with measurement; patients with pheochromocytoma almost always have increases in catecholamines or metanephrines 2 or 3 times higher than upper reference limits [30]. In cases in which it is otherwise impossible to distinguish increased catecholamine release due to sympathetic activation from increased catecholamine release due to pheochromocytoma, a clonidine suppression test can be performed [36, 37].

Provocative testing using glucagon, histamine, metoclopramide, or naloxone, followed by timed plasma catecholamine measurement was used in the past to increase the sensitivity of testing. However, this practice adds no value to current methods of testing, has the potential to be dangerous, and has therefore become obsolete [38].

Chromogranin A is often elevated in patients with neuroendocrine tumors, but has a sensitivity as low as 65% in patients with pheochromocytoma, and therefore is not useful in making a diagnosis [39]. However, it can be obtained as a baseline tumor marker and incorporated into follow-up, particularly in patients judged to be at relatively high risk for recurrence or metastasis.

Localization Studies

Once the biochemical diagnosis of pheochromocytoma is confirmed, localization studies are performed for operative planning. Computed tomography (CT) or magnetic resonance imaging (MRI) of the abdomen and pelvis (at least through the level of the aortic bifurcation) are the most commonly used localization studies. Both have similar sensitivity (90–100%) and specificity (70–80%) [40]. CT (Fig. 13.2a) provides excellent anatomic detail, although intravenous ionic contrast can occasionally precipitate a hypertensive crisis, and therefore patients typically require α-adrenergic blockade prior to undergoing CT imaging. There is some evidence that hypertensive crisis does not occur with the nonionic contrast medium that is most commonly used today [41]. MRI (Fig. 13.2b) provides good anatomic and some functional imaging, in that pheochromocytomas and extra-adrenal paragangliomas display a characteristic high-intensity signal on T2-weighted images, and no adrenergic blockade is necessary prior to administration of gadolinium [40].

Additional functional imaging may be considered if initial CT or MRI does not localize the tumor or in patients who are likely to have multifocal disease, malignant disease, or recurrent disease. ^{123}I-metaiodobenzylguanidine (MIBG) scintigraphy coupled with CT imaging provides functional and anatomic information and has good sensitivity (80–90%) and specificity (95–100%) [40]. ^{131}I-MIBG can be used if ^{123}I-MIBG is not available, although the image quality is not as high [42]. Certain medications (e.g., labetalol, tricyclic antidepressants, calcium-channel blockers) can interfere with tumor uptake and/or retention of radiolabeled MIBG and should

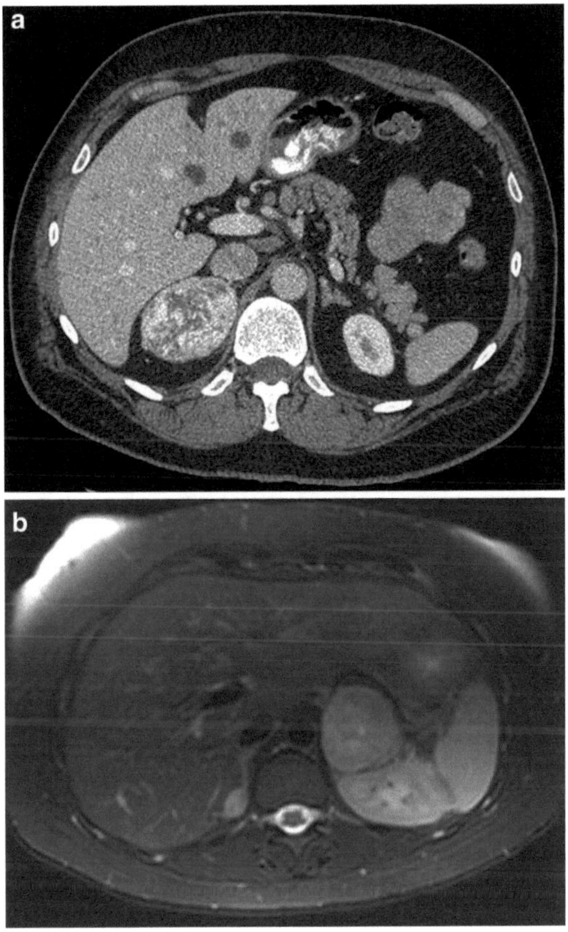

Fig. 13.2 (**a**) CT scan demonstrating right pheochromocytoma, the liver contains cysts; (**b**) T2-weighted magnetic resonance imaging (MRI) depicting bilateral pheochromocytoma in a patient with MEN2A

be held prior to imaging [43]. Other functional imaging alternatives include ^{111}In-octreotide scintigraphy and ^{18}F-fluorodeoxyglucose positron emission tomography (^{18}F-FDG-PET), both of which can be coupled with CT for additional anatomic detail. With thoughtful use of available imaging modalities, it is rare for localization of a pheochromocytoma to be unsuccessful.

Genetic Testing

Since 2002, when Neumann et al. [15] published their data suggesting that the incidence of hereditary pheochromocytoma and extra-adrenal paraganglioma is higher than previously thought (up to 24.6% of apparently sporadic cases), it has been proposed that all patients diagnosed with a pheochromocytoma or paraganglioma should undergo genetic testing [14, 23]. Genetic testing permits earlier identification of a hereditary syndrome, which in turn allows earlier screening for other associated tumors and identification of family members at risk. In addition, because some patients with a hereditary syndrome are more likely to have multifocal, malignant, or recurrent disease, knowledge of the genetic mutation allows for increased vigilance in these patients during preoperative localization or postoperative surveillance. However, certain subgroups of patients have a very low risk of having an inherited syndrome; for example, the risk of a hereditary syndrome in patients diagnosed with pheochromocytoma after age 50 is less than 2% [15]. Therefore, testing all patients diagnosed with a pheochromocytoma or paraganglioma may not be practical or cost-effective from a population standpoint.

It is currently recommended that every patient diagnosed with a pheochromocytoma or extra-adrenal paraganglioma first undergo a risk evaluation by a certified genetics counselor. Genetic testing is recommended for patients with a personal or family history of clinical features suggestive of a hereditary PGL syndrome (Tables 13.1 and 13.3), patients with bilateral or multifocal tumors, patients with sympathetic extra-adrenal paragangliomas, patients with malignant extra-adrenal paragangliomas, and patients diagnosed before age 40. Genetic testing can be considered in patients between 40 and 50 years of age with a unilateral pheochromocytoma and no personal or family history to suggest hereditary disease. Genetic testing is not recommended in patients over age 50 with a unilateral pheochromocytoma and no personal or family history to suggest hereditary disease.

Most patients do not need to be tested for all genes currently clinically available. Genetic testing for NF1 is almost never necessary because patients can be readily identified on physical exam. Table 13.4 depicts an algorithm for genetic testing. The order in which the various genetic tests should be considered takes into account the age of the patient, location and number of tumors, presence of metastases, biochemical profile, and quality of family history information. It is important to recognize that currently available genetic testing cannot identify all patients with a hereditary form of pheochromocytoma.

Table 13.4 Algorithm for genetic testing in pheochromocytoma or extra-adrenal paraganglioma [14, 16, 87]

Patients with no known hereditary syndrome[a]		
Presentation	Subgroup	Order of testing
Unilateral pheochromocytoma	Age <20 years	*VHL>RET>SDHB=SDHD*
	Age 20–50 years	*SDHB>VHL>SDHD>>RET*
	Age >50 years	Testing not recommended
Bilateral pheochromocytoma	Increased norepinephrine and/ or normetanephrine	*VHL>>SDHB=SDHD>RET*
	Increased epinephrine and/ or metanephrine	*RET>>SDHB=SDHD>VHL*
Sympathetic extra-adrenal paraganglioma	Age <20 years	*VHL>SDHB>SDHD*
	Age ≥20 years	*SDHB>VHL>SDHD*
Malignant disease		*SDHB >>>VHL>SDHD*

[a]May alter order of testing if suspicion exists for a specific hereditary disease

If a mutation is identified, predictive genetic testing should be offered to asymptomatic at-risk family members. Genetic testing should always be preceded by careful genetic counseling, since there are no evidence-based screening guidelines proven to decrease disease-related morbidity or mortality. Of note, *SDHD* and *SDH5* gene mutations are inherited with parent-of-origin effect: only individuals with a paternally inherited mutation are at risk to develop disease, whereas maternally inherited mutations are not associated with disease risk but can be passed to future generations. Therefore, individuals at risk to inherit a *SDHD* or *SDH5* mutation from their mother should be offered genetic testing only when they reach adulthood, since the information is mainly for reproductive risk knowledge and not for early screening and prevention.

Management

Preoperative Management

In 1951, Priestley and colleagues first reported a dramatic decrease in intraoperative mortality that accompanied their use of preoperative and intraoperative medications for blood pressure control [7]. Today, surgical resection of a pheochromocytoma is associated with perioperative mortality of less than 3% and intraoperative mortality of less than 1% [44, 45]. Careful preoperative preparation is essential in order to prevent the potentially life-threatening cardiovascular catastrophes that can occur as a result of excess catecholamine secretion during surgery, including hypertensive crisis, cardiac arrhythmia, myocardial infarction, and pulmonary edema.

α-Adrenergic blockade is essential to preoperative medical preparation. Phenoxybenzamine, a nonselective α-antagonist, is the usual drug of choice; it may be started at a dose of 10 mg orally twice daily and increased every 2–3 days by 10–20 mg/day to a maximum dose of 1 mg/kg/day until adequate α-blockade is reached. The selective α1-antagonists prazosin [46] and doxazosin [47] are alternatives to phenoxybenzamine and have the theoretical benefit that they are shorter acting, and therefore the duration of postoperative hypotension is theoretically lessened. However, there is less overall experience with the use of selective α1-antagonists compared with phenoxybenzamine. Metyrosine, which blocks catecholamine synthesis, and/or calcium-channel blockers (such as nifedipine) may be useful as adjuncts, but are not effective alone. A preoperative treatment period of 1–3 weeks is usually sufficient; the presence of orthostatic hypotension indicates that α-blockade is adequate. As α-blockade increases, restoration of fluid and electrolytes by salt and volume loading is important in order to reduce excessive orthostatic hypotension both pre- and postoperatively. In addition, the tachyarrhythmia that may develop with α-blockade can be treated with β-blockade *after several days* of α-blockade. It is critical that β-blockade never be initiated before α-blockade; doing so blocks β-receptor-mediated vasodilation and leaves α-receptor-mediated vasoconstriction unopposed, which can result in a life-threatening crisis.

Operative Management

Definitive treatment for pheochromocytoma and extra-adrenal paraganglioma is surgical resection. Preoperative imaging and localization studies are critically important to selection of the ideal operative approach.

When preoperative imaging reveals a benign-appearing pheochromocytoma (less than 5 cm, no evidence of invasion into adjacent structures, and no evidence of regional or metastatic disease) and a normal contralateral adrenal gland, minimally invasive adrenalectomy is the preferred approach. Advantages of a minimally invasive approach compared to an open procedure include faster recovery, less discomfort, and a superior cosmetic result. Anterior laparoscopic adrenalectomy was first described by Gagner et al. [48], and it has become the most commonly used approach to adrenalectomy worldwide. Posterior retroperitoneoscopic adrenalectomy was first described by Mercan et al. [49] and has been popularized by Walz and his group in Essen, Germany [50]. Advantages to a posterior approach compared to an anterior approach include the ability to avoid intraabdominal adhesions from prior surgery and less cardiopulmonary fluctuations as a result of insufflation of the operating space. In addition, a posterior approach can be technically easier than an anterior approach in patients with moderate obesity, and a bilateral adrenalectomy can be performed without repositioning the patient [51]. The main disadvantage of any minimally invasive approach to pheochromocytoma is that it is often impossible to ligate the adrenal vein early in the procedure, which has been the standard for open adrenalectomy because it minimizes excess catecholamine secretion; in addition, a minimally invasive approach may involve greater tumor manipulation (and greater potential for catecholamine release) compared to an open approach. However, both anterior laparoscopic as well as retroperitoneoscopic adrenalectomy have been demonstrated to be safe for the majority of patients with modestly sized, clinically benign pheochromocytoma [50, 52].

An open approach is generally necessary when preoperative imaging suggests malignancy, an extra-adrenal paraganglioma, or multifocal disease. Although extra-adrenal paragangliomas are often located adjacent to major blood vessels, they are usually not invasive, and careful dissection can preserve the vascular anatomy while completely removing the tumor.

The operative management of patients with pheochromocytoma in the setting of the hereditary syndromes MEN2 and VHL is controversial. In both of these syndromes, pheochromocytoma is bilateral in at least 50% of patients. For this reason, traditional teaching advocated bilateral total adrenalectomy in MEN2 or VHL patients, including those who presented with unilateral pheochromocytoma – the contralateral gland was certain to have some degree of medullary hyperplasia, and thus prophylactic adrenalectomy was thought necessary to reduce the risk of recurrence and the possibility of future malignancy. However, malignancy is uncommon in both MEN2 and VHL, whereas bilateral total adrenalectomy commits patients to lifelong steroid dependence and results in acute adrenal insufficiency (Addisonian crisis) in approximately 25% of patients [53, 54]. Increased awareness of the complications associated with bilateral total adrenalectomy has led to a movement toward preservation of adrenal tissue in patients with MEN2 and VHL: patients who initially present with unilateral pheochromocytoma undergo unilateral adrenalectomy, and patients who present with bilateral pheochromocytoma or who develop pheochromocytoma in their remaining adrenal gland undergo cortical-sparing adrenalectomy [53]. Adrenal cortical reserve is tested postoperatively using the cosyntropin stimulation test, and patients with inadequate function receive replacement steroids. This strategy has been demonstrated to eliminate the need for steroid replacement in approximately 60% of patients, with a recurrence rate of 14%, and no patients having developed metastatic pheochromocytoma [55]. Insufficient data exists to extend this approach to other hereditary PGL syndromes; adrenal preservation is not recommended in patients with SDHB mutations and bilateral disease, because of the high risk of malignancy.

Even after optimal preoperative medical management, the intraoperative anesthetic management of patients with pheochromocytoma and sympathetic extra-adrenal paraganglioma can be challenging because α-blockade is rarely complete. Establishment of large-bore intravenous access and an arterial line is routine, with placement of a central venous catheter or a pulmonary artery catheter as indicated (e.g., in a patient with coexisting cardiovascular disease). Hypertension can be controlled with intravenous infusions of phentolamine, sodium nitroprusside, or a short-acting calcium-channel blocker such as nicardipine. Tachyarrhythmias can be treated with a short-acting β-blocker such as esmolol. After tumor removal, a precipitous fall in blood pressure may require rapid volume replacement and intravenous vasoconstrictors such as norepinephrine or phenylephrine.

Postoperative Management

Postoperatively, patients should be kept in a monitored environment for 24 h because of the risks of postoperative hypotension and hypoglycemia. Postoperative hypotension results from the abrupt decrease in circulating catecholamines after tumor resection in the presence of α-adrenergic blockade (phenoxybenzamine) that has not yet been cleared from the patient's circulation. Hypoglycemia may result from the sudden recovery of insulin secretion after tumor removal.

Interpretation of Pathology

Pathology typically reveals a classic pattern of "zellballen," with characteristic small nests of uniform polygonal cells (Fig. 13.3). A diagnosis of malignancy can only be made by documenting the presence of tumor deposits in tissues that do not normally contain chromaffin cells. Regional or distant metastatic disease is identified on initial pathology in 3–8% of patients, either by documenting tumor cells in lymph nodes or blood vessels adjacent to the pheochromocytoma or paraganglioma, or through the biopsy of an abnormal lesion distant from the primary tumor site (e.g., liver nodule) [56–58].

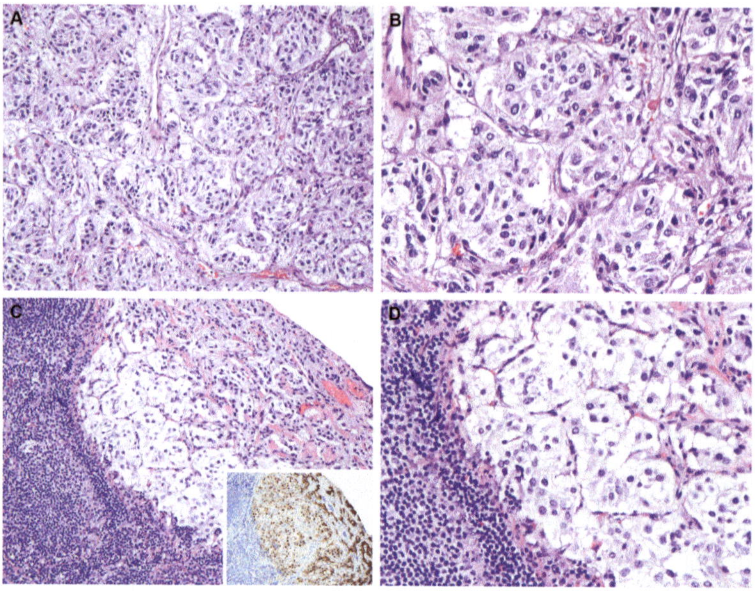

Fig. 13.3 (**a**) Paraganglioma, H&E ×100; (**b**) High-power view demonstrating groups of cells surrounded by capillaries: "Zellballen" appearance, H&E ×200; (**c**) Paraganglioma metastatic to a lymph node, H&E ×100; *inset* demonstrates positive immunohistochemical stain for chromogranin, ×40; (**d**) High-power view, H&E ×200. Photomicrographs kindly provided by Dr. Mahmoud Goodarzi, Department of Pathology, The University of Texas M. D. Anderson Cancer Center

Pathologic features sometimes associated with malignancy include large tumor size, increased number of mitoses, DNA aneuploidy, and extensive tumor necrosis. However, in the absence of clearly documented malignancy, no histopathologic feature, either alone or in combination with other histopathologic, clinical, or biochemical features, has been shown to reliably predict the biologic behavior of pheochromocytoma [57–61]. Therefore, even when no definite malignancy is identified, pathology generally offers insufficient prognostic information regarding the likelihood of recurrence or metastasis, and these lesions cannot be considered "benign" by default [62].

Follow-Up and Surveillance

Long-term follow-up is essential for patients with pheochromocytoma or extra-adrenal paraganglioma, even if initial pathology demonstrates no evidence of malignancy. Recurrence rates range from 6.5 to 16.5% in patients with apparently "benign" pathology, and recurrences can occur more than 15 years after initial surgery [56, 63, 64]. Recurrence is more likely in patients with extra-adrenal disease (33%) than in patients whose disease is confined to the adrenal gland (14%), and is more likely in patients with hereditary syndromes (33%) than in patients with sporadic disease (13%) [65]. Approximately 50% of patients who recur develop distant metastasis [64]. The 5-year survival in the setting of metastatic disease is 40–45% [66].

Surveillance for patients who have undergone complete surgical resection for a solitary sporadic pheochromocytoma with no malignancy identified on their pathology should include biochemical testing (plasma metanephrines or 24-h urinary catecholamines) 2 weeks postoperatively, and then annually for life. If there is evidence of excess catecholamine production on biochemical screening, imaging (CT or MRI, and radiolabeled-MIBG) should be performed for localization and to evaluate for metastatic disease. Patients who have undergone complete surgical resection of a sporadic noncatecholamine-producing tumor (usually a parasympathetic paraganglioma of the head and neck or thorax) should undergo annual imaging with CT or MRI and periodic imaging with radiolabeled-MIBG to evaluate for recurrence or metastasis.

Surveillance for patients who have undergone complete surgical resection for pheochromocytoma and/or extra-adrenal paraganglioma in the setting of a hereditary syndrome also includes lifelong annual biochemical screening, in addition to routine screening for other tumors involved in their specific syndrome. For carriers of MEN2 and VHL, imaging should be performed if biochemical testing is positive. For carriers of SDH mutations, periodic imaging with CT or MRI and radiolabeled-MIBG should be considered to evaluate for noncatecholamine-producing tumors [67].

Current recommendations for patients identified as mutation carriers because of predictive gene testing, or patients who are at risk for a hereditary syndrome but who have not undergone genetic testing, are for screening with lifelong annual biochemical testing. For carriers of MEN2, recent American Thyroid Association Guidelines suggest that screening should begin at age 8 for *RET* mutations involving codons 918, 630, and 634, and screening should begin at age 20 for other *RET* mutations [68]. For carriers of other hereditary syndromes, it is reasonable to begin biochemical screening at 10 years of age. For carriers of MEN2 and VHL, imaging should be performed if biochemical testing is positive. For carriers of SDH mutations, periodic imaging with CT or MRI and radiolabeled-MIBG should be considered to evaluate for noncatecholamine-producing tumors [67].

There are no established standards for incorporating chromogranin A levels into the follow-up of patients with pheochromocytoma or paraganglioma. However, it is reasonable to consider at least an annual chromogranin A level in patients with baseline presurgical elevation of this maker, and in patients judged at relatively high risk for the development of recurrence or metastasis (i.e., documented inherited tumor syndrome, large tumor, regional or distant metastasis at presentation). It is important to note that impaired renal or hepatic function, as well as the use of proton pump inhibitors, may cause an artifactual elevation of chromogranin A.

Hypertension is cured in the majority of patients who undergo complete resection of a catecholamine-producing tumor. However, hypertension can persist postoperatively, especially if the patient experienced sustained hypertension as opposed to paroxysmal hypertension at the time of diagnosis. The incidence of postoperative hypertension in this patient population is approximately 25% at 5 years and almost 50% at 10 years [56].

Metastatic Disease

Patients with known or suspected malignancy should undergo staging with CT or MRI as well as functional imaging such as ^{123}I-MIBG. The most common sites of metastasis from a pheochromocytoma or extra-adrenal paraganglioma are the bones, lungs, liver, and lymph nodes.

There is no effective treatment for metastatic pheochromocytoma or paraganglioma. If the primary tumor was functioning, recurrent tumor is also likely to secrete catecholamines, and patients are often quite symptomatic. For resectable disease, including metastases that are limited in number, surgery is the mainstay of therapy, and can offer palliation of symptoms and occasional long-term remission. In the setting of unresectable disease, surgical debulking is sometimes indicated for symptom palliation.

Medical therapy for metastatic pheochromocytoma or paraganglioma has been generally disappointing. The best-established cytotoxic chemotherapy regimen is the Averbuch protocol: a combination of cyclophosphamide, vincristine, and dacarbazine (CVD) [66]. Results of this treatment in 18 patients demonstrated a complete response rate of 11%, a partial response rate of 44%, and a biochemical response in 72% of patients. Median survival was 3.3 years [69]. Modifications to this regimen (e.g., the addition of anthracyclines), or other cytotoxic regimens (such as combination temozolomide and thalidomide), have been reported [70, 71]. However, there is limited data to support their use, and in general, side effects appear to outweigh any benefit of modified or other regimens.

Approximately 60% of sites of metastasis are MIBG-avid; [72] therefore, ^{131}I-MIBG radiotherapy has been evaluated as a treatment modality. Overall, ^{131}I-MIBG therapy is associated with occasional (<5%) complete responses, and up to 45% partial responses, with a duration of therapy of approximately 2 years [73, 74]. Recent data using high-dose ^{131}I-MIBG in 30 patients demonstrated a sustained complete remission in 13%, a sustained partial remission in 50%, and an estimated 5-year survival of 75% in this group of patients. Bone marrow suppression was the main toxicity reported, and occurred in up to 80% of patients [72]. Thus, it appears that high-dose ^{131}I-MIBG therapy offers some promise, but more data is needed. Therapeutic agents using other radiolabeled particles, such as radiolabeled somatostatin analogs, are also under investigation; protocol-based treatment with these agents can be considered for metastases that do not take up MIBG.

Novel targeted therapies are emerging as potential treatment strategies for metastatic pheochromocytoma or paraganglioma. Somewhat disappointing initial results have been reported with the mammalian target of rapamycin (mTOR) inhibitor everolimus [75]; results with the tyrosine kinase inhibitor sunitinib have been more encouraging, although in a very small number of treated patients [76, 77].

Palliation of symptoms remains the primary focus of treatment for most patients with metastatic disease. Phenoxybenzamine is as effective for control of symptoms related to catecholamine overproduction for patients with metastatic disease as it is for patients with primary disease, and metyrosine can be added if needed.

Other palliative treatment modalities include external beam radiation therapy for palliation of bone metastases, and embolization or other ablative techniques (e.g., radiofrequency ablation) to reduce bulky hepatic metastases.

Pheochromocytoma and Pregnancy

Pheochromocytoma is diagnosed during approximately 0.007% of pregnancies [78]. Although this situation is very rare, it deserves special mention because women with hereditary conditions that increase their risk of developing pheochromocytoma are often also of child-bearing age and the consequences of undiagnosed pheochromocytoma during pregnancy can be catastrophic. Prenatal diagnosis dramatically decreases the mortality rate of the mother and the infant [79]. Before 1970, a prenatal diagnosis was made in approximately 25% of cases, with a resulting mortality rate of 50% in both mother and neonate [80, 81]. Data from the 1980s to 1990s has revealed a prenatal diagnosis rate of over 80%, with maternal and neonatal mortality rates of 6 and 15%, respectively [80, 82]. Therefore, the diagnosis should be considered in any patient who develops hypertension without preeclampsia during pregnancy. Pregnancy does not alter levels of catecholamines in normal patients [83]; thus, the usual biochemical tests are valid. MRI is the preferred localization study because it does not involve ionizing radiation. As soon as the diagnosis is made, α-adrenergic blockade should be initiated. Phenoxybenzamine is safe to use in pregnancy, but β-blockers have been associated with intrauterine growth retardation, and therefore should only be initiated if needed [84, 85]. Definitive management depends upon the location of the tumor and the gestational age of the fetus at the time of diagnosis. Surgical resection of the tumor can often be performed safely during the second trimester; alternatively, a combined cesarean section and tumor resection can be undertaken when the fetus is ready to be delivered. In rare cases, surgical resection can be delayed until a short time after delivery [86]. Careful monitoring throughout the pregnancy, and the availability of an experienced team of surgeons, anesthesiologists, obstetricians, and neonatologists, are essential to the successful management of pheochromocytoma in pregnancy.

Summary

Pheochromocytomas and extra-adrenal paragangliomas are rare neuroendocrine tumors of the adrenal glands or extra-adrenal sympathetic and parasympathetic paraganglia. Most secrete catecholamines with the potential for devastating cardiovascular consequences. Patients typically present with paroxysmal episodes of hypertension, palpitations, headache, pallor, and diaphoresis. Diagnosis is confirmed by biochemical testing followed by imaging studies for localization. An underlying genetic basis for the disease should be considered. Surgery is the cornerstone of treatment, and *must* be preceded by appropriate α-adrenergic blockade. Prognosis in the setting of completely resected sporadic disease is excellent; however, long-term follow-up is essential. No good therapy exists for metastatic disease, although new targeted therapies may offer promise.

References

1. DeLellis R, Lloyd RV, Heitz PU, Eng C, editors. World Health Organization classification of tumors: pathology and genetics of tumours of endocrine organs. Lyon, France: IARC Press; 2004.
2. Frankel F. Ein fall von doppelseitigen vollig latent verlaufen nebennierentumor und gleichseitiger nephritis mit veranderungen am circulation sappart und retinitis. Virchows Arch A. 1886;103:244.
3. Poll H. Die vergleichende Entwicklung der nebennierensysteme. In: Hertwig O, editor. Handbuch der Entwicklungsgeschichte des Menschen und der Wirbeltiere. Jena, Germany: Gustave Fischer; 1905. p. 443–8.
4. Pick L. Das Ganglioma embryonale sympathicum (sympathoma embryonale), eine typische bosartige geschwuestform des sympathischen nervensystems. Berl Klin Wochenschr. 1912;49:16–22.
5. Welbourn RB. Early surgical history of phaeochromocytoma. Br J Surg. 1987;74(7):594–6.
6. Graham JB. Pheochromocytoma and hypertension; an analysis of 207 cases. Int Abstr Surg. 1951;92(2):105–21.
7. Kvale WF, Manger WM, Priestley JT, Roth GM. Pheochromocytoma. Circulation. 1956;14(4 Part 1):622–30.
8. Beard CM, Sheps SG, Kurland LT, Carney JA, Lie JT. Occurrence of pheochromocytoma in Rochester, Minnesota, 1950 through 1979. Mayo Clin Proc. 1983;58(12):802–4.
9. Stenstrom G, Svardsudd K. Pheochromocytoma in Sweden 1958–1981. An analysis of the National Cancer Registry Data. Acta Med Scand. 1986;220(3):225–32.
10. Sinclair AM, Isles CG, Brown I, Cameron H, Murray GD, Robertson JW. Secondary hypertension in a blood pressure clinic. Arch Intern Med. 1987;147(7):1289–93.
11. Anderson Jr GH, Blakeman N, Streeten DH. The effect of age on prevalence of secondary forms of hypertension in 4429 consecutively referred patients. J Hypertens. 1994;12(5):609–15.
12. Omura M, Saito J, Yamaguchi K, Kakuta Y, Nishikawa T. Prospective study on the prevalence of secondary hypertension among hypertensive patients visiting a general outpatient clinic in Japan. Hypertens Res. 2004;27(3):193–202.
13. Young WF, Jr. Management approaches to adrenal incidentalomas. A view from Rochester, Minnesota. Endocrinol Metab Clin North Am. 2000;29(1):159–85, x.
14. Amar L, Bertherat J, Baudin E, et al. Genetic testing in pheochromocytoma or functional paraganglioma. J Clin Oncol. 2005;23(34):8812–8.
15. Neumann HP, Bausch B, McWhinney SR, et al. Germ-line mutations in nonsyndromic pheochromocytoma. N Engl J Med. 2002;346(19):1459–66.
16. Jimenez C, Cote G, Arnold A, Gagel RF. Review: Should patients with apparently sporadic pheochromocytomas or paragangliomas be screened for hereditary syndromes? J Clin Endocrinol Metab. 2006;91(8):2851–8.
17. Dackiw AP, Cote GJ, Fleming JB, et al. Screening for MEN1 mutations in patients with atypical endocrine neoplasia. Surgery. 1999;126(6):1097–103; discussion 1103–1094.
18. Zoller ME, Rembeck B, Oden A, Samuelsson M, Angervall L. Malignant and benign tumors in patients with neurofibromatosis type 1 in a defined Swedish population. Cancer. 1997;79(11):2125–31.

19. Walther MM, Herring J, Enquist E, Keiser HR, Linehan WM. von Recklinghausen's disease and pheochromocytomas. J Urol. 1999;162(5):1582–6.
20. Eng C, Clayton D, Schuffenecker I, et al. The relationship between specific RET proto-oncogene mutations and disease phenotype in multiple endocrine neoplasia type 2. International RET mutation consortium analysis. JAMA. 1996;276(19):1575–9.
21. Maher ER, Webster AR, Richards FM, et al. Phenotypic expression in von Hippel-Lindau disease: correlations with germline VHL gene mutations. J Med Genet. 1996;33(4):328–32.
22. Hao HX, Khalimonchuk O, Schraders M, et al. SDH5, a gene required for flavination of succinate dehydrogenase, is mutated in paraganglioma. Science. 2009;325(5944):1139–42.
23. Neumann HP, Pawlu C, Peczkowska M, et al. Distinct clinical features of paraganglioma syndromes associated with SDHB and SDHD gene mutations. JAMA. 2004;292(8):943–51.
24. Ricketts C, Woodward ER, Killick P, et al. Germline SDHB mutations and familial renal cell carcinoma. J Natl Cancer Inst. 2008;100(17):1260–2.
25. Vanharanta S, Buchta M, McWhinney SR, et al. Early-onset renal cell carcinoma as a novel extraparaganglial component of SDHB-associated heritable paraganglioma. Am J Hum Genet. 2004;74(1):153–9.
26. Carney JA. Gastric stromal sarcoma, pulmonary chondroma, and extra-adrenal paraganglioma (Carney Triad): natural history, adrenocortical component, and possible familial occurrence. Mayo Clin Proc. 1999;74(6):543–52.
27. Carney JA, Stratakis CA. Familial paraganglioma and gastric stromal sarcoma: a new syndrome distinct from the Carney triad. Am J Med Genet. 2002;108(2):132–9.
28. Pasini B, McWhinney SR, Bei T, et al. Clinical and molecular genetics of patients with the Carney-Stratakis syndrome and germline mutations of the genes coding for the succinate dehydrogenase subunits SDHB, SDHC, and SDHD. Eur J Hum Genet. 2008;16(1): 79–88.
29. Dluhy RG. Pheochromocytoma – death of an axiom. N Engl J Med. 2002;346(19):1486–8.
30. Lenders JW, Eisenhofer G, Mannelli M, Pacak K. Phaeochromocytoma. Lancet. 2005; 366(9486):665–75.
31. La Batide-Alanore A, Chatellier G, Plouin PF. Diabetes as a marker of pheochromocytoma in hypertensive patients. J Hypertens. 2003;21(9):1703–7.
32. Berne R, Levy MN. Physiology. 3rd ed. St. Louis, MO: Mosby Year Book; 1993.
33. Eisenhofer G, Walther MM, Huynh TT, et al. Pheochromocytomas in von Hippel-Lindau syndrome and multiple endocrine neoplasia type 2 display distinct biochemical and clinical phenotypes. J Clin Endocrinol Metab. 2001;86(5):1999–2008.
34. Lenders JW, Pacak K, Walther MM, et al. Biochemical diagnosis of pheochromocytoma: which test is best? JAMA. 2002;287(11):1427–34.
35. Sawka AM, Jaeschke R, Singh RJ, Young Jr WF. A comparison of biochemical tests for pheochromocytoma: measurement of fractionated plasma metanephrines compared with the combination of 24-hour urinary metanephrines and catecholamines. J Clin Endocrinol Metab. 2003;88(2):553–8.
36. Bravo EL, Tarazi RC, Fouad FM, Vidt DG, Gifford Jr RW. Clonidine-suppression test: a useful aid in the diagnosis of pheochromocytoma. N Engl J Med. 1981;305(11):623–6.
37. Eisenhofer G, Goldstein DS, Walther MM, et al. Biochemical diagnosis of pheochromocytoma: how to distinguish true- from false-positive test results. J Clin Endocrinol Metab. 2003;88(6):2656–66.
38. Young Jr WF. Phaeochromocytoma: how to catch a moonbeam in your hand. Eur J Endocrinol. 1997;136(1):28–9.
39. Bernini GP, Moretti A, Ferdeghini M, et al. A new human chromogranin 'A' immunoradiometric assay for the diagnosis of neuroendocrine tumours. Br J Cancer. 2001;84(5):636–42.
40. Ilias I, Pacak K. Current approaches and recommended algorithm for the diagnostic localization of pheochromocytoma. J Clin Endocrinol Metab. 2004;89(2):479–91.
41. Mukherjee JJ, Peppercorn PD, Reznek RH, et al. Pheochromocytoma: effect of nonionic contrast medium in CT on circulating catecholamine levels. Radiology. 1997;202(1): 227–31.

42. Furuta N, Kiyota H, Yoshigoe F, Hasegawa N, Ohishi Y. Diagnosis of pheochromocytoma using [123I]-compared with [131I]-metaiodobenzylguanidine scintigraphy. Int J Urol. 1999;6(3):119–24.
43. Solanki KK, Bomanji J, Moyes J, Mather SJ, Trainer PJ, Britton KE. A pharmacological guide to medicines which interfere with the biodistribution of radiolabelled meta-iodobenzylguanidine (MIBG). Nucl Med Commun. 1992;13(7):513–21.
44. Kinney MA, Warner ME, vanHeerden JA, et al. Perianesthetic risks and outcomes of pheochromocytoma and paraganglioma resection. Anesth Analg. 2000;91(5):1118–23.
45. Plouin PF, Duclos JM, Soppelsa F, Boublil G, Chatellier G. Factors associated with perioperative morbidity and mortality in patients with pheochromocytoma: analysis of 165 operations at a single center. J Clin Endocrinol Metab. 2001;86(4):1480–6.
46. Cubeddu LX, Zarate NA, Rosales CB, Zschaeck DW. Prazosin and propranolol in preoperative management of pheochromocytoma. Clin Pharmacol Ther. 1982;32(2):156–60.
47. Prys-Roberts C, Farndon JR. Efficacy and safety of doxazosin for perioperative management of patients with pheochromocytoma. World J Surg. 2002;26(8):1037–42.
48. Gagner M, Lacroix A, Bolte E. Laparoscopic adrenalectomy in Cushing's syndrome and pheochromocytoma. N Engl J Med. 1992;327(14):1033.
49. Mercan S, Seven R, Ozarmagan S, Tezelman S. Endoscopic retroperitoneal adrenalectomy. Surgery. 1995;118(6):1071–5; discussion 1075–6.
50. Walz MK, Alesina PF, Wenger FA, et al. Posterior retroperitoneoscopic adrenalectomy – results of 560 procedures in 520 patients. Surgery. 2006;140(6):943–8; discussion 948–50.
51. Callender GG, Kennamer DL, Grubbs EG, Lee JE, Evans DB, Perrier ND. Posterior retroperitoneoscopic adrenalectomy. Adv Surg. 2009;43:147–57.
52. Gagner M, Breton G, Pharand D, Pomp A. Is laparoscopic adrenalectomy indicated for pheochromocytomas? Surgery. 1996;120(6):1076–9; discussion 1079–80.
53. Lee JE, Curley SA, Gagel RF, Evans DB, Hickey RC. Cortical-sparing adrenalectomy for patients with bilateral pheochromocytoma. Surgery. 1996;120(6):1064–70; discussion 1070–1061.
54. de Graaf JS, Dullaart RP, Zwierstra RP. Complications after bilateral adrenalectomy for phaeochromocytoma in multiple endocrine neoplasia type 2 – a plea to conserve adrenal function. Eur J Surg. 1999;165(9):843–6.
55. Yip L, Lee JE, Shapiro SE, et al. Surgical management of hereditary pheochromocytoma. J Am Coll Surg. 2004;198(4):525–34; discussion 534–525.
56. Plouin PF, Chatellier G, Fofol I, Corvol P. Tumor recurrence and hypertension persistence after successful pheochromocytoma operation. Hypertension. 1997;29(5):1133–9.
57. Thompson LD. Pheochromocytoma of the Adrenal gland Scaled Score (PASS) to separate benign from malignant neoplasms: a clinicopathologic and immunophenotypic study of 100 cases. Am J Surg Pathol. 2002;26(5):551–66.
58. Nativ O, Grant CS, Sheps SG, et al. The clinical significance of nuclear DNA ploidy pattern in 184 patients with pheochromocytoma. Cancer. 1992;69(11):2683–7.
59. Wu D, Tischler AS, Lloyd RV, et al. Observer variation in the application of the Pheochromocytoma of the Adrenal Gland Scaled Score. Am J Surg Pathol. 2009;33(4):599–608.
60. Kimura N, Watanabe T, Noshiro T, Shizawa S, Miura Y. Histological grading of adrenal and extra-adrenal pheochromocytomas and relationship to prognosis: a clinicopathological analysis of 116 adrenal pheochromocytomas and 30 extra-adrenal sympathetic paragangliomas including 38 malignant tumors. Endocr Pathol. Spring 2005;16(1):23–32.
61. Linnoila RI, Keiser HR, Steinberg SM, Lack EE. Histopathology of benign versus malignant sympathoadrenal paragangliomas: clinicopathologic study of 120 cases including unusual histologic features. Hum Pathol. 1990;21(11):1168–80.
62. Tischler AS. Pheochromocytoma and extra-adrenal paraganglioma: updates. Arch Pathol Lab Med. 2008;132(8):1272–84.
63. van Heerden JA, Roland CF, Carney JA, Sheps SG, Grant CS. Long-term evaluation following resection of apparently benign pheochromocytoma(s)/paraganglioma(s). World J Surg. 1990;14(3):325–9.

64. Amar L, Servais A, Gimenez-Roqueplo AP, Zinzindohoue F, Chatellier G, Plouin PF. Year of diagnosis, features at presentation, and risk of recurrence in patients with pheochromocytoma or secreting paraganglioma. J Clin Endocrinol Metab. 2005;90(4):2110–6.
65. Brunt LM, Lairmore TC, Doherty GM, Quasebarth MA, DeBenedetti M, Moley JF. Adrenalectomy for familial pheochromocytoma in the laparoscopic era. Ann Surg. 2002;235(5):713–20; discussion 720–711.
66. Averbuch SD, Steakley CS, Young RC, et al. Malignant pheochromocytoma: effective treatment with a combination of cyclophosphamide, vincristine, and dacarbazine. Ann Intern Med. 1988;109(4):267–73.
67. http://www.genetests.org. Accessed 12 May 2009.
68. Kloos RT, Eng C, Evans DB, et al. Medullary thyroid cancer: management guidelines of the American Thyroid Association. Thyroid. 2009;19(6):565–612.
69. Huang H, Abraham J, Hung E, et al. Treatment of malignant pheochromocytoma/paraganglioma with cyclophosphamide, vincristine, and dacarbazine: recommendation from a 22-year follow-up of 18 patients. Cancer. 2008;113(8):2020–8.
70. Nakane M, Takahashi S, Sekine I, et al. Successful treatment of malignant pheochromocytoma with combination chemotherapy containing anthracycline. Ann Oncol. 2003;14(9):1449–51.
71. Kulke MH, Stuart K, Enzinger PC, et al. Phase II study of temozolomide and thalidomide in patients with metastatic neuroendocrine tumors. J Clin Oncol. 2006;24(3):401–6.
72. Fitzgerald PA, Goldsby RE, Huberty JP, et al. Malignant pheochromocytomas and paragangliomas: a phase II study of therapy with high-dose 131I-metaiodobenzylguanidine (131I-MIBG). Ann N Y Acad Sci. 2006;1073:465–90.
73. Buscombe JR, Cwikla JB, Caplin ME, Hilson AJ. Long-term efficacy of low activity meta-[131I]iodobenzylguanidine therapy in patients with disseminated neuroendocrine tumours depends on initial response. Nucl Med Commun. 2005;26(11):969–76.
74. Scholz T, Eisenhofer G, Pacak K, Dralle H, Lehnert H. Clinical review: current treatment of malignant pheochromocytoma. J Clin Endocrinol Metab. 2007;92(4):1217–25.
75. Druce MR, Kaltsas GA, Fraenkel M, Gross DJ, Grossman AB. Novel and evolving therapies in the treatment of malignant phaeochromocytoma: experience with the mTOR inhibitor everolimus (RAD001). Horm Metab Res. 2009;41(9):697–702.
76. Jimenez C, Cabanillas ME, Santarpia L, et al. Use of the tyrosine kinase inhibitor sunitinib in a patient with von Hippel-Lindau disease: targeting angiogenic factors in pheochromocytoma and other von Hippel-Lindau disease-related tumors. J Clin Endocrinol Metab. 2009;94(2):386–91.
77. Joshua AM, Ezzat S, Asa SL, et al. Rationale and evidence for sunitinib in the treatment of malignant paraganglioma/pheochromocytoma. J Clin Endocrinol Metab. 2009;94(1):5–9.
78. Harrington JL, Farley DR, van Heerden JA, Ramin KD. Adrenal tumors and pregnancy. World J Surg. 1999;23(2):182–6.
79. Freier DT, Thompson NW. Pheochromocytoma and pregnancy: the epitome of high risk. Surgery. 1993;114(6):1148–52.
80. Mannelli M, Bemporad D. Diagnosis and management of pheochromocytoma during pregnancy. J Endocrinol Invest. 2002;25(6):567–71.
81. Schenker JG, Granat M. Phaeochromocytoma and pregnancy – an updated appraisal. Aust N Z J Obstet Gynaecol. 1982;22(1):1–10.
82. Ahlawat SK, Jain S, Kumari S, Varma S, Sharma BK. Pheochromocytoma associated with pregnancy: case report and review of the literature. Obstet Gynecol Surv. 1999;54(11):728–37.
83. Jaffe RB, Harrison TS, Cerny JC. Localization of metastatic pheochromocytoma in pregnancy by caval catheterization. Including urinary catecholamine values in uncomplicated pregnancies. Am J Obstet Gynecol. 1969;104(7):939–44.
84. Butters L, Kennedy S, Rubin PC. Atenolol in essential hypertension during pregnancy. BMJ. 1990;301(6752):587–9.
85. Montan S, Ingemarsson I, Marsal K, Sjoberg NO. Randomised controlled trial of atenolol and pindolol in human pregnancy: effects on fetal haemodynamics. BMJ. 1992;304(6832):946–9.

86. Junglee N, Harries SE, Davies N, Scott-Coombes D, Scanlon MF, Rees DA. Pheochromocytoma in pregnancy: when is operative intervention indicated? J Womens Health (Larchmt). 2007;16(9):1362–5.
87. Bryant J, Farmer J, Kessler LJ, Townsend RR, Nathanson KL. Pheochromocytoma: the expanding genetic differential diagnosis. J Natl Cancer Inst. 2003;95(16):1196–204.

Chapter 14
Merkel Cell Carcinoma

Leonid Izikson and Nathalie C. Zeitouni

Abstract Merkel cell carcinoma is a rare and aggressive neuroendocrine malignancy. In this chapter, we summarize the current knowledge regarding its epidemiology, pathogenesis, clinical features, histopathologic features, clinical staging, and prognosis. Furthermore, we review the evidence for various therapeutic approaches, including surgery, radiation therapy, and chemotherapy.

Keywords Merkel cell carcinoma • Oncogenic transformation • Staging • Treatment

Introduction

Merkel cell carcinoma (MCC) is a rare and highly aggressive cutaneous malignancy of neuroendocrine origin. It was first described in 1972 by Toker [1] as a "trabecular carcinoma of the skin" in five patients with unusual skin tumors, marked histologically by anastomosing cell trabeculae and cell nests in the dermis. Subsequently, these were classified by Tang and Toker [2] as "neuroendocrine carcinoma" based on the identification of electron-dense neurosecretory granules within tumor cells.

While the cellular ontogeny of MCC remains unproven, most authors believe it derives from skin-resident Merkel cells. Merkel cells, first described in 1875 by Friedrich Sigmund Merkel, are found in the basal epidermis of normal skin, where they are associated with touch domes and function as mechanoreceptors [3, 4]. They are the only type of skin cells which form neuroendocrine granules and belong to the amine precursor and decarboxylation system. Accordingly, it has been postulated

N.C. Zeitouni (✉)
Department of Dermatology, Roswell Park Cancer Institute and University at Buffalo, Elm and Carlton Streets, Buffalo, NY 14263, USA
e-mail: nathalie.zeitouni@roswellpark.org

J.C. Yao et al. (eds.), *Neuroendocrine Tumors*, Current Clinical Oncology,
DOI 10.1007/978-1-60327-997-0_14, © Springer Science+Business Media, LLC 2011

that MCC derive from Merkel cells [5], where presumed target cells for oncogenic transformation are not terminally differentiated cells, but adult stem or progenitor cells [5]. Despite ultrastructural similarities to Merkel cells, there is discrepancy between the deep location of MCC and the more superficial location of normal Merkel cells [4]. To date, the issue of whether MCC actually derive from Merkel cells or simply simulate their features has not been resolved definitively [3].

Epidemiology

MCC is a rare tumor. In the US, the incidence is 1,500 new cases per year, and is predicted to increase [5, 6]. Its incidence is greater than that of cutaneous T cell lymphoma [5], and the incidence rate of MCC has risen sharply in the past two decades [7]. Some of the increase in the incidence rate for MCC is likely related to improved diagnostic tools (e.g., availability of histochemical reagents for more definitive distinction from histologic mimics) [3].

In an analysis of MCC cases identified using the US surveillance, epidemiology, and end results (SEER) program from 1986 to 2001, Hodgson found that the rate of MCC tripled from 0.15 cases per 100,000 in 1986 to 0.44 cases per 100,000 in 2001. The estimated annual percentage change for the time period was a statistically significant 8.08%. Comparatively, the increase in melanoma incidence rates has been 3% over the same 15 year period [7]. Both male and female rates have increased significantly, with the rates in males almost threefold higher than in females. Age-specific incidence was highest in the elderly, with 4.28 per 100,000 in the 85+ age group [7]. Since 80+ years old individuals are the fastest-growing segment of the US population [7], the incidence rates of MCC is predicted to increase in the coming years.

MCC primarily affects elderly patients, with the mean age at initial diagnosis of 69 years [8]. Over 90% of the patients with MCC are white, with a male predominance [3, 7, 8]. Only 5% of MCC occurs before age 50 [9]. There is a high degree of association between MCC and squamous cell carcinoma (SCC), basal cell carcinoma (BCC), SCCIS, internal malignancies, and hematologic malignancies [5].

Immunosuppression is an important risk factor for MCC, and MCC occurs much more frequently in patients with HIV infection, CLL, and solid organ transplants [8–12]. Heath et al. [8] found that 7.8% of 195 MCC patients had some form of immunosuppression, a 16-fold higher frequency than expected in the general US population. CLL was particularly over-represented (4.1%). Engels et al. [10] found a relative risk of 13.4 (95% CI 4.9–29.1) for MCC in HIV population compared with the general population. Izikson et al. have found that there is an increased risk of MCC in HIV patients, with a trend toward male predominance and earlier age of disease onset in HIV-associated MCC. There was no clear relationship between CD4 counts and the duration between HIV and MCC diagnosis or length of survival [12]. Immunosuppressed patients tend to develop MCC at an earlier age [10, 13] and present with more advanced disease, with 67% of immunocompromised patients showing either nodal or distant metastatic disease compared to 42% in the immunocompetent group [8]. Interestingly, Friedlaender et al. [11] described temporary regression of MCC metastases after discontinuation of cyclosporine in a kidney transplant patient.

Pathogenesis

Although the pathogenesis of MCC has not been fully elucidated, recent discovery of a new Merkel cell polyomavirus (MCPyV) linked to MCC provides strong arguments in favor of an infectious cause with a viral-induced oncogenesis [14, 15]. Feng et al. [14] were the first to discover the presence of MCPyV in a majority of MCC tumors. Using digital transcriptome subtraction analysis of MCC tissues, they detected a fusion transcript between a previously undescribed viral T antigen and a human receptor tyrosine phosphatase. This led to subsequent identification and sequence analysis of the 5,387-base-pair genome of a previously unknown MCPyV. MCPyV sequences were detected in 8 of 10 (80%) MCC tumors but only 5 of 59 (8%) control tissues from various body sites and 4 of 25 (16%) control skin tissues. In six of eight MCPyV-positive MCCs, viral DNA was integrated within the tumor genome in a clonal pattern, suggesting that MCPyV infection and integration preceded clonal expansion of the tumor cells [14].

Subsequently, other groups have confirmed the presence of MCPyV in MCC [16–18]. Garneski et al. [16] have found that 16 of 37 MCC tumor tissues were positive for MCPyV DNA (43%); and Becker et al. [17] have found MCPyV in 45 of 53 MCC tumors (84.9%) from European patients. Furthermore, Busam et al. [18] have found that 15 of 17 (88%) MCC were positive for MCPyV by PCR, and 93% stained positive with a novel monoclonal antibody CM2B4, generated against a predicted antigenic epitope on the MCPyV T antigen. Additionally, Tolstov et al. [19] have shown that among 21 MCC patients with MCPyV-positive tumors, all (100%) had high serum MCV IgG but not high MCV IgM levels, and MCC patients had a markedly elevated MCPyV IgG response compared with control patients. Finally, Shuda et al. [20, 21] have provided a molecular basis for MCPyV involvement in MCC oncogenesis. They identified a signature mutation in MCC tumor-derived large T antigen genomic sequences [20] and showed that MCPyV large T antigen localized to nuclei of tumor cells from MCC [21].

However, the presence of viral DNA in MCC, positive staining with an anti-large T antigen antibody, or presence of anti-viral antibodies in MCC patients do not in themselves prove a causal relationship. Additional arguments against a causative relationship between MCPyV and MCC include the existence of MCV-negative MCCs and lack of tumor clusters among close relatives that might be expected with a viral infection [15]. Further studies to evaluate the role of viral oncogenesis in MCC are ongoing.

Many have also suggested a role for UV radiation-induced carcinogenesis in the evolution of MCC because the majority (81%) of MCCs occur on sun-damaged sites, frequently co-occur in conjunction with actinic keratosis (AK), SCC, or BCC, and the incidence of MCC correlates with regional solar UVB indices [3, 5, 22]. Lunder and Stern [23] reported that the incidence of MCC is about 100 times higher among patients treated with PUVA than that expected in the general population. Additionally, UVB specific mutations have been observed in the p53 and H-ras genes of MCC similar to SCC [3, 24]. However, MCC can arise in the absence of significant UV exposure. Importantly, 5% of patients in the study by Heath et al. [8] had tumors on highly sun-protected sites (buttock or vulva), and 14% had tumors on partially protected sites (abdomen, thighs and hair-bearing scalp).

Multiple studies have examined the contributions of various molecular oncogenic pathways in MCC. Interestingly, the "mitogenic" Raf/MEK/ERK cascade for tumorigenesis activated by Ras is generally inactive in MCC and distinguishes it from many other tumors, such as melanoma. However, it is likely that the molecular pathogenesis involves the Ras-activated PI3K/AKT signaling pathway [5]. Recently, a genomic analysis of MCC revealed frequent aberrations, such as extra copies of chromosomes 1, 3q, 5p, and 6 and lost chromosomes 3p, 4, 5q, 7, 10, and 13 [25]. 26% of tumors showed a deletion of 5q12-21, 26% of tumors showed a deletion of 13q14-21 that contains the well-characterized tumor suppressor RB1, and 36% of tumors showed a previously unreported focal amplification at 1p34 that centers on L-Myc (MYCL1), a protein with transforming activity related to the c-Myc proto-oncogene, which is also amplified in the closely related small cell lung cancer [25]. MCC pathogenesis also involves defective antigen presentation, induction of immunosuppressive cytokines such as IL-10 and TNF, the isomerization of *trans*- to *cis*-urocanic acid, and the formation of ROS [5].

Clinical Features

The clinical features of MCC are not distinctive. MCC usually presents as a nonspecific rapidly growing erythematous or violaceous papule or nodule with a smooth, shiny surface (Fig. 14.1) on sun damaged skin that develops over weeks to months [3, 5]. Tumor cell doubling times of 5–12 days are characteristic, but doubling can occur within 1–5 days in aggressive subtypes [4]. However, some tumors tend to grow slowly [3, 8]. MCC usually grows in a spherical and infiltrating fashion superficially and deeply, so that intact epidermis is stretched [5]. Tumors are usually 1–2 cm in diameter and asymptomatic [4, 8]. Additional presentations include a plaque, deep-seated nodule, or a cystic structure [3]. Some MCCs associated with SCC tend to resemble SCC in their clinical appearance, and more frequently show a scale, crust, and/or ulceration [26]. However, ulcerations are very rare and found primarily in very advanced tumors. Such lesions may also become large and painful [3, 4]. Satellite metastases can also occur early in the course of disease [4, 5]. Immunosuppressed patients present with more advanced disease [8].

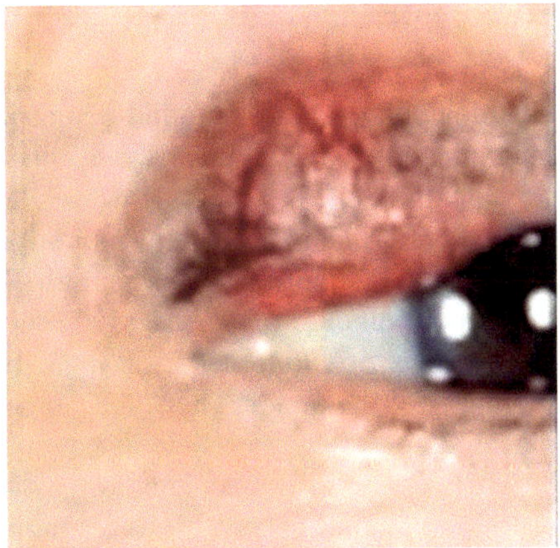

Fig. 14.1 Merkel cell carcinoma (MCC) presenting as an asymptomatic erythematous nodule of the upper eyelid

While the overwhelming majority of lesions appear on sun-exposed skin, up to 19% presented on the buttock or other minimally sun-exposed areas in one study [8]. Most commonly tumors present on the head and neck region. Sun-exposed extremities are the next most common location [8]. MCC can also present as a plaque on the trunk [5], but truncal tumors are rare overall [3]. A few cases have also been reported on genitalia and mucosa [4, 8].

MCC is rarely recognized as such. Clinically, biopsies are submitted to rule out BCC, adnexal tumor, SCC, cyst, lipoma, amelanotic melanoma, cutaneous lymphoma or others [3, 4]. In the study by Heath et al. [8], a cyst or acneiform lesion was the single most common presumptive diagnosis (32%), followed by lipoma (6%), dermatofibroma or fibroma (4%) and vascular lesion (4%). Malignant diagnoses comprised an additional 36% of the clinical impressions, with non melanoma skin cancer being the most common of these (19%), followed by lymphoma (6%), metastatic carcinoma (2%), and sarcoma (2%). The correct clinical diagnosis of MCC was made presumptively in only two cases (1%).

Heath et al. have also identified several tumor characteristics that may aid a clinician in suspecting MCC, summarized as AEIOU (Asymptomatic, Expanding Rapidly, Immunosuppressed, Older than age 50 years, UV exposed). Notably, they found that the lack of tenderness (found in 88% of MCC patients) is an important feature in MCC compared to many other lesions that are rapidly growing and red or pink [8].

The majority of patients (70% in the largest published series) present with a localized skin tumor and clinically negative nodes [3, 27]; at the time of diagnosis, 30% have metastatic disease. Most of these have nodal and/or cutaneous metastases. A subset of patients (3–20%) present with metastases, usually to the lymph node, without a known primary MCC. This is most likely due to regression of the skin tumor [3]. Hence, a careful skin and lymphatic exam is essential to establish whether there is tumor spread [4]. In most patients, MCC will progress and metastasize, but spontaneous resolution has been reported in some cases [4].

Histologic Features

Histologically, MCC is found primarily within the dermis [15]. At scanning magnification, MCC typically presents as a "blue" cell tumor in the dermis and/or subcutis [3] (Fig. 14.2). However, epidermal involvement can be present in 8%, where it manifests as bowenoid dysplasia [28]. MCC may be fairly circumscribed, but more often shows an infiltrative growth pattern at its periphery. Often the tumor cells are dispersed as sheets lacking a distinct architectural arrangement. Rows of single cells, or small balls of cells, are commonly seen at the periphery of the tumor. The "blue" appearance is due to cells with minimal cytoplasm [3].

MCC exists in three main forms: intermediate type (80%), trabecular type (10%), and small cell type (10%), though tumors usually demonstrate a mix of these three patterns. The intermediate type demonstrates large nests of neoplastic cells [5, 15]. The trabecular "organoid" type demonstrates bridged strands of tumor cells throughout the dermis forming clusters and pseudorosettes [3, 15]. It is typically found in the periphery and often associated with adnexal structures, especially hair follicles. The small cell type demonstrates more loosely organized sheets of tumor cells among collagen strands, reminiscent of other small cell tumor types [15].

Areas of squamous differentiation, focal necrosis, lymphocytic inflammatory cell infiltrate of variable density may be present, and lymphatic tumor emboli are commonly identified at the periphery of many tumors [3, 15]. Mitotic figures and

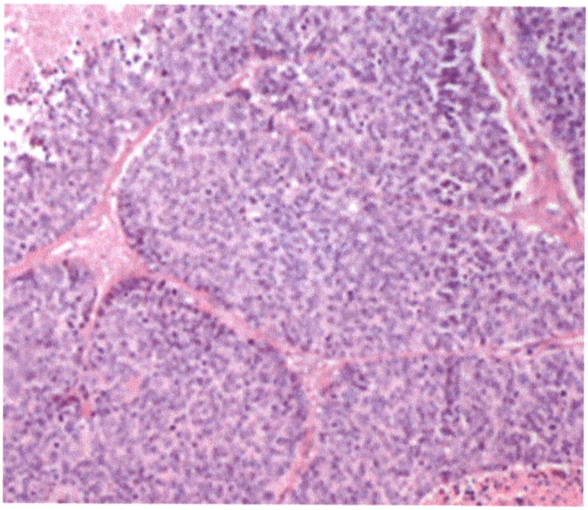

Fig. 14.2 A characteristic histologic pattern of MCC in the dermis and subcutis (intermediate type), demonstrating large nests of small blue neoplastic cells

apoptotic bodies tend to be numerous, as the mitotic index is very high, and many atypical mitoses are seen [3, 5]. Also, there may be an associated increase in the vascularity of the peritumoral or intratumoral stroma and amyloid deposition [3]. Rare findings include stromal desmoplasia and amyloid deposits [15].

While the majority of MCCs develop de novo and are histologically pure, a subset of MCCs can occur in association with other non-neuroendocrine carcinomas, most often SCCs, rarely basal cell carcinoma, or other miscellaneous adnexal tumors, or cysts. These most likely represent collision tumors. However, a subset of MCCs may represent biphenotypic (combined) carcinomas, at least for SCCs, given the intimate admixture of squamous and neuroendocrine tumor components and the presence of transition areas in some such lesions. Some cases can also demonstrate glandular and melanocytic differentiation [15]. Rarely, MCC can be associated with a sarcomatoid component, such as an atypical fibroxanthoma, fibrosarcoma, leiomyosarcoma, or rhabdomyosarcoma, or exhibit paraganglioma-like features [3].

The MCC tumor cells themselves are small, basophilic, round to oval blue cells. They contain vesicular hyperchromaic nuclei, multiple nucleoli, and multiple mitoses [15]. The nuclei have finely granular "salt and pepper" chromatin pattern [3]. Cell borders are poorly defined and cytoplasm is scant [15]. At times, a significant proportion of MCC cells display features identical to small cell lung carcinoma. These include small cell size, dense hyperchromatic nucleus, nuclear molding, and associated crush artifact [3]. MCC may simulate a lymphoma when MCC cells show a more discohesive growth pattern and round nuclear contours. The cytoplasm may be unusually abundant ("plasmacytoid"), or the tumor cells may show clear cell, anaplastic or spindle cell features [3].

Electron microscopy (EM) demonstrates membrane-bound dense core neuroendocrine cytoplasmic granules (diameter about 100 nm), as well as abundant paranuclear intermediate filaments in round groups, and a lobular nucleus [3, 15]. The availability of antibodies to detect the contents of neurosecretory granules and paranuclear intermediate filaments by immunohistochemistry (IH) and immunofluorescence (IF) has rendered EM unnecessary for the diagnosis of MCC [3].

The histologic differential diagnosis of small blue cells includes small cell lung carcinoma, cutaneous large cell carcinoma, neuroblastoma, high grade neuroendocrine tumors, amelanotic melanoma, small cell melanoma, sweat gland carcinoma, other primary cutaneous tumors, such as carcinomas with basaloid or small cell features (BCC), pilomatrix carcinoma, Langerhans cell histiocytosis, Ewing's sarcoma, and lymphoma [3, 15]. On occasion, the distinction may be difficult on a small biopsy sample, but attention to the presence or absence of characteristic nuclear features associated with MCC and the use of IH markers should lead to the correct diagnosis [3].

Differentiation of MCC from its mimics can be accomplished in most cases by IH and IF studies. Most MCC are positive for CK-20, NSE, and EMA [15]. CK-20 staining, positive in 75–100% of the cases, usually shows a paranuclear dot pattern, but a dot-like pattern is not always seen. Occasionally, the staining pattern can be mixed membranous or diffuse cytoplasmic. Rarely, a membranous pattern dominates. [3]. Although often negative for CK-7, up to a quarter of MCCs has been reported to stain for this type of cytokeratin [3]. MCC also express other neuroendocrine markers, including chromogranin, synaptophysin, somatostatin, calcitonin, and VIP, as well as the neural markers CD56 and neurofilament protein (NF) [3, 15]. Although CD117 is commonly positive in MCC, activating c-kit mutations have not been observed [3]. In contrast to the majority of pulmonary and a subset of extrapulmonary (noncutaneous) neuroendocrine carcinomas, MCCs are usually negative for TTF-1 [3]. Characteristically, MCC do not express S-100, CD45 (leukocyte common antigen), and laminin [15].

Recently, Busam et al. [18] found that 93% of MCC stained positive with a monoclonal antibody CM2B4, generated against a predicted antigenic epitope on the MCPyV T antigen. Skin tumors with a combined squamous and neuroendocrine phenotype and all pulmonary neuroendocrine carcinomas failed to react with CM2B4. Hence, this antibody can be useful in distinguishing most MCC from pulmonary neuroendocrine carcinomas [18].

Staging

In MCC, as in all malignancies, stage of disease is the most important prognostic factor. Currently, many centers use a modified four-tiered basic clinical staging system based on whether MCC is restricted to the primary skin site, involves regional nodes, or has spread beyond the regional nodal basin, provided below [3]. Although there is no universally implemented and accepted staging system in current use, the American Joint Commission on Cancer has devised a consensus system for MCC that builds on the four-tiered system and takes histologic findings of the sentinel lymph node (SLN) status into account (Box 14.1) [3]. A proposed new staging system taking into account the size and nature of the primary tumor, nature of lymph node involvement, and nature of any metastatic disease, has been devised [29].

SLN mapping and biopsy are essential for accurate staging of disease, as sentinel node status is a powerful predictor of disease recurrence and disease-specific survival [3, 30]. If no obvious tumor is found on the initial levels of a bisected SLN, additional levels and immunostains for CK-20 or Cam 5.2 can help to identify small metastatic deposits [3, 31]. Approximately 20–30% of MCC patients with clinically negative nodes are found to have a histologically positive SLN. Patients with a histologically negative SLN have a better prognosis than those with microscopic tumor deposits [3]. Radiographic imaging, such as chest X-ray and CT scan, is necessary to establish staging and rule out the possibility of a primary SCLC [4]. PET and 18-flurodeoxyglucose-PET has been shown as more sensitive than CT and may be considered [4]. The value of the recently introduced Gallium-DOTATOC PET is currently being studied in MCC [5].

Box 14.1. Four-Tiered Clinical Staging System (AJCC) [32]

Anatomic Stage • Prognostic Groups

Patients with primary MCC with no evidence of regional or distant metastases (either clinically or pathologically) are divided into two stages: Stage I for primary tumors ≤2 cm in size and Stage II for primary tumors >2 cm in size. Stages I and II are further divided into A and B substages based on method of nodal evaluation. Patients who have pathologically proven node negative disease (by microscopic evaluation of their draining lymph nodes) have improved survival (substaged as A) compared to those who are only evaluated clinically (substaged as B). Stage II has an additional substage (IIC) for tumors with extracutaneous invasion (T4) and negative node status regardless of whether the negative node status was established microscopically or clinically. Stage III is also divided into A and B categories for patients with microscopically positive and clinically occult nodes (IIIA) and macroscopic nodes (IIIB). There are no subgroups of stage IV MCC.

Stage 0	Tis	N0	M0
Stage IA	T1	pN0	M0
Stage IB	T1	cN0	M0
Stage IIA	T2/T3	pN0	M0
Stage IIB	T2/T3	cN0	M0
Stage IIC	T4	N0	M0
Stage IIIA	Any T	N1a	M0
Stage IIIB	Any T	N1b/N2	M0
Stage IV	Any T	Any N	M1

Prognosis and Follow-Up

Despite its reputation as an extremely aggressive malignancy with almost universal lethality, overall survival rates for MCC have been reported between 30 and 75% in the literature. Delineating the natural course of disease has been fraught with a plethora of difficulties, including disparate methods for staging used in various studies, low numbers of patients with limited follow-up, and lack of stage-specific survival data [30]. In 2005, Allen et al. found a 64% disease-specific 5-year survival rate among 251 patients treated at the MSKCC between 1970 and 2002. They found that disease stage was the only independent predictor of survival. Accordingly, survival was 81% in stage I disease, 67% in stage II disease, 52% in stage II disease, and 11% in stage IV disease. Disease recurred in 43% of the patients, and median time to recurrence was 9 months. Local recurrence developed in 8% after margin-negative excision [30].

Other unfavorable clinical and histologic prognostic factors, in addition to advanced stage of disease and increased tumor thickness, include male gender, tumor location on the head and neck region or the trunk, the presence of immunosuppression [5], lymphovascular invasion by the tumor, infiltrative tumor growth pattern [33], absence of tumor infiltrating lymphocytes, poorly differentiated cell type (small cell), and overexpression of p63 or survivin [5]. Patients with small circumscribed tumors limited to the dermis have a much better prognosis than those with diffusely infiltrative subcutaneous tumors associated with lymphatic tumor emboli [33].

Regional disease is found in 30% of cases at presentation and another 20% during the course of disease [4]. MCC has a tendency to invade dermal lymphatics early in disease progression, and this may lead to local micrometastases in skin areas adjacent to the primary tumor, contributing to the difficulty of establishing true negative margins. Subclinical spread is likely responsible for the relatively high 30% local recurrence rate [4]. Metastases eventually occur in 50% of the patients, most commonly to skin, lymph nodes, liver, bone, lung, and brain [4].

Patients should be followed closely and restaged based on clinical findings and further imaging or biopsies. The national Comprehensive Cancer Network recommends a physical exam with a complete skin check, in addition to optional CXR and serum LDH, every 1–3 month for 1 year, then every 3–6 month for 1 year, followed by annual physical exams. Patient education and monthly self examination are also important for comprehensive care [4]. Clinical examination should include a thorough inspection of skin and palpation of lymph nodes. The value of imaging and measurements of serum markers (chromogranin A or NSE) remains unclear [5].

Therapy

Although many therapies have been attempted for MCC, no definitive and universally employed management algorithm has been developed [34]. To date, there have been no prospective, randomized, double-blinded studies to address therapies for MCC. Accordingly, treatment guidelines are established and continually updated by an interdisciplinary consensus [5]. Current strategies include surgical excision with wide margins vs. Mohs surgery with clear margins, followed by SNLB, definitive lymph node dissection, irradiation, or chemotherapy [34].

Surgical excision is the mainstay of treatment for patients with MCC [3]. Most experts agree that the initial management of MCC is wide local excision with 2–3 cm margins [34]. Narrower margins may be acceptable for head and neck, as no difference in locoregional control or survival was found among groups with surgical margins smaller than 1 cm, 1–2 cm, and larger than 2 cm on the head and neck [35]. Mohs surgery can also be an effective approach for achieving local control [36–40], and in the treatment of MCC in other cosmetically sensitive locations [41].

Due to the propensity of MCC for regional lymphatic spread and its recurrence in the lymphatics, effective management of the lymph node basin is critical [34]. A SNLB should be performed, ideally at the time of excision. When SNL is positive for micrometastases, a complete lymphadenectomy of the basin is indicated [5]. While some have advocated elective LND because it is associated with increased time to recurrence, it has never been shown to improve survival and carries significant morbidity [34]. Most do not recommend elective LND, but reserve it for management of patients who have positive SNL or clinically positive lymph nodes [34].

Since MCC is highly radiosensitive, radiation therapy also plays an important role in the management of patients with MCC [3, 5]. Most experts have found that adjuvant radiotherapy following surgical excision is an effective combination for achieving locoregional control [5, 34, 42]. Overall, the use of radiation therapy was associated with an improved survival for patients with all sizes of tumors, but particularly in patients with primary lesions larger than 2 cm [42]. Currently, adjuvant radiation is undertaken for patients at high risk as defined by some investigators: lesions larger than 1.5 cm, vascular invasion, perineural invasion, microscopic positive margins, residual disease, and/or regional lymph node involvement [43]. However, Boyer et al. [40] have found that adjuvant radiation appears unessential to secure local control of primary MCC lesions completely excised with Mohs micrographic surgery, and Allen et al. [30] have found that the use of adjuvant radiotherapy to the nodal basin was not associated with a decrease in nodal recurrence. Still, most centers currently use post-operative radiation therapy. Additionally, radiation therapy can be beneficial for unresectable tumors or recurrent tumors [3].

For stage 1 disease, 4,500–6,000 cGy over 5–6 weeks to the tumor site with 3–5 cm margins is recommended. For stage 1 tumors that show aggressive features in histology or size, consideration should be made to include in transit lymphatics and the draining lymph node basin [4]. In stage 2 disease, radiation therapy is recommended for the primary tumor bed, in transit lymphatics, and the draining lymph node after complete LND. Radiation doses greater than 5,000 Gy may be required for bulky disease [4]. Still, local recurrence of MCC is 30–75%, mostly within 2 years after initial diagnosis. In this setting, aggressive management includes repeated excision, lymphadenectomy, irradiation, and chemotherapy, but the results are quite poor [34].

MCC is considered a chemosensitive tumor, and chemotherapy is an option for palliative therapy of patients with stage IV disease [3, 5]. These patients with distant metastatic disease represent 1/3 of the cases and have a median survival of 9 months [4]. Chemotherapy can also be used in the setting of locally advanced disease and recurrence [34], and for therapy of in-transit metastases on the extremities using the isolated limb perfusion (ILP) and infusion (ILI) methods [44, 45].

For the treatment of in-transit MCC, high dosage concentrated melphalan administered via ILP or ILI methods was found to be beneficial [44, 45]. These techniques allow for delivery of up to 25 times the allotted systemic dosage of chemotherapeutics to a limited area, thereby eradicating the tumor more effectively while minimizing systemic toxicities [44]. As a result of ILP or ILI with melphalan, either alone or in combination with systemic tumor necrosis factor alpha, actinomycin D, interferon gamma, or nitrogen mustard, all patients avoided limb amputation, with the average survival of 37 months post-treatment. Although ILP or ILI did not increase overall patient survival, these approaches nevertheless allowed for improved locoregional control of disease and limb preservation with limited systemic toxicities (personal observation, NCZ).

Overall, two-thirds of MCC respond to systemic chemotherapy, but disease often recurs within a few months [3] and chemotherapy has not been shown to improve overall survival rate [5]. Additionally, chemotherapy toxicities require careful patient selection. To date, no standardized evidence-based optimal chemotherapy regimen exists for MCC [5, 34], and an adequate study to assess survival in patients treated with chemotherapy has not been carried out. Because of morphologic similarities to small cell lung cancer, similar regimens have been used for MCC, including anthracyclines, anti-metabolites, bleomycin, cyclophosphamide, and platinum derivatives including cisplatin, carboplatin, etoposide, or topotecal [4, 5]. Chemotherapy with doxorubicin used in patients with established metastatic disease has not been associated with increased survival [4]. Due to the rarity of MCC, prospective randomized studies of adjuvant therapy are lacking [30].

In sum, on the basis of outcomes from available literature, Ruan and Reeves recommend the following therapeutic approach for MCC: surgical excision of the primary tumor with 2–3 cm margins and consideration of adjuvant irradiation; SNLB for patients with no clinical nodal disease; definitive LND for patients with nodal disease; radiotherapy for locoregional control in node-positive cases, locally advanced disease, or local recurrence; and possible systemic chemotherapy for recurrence, locally advanced disease, and distant metastases [34].

The potential virally mediated oncogenesis of MCC opens the possibility that new regimens, including antiviral interferons and other immunotherapies, may be useful. Anecdotal case reports reveal successful use of TNF-α, IFN-α, anti CD56 Abs, and vaccines [5]. However, Imatinib, a Kit inhibitor, as well as Oblimersen, an antisense oligonucleotide against bcl-2 (an anti-apoptotic protein), have not shown clinical efficacy against MCC [5].

References

1. Toker C. Trabecular carcinoma of the skin. Arch Dermatol. 1972;105(1):107–10.
2. Tang CK, Toker C. Trabecular carcinoma of the skin: an ultrastructural study. Cancer. 1978;42(5):2311–21.
3. Pulitzer MP, Amin BD, Busam KJ. Merkel cell carcinoma: review. Adv Anat Pathol. 2009;16(3):135–44.
4. Swann MH, Yoon J. Merkel cell carcinoma. Semin Oncol. 2007;34(1):51–6.
5. Becker JC, Kauczok CS, Ugurel S, Eib S, Bröcker EB, Houben R. Merkel cell carcinoma: molecular pathogenesis, clinical features and therapy. J Dtsch Dermatol Ges. 2008;6(9): 709–19.
6. Lemos B, Nghiem P. Merkel cell carcinoma: more deaths but still no pathway to blame. J Invest Dermatol. 2007;127(9):2100–3.

7. Hodgson NC. Merkel cell carcinoma: changing incidence trends. J Surg Oncol. 2005;89(1):1–4.
8. Heath M, Jaimes N, Lemos B, Mostaghimi A, Wang LC, Peñas PF, et al. Clinical characteristics of Merkel cell carcinoma at diagnosis in 195 patients: the AEIOU features. J Am Acad Dermatol. 2008;58(3):375–81.
9. Miller RW, Rabkin CS. Merkel cell carcinoma and melanoma: etiological similarities and differences. Cancer Epidemiol Biomarkers Prev. 1999;8(2):153–8.
10. Engels EA, Frisch M, Goedert JJ, Biggar RJ, Miller RW. Merkel cell carcinoma and HIV infection. Lancet. 2002;359(9305):497–8.
11. Friedlaender MM, Rubinger D, Rosenbaum E, Amir G, Siguencia E. Temporary regression of Merkel cell carcinoma metastases after cessation of cyclosporine. Transplantation. 2002;73(11):1849–50.
12. Izikson L, Nornhold E, Iyer JG, Nghiem P, Zeitouni NC. Merkel cell carcinoma associated with HIV: Review of 14 patients. AIDS. 2011;25(1):119–21.
13. Penn I, First MR. Merkel's cell carcinoma in organ recipients: report of 41 cases. Transplantation. 1999;68(11):1717–21.
14. Feng H, Shuda M, Chang Y, Moore PS. Clonal integration of a polyomavirus in human Merkel cell carcinoma. Science. 2008;319(5866):1096–100.
15. Dubina M, Goldenberg G. Viral-associated nonmelanoma skin cancers: a review. Am J Dermatopathol. 2009;31(6):561–73.
16. Garneski KM, Warcola AH, Feng Q, Kiviat NB, Leonard JH, Nghiem P. Merkel cell polyomavirus is more frequently present in North American than Australian Merkel cell carcinoma tumors. J Invest Dermatol. 2009;129(1):246–8.
17. Becker JC, Houben R, Ugurel S, Trefzer U, Pföhler C, Schrama D. MC polyomavirus is frequently present in Merkel cell carcinoma of European patients. J Invest Dermatol. 2009;129(1):248–50.
18. Busam KJ, Jungbluth AA, Rekthman N, Coit D, Pulitzer M, Bini J, et al. Merkel cell polyomavirus expression in Merkel cell carcinomas and its absence in combined tumors and pulmonary neuroendocrine carcinomas. Am J Surg Pathol. 2009;33(9):1378–85.
19. Tolstov YL, Pastrana DV, Feng H, Becker JC, Jenkins FJ, Moschos S, et al. Human Merkel cell polyomavirus infection II. MCV is a common human infection that can be detected by conformational capsid epitope immunoassays. Int J Cancer. 2009;125(6):1250–6.
20. Shuda M, Feng H, Kwun HJ, Rosen ST, Gjoerup O, Moore PS, et al. T antigen mutations are a human tumor specific signature for Merkel cell polyomavirus. Proc Natl Acad Sci U S A. 2008;105(42):16272–7.
21. Shuda M, Arora R, Kwun HJ, Feng H, Sarid R, Fernández-Figueras MT, et al. Human Merkel cell polyomavirus infection I. MCV T antigen expression in Merkel cell carcinoma, lymphoid tissues and lymphoid tumors. Int J Cancer. 2009;125(6):1243–9.
22. Agelli M, Clegg LX. Epidemiology of primary Merkel cell carcinoma in the United States. J Am Acad Dermatol. 2003;49(5):832–41.
23. Lunder EJ, Stern RS. Merkel-cell carcinomas in patients treated with methoxsalen and ultraviolet A radiation. NEJM. 1998;339(17):1247–8.
24. Popp S, Waltering S, Herbst C, Moll I, Boukamp P. UV-B-type mutations and chromosomal imbalances indicate common pathways for the development of Merkel and skin squamous cell carcinomas. Int J Cancer. 2002;99(3):352–60.
25. Paulson KG, Lemos BD, Feng B, Jaimes N, Peñas PF, Bi X, et al. Array-CGH reveals recurrent genomic changes in Merkel cell carcinoma including amplification of L-Myc. J Invest Dermatol. 2009;129(6):1547–55.
26. Walsh NM. Primary neuroendocrine (Merkel cell) carcinoma of the skin: morphologic diversity and implications thereof. Hum Pathol. 2001;32(7):680–9.
27. Medina-Franco H, Urist MM, Fiveash J, Heslin MJ, Bland KI, Beenken SW. Multimodality treatment of Merkel cell carcinoma: case series and literature review of 1024 cases. Ann Surg Oncol. 2001;8(3):204–8.
28. Smith KJ, Skelton III HG, Holland TT, Morgan AM, Lupton GP. Neuroendocrine (Merkel cell) carcinoma with an intraepidermal component. Am J Dermatopathol. 1993;15(6):528–33.

29. Lemos BD, Storer BE, Iyer JG, et al. Pathologic nodal evaluation improves prognostic accuracy in merkel cell carcinoma: Analysis of 5823 cases as the basis of the first consensus staging system. J Am Acad Dermatol. 2010;63(5):751–61.
30. Allen PJ, Bowne WB, Jaques DP, Brennan MF, Busam K, Coit DG. Merkel cell carcinoma: prognosis and treatment of patients from a single institution. J Clin Oncol. 2005;23(10): 2300–9.
31. Bichakjian CK, Lowe L, Lao CD, Sandler HM, Bradford CR, Johnson TM, et al. Merkel cell carcinoma: critical review with guidelines for multidisciplinary management. Cancer. 2007;110(1):1–12.
32. Warner CL, Cockerell CJ. The new seventh edition American Joint Committee on cancer staging of cutaneous non-melanoma skin cancer: a critical review. Am J Clin Dermatol. 2011;12(3):147–154.
33. Andea AA, Coit DG, Amin B, Busam K. Merkel cell carcinoma: histologic features and prognosis. Cancer. 2008;113(9):2549–58.
34. Ruan JH, Reeves M. Merkel cell carcinoma treatment algorithm. Arch Surg. 2009;144(6): 582–5.
35. Gillenwater AM, Hessel AC, Morrison WH, Burgess M, Silva EG, Roberts D, et al. Merkel cell carcinoma of the head and neck: effect of surgical excision and radiation on recurrence and survival. Arch Otolaryngol Head Neck Surg. 2001;127(2):149–54.
36. O'Connor WJ, Roenigk RK, Brodland DG. Merkel cell carcinoma. Comparison of Mohs micrographic surgery and wide excision in eighty-six patients. Dermatol Surg. 1997;23(10):929–33.
37. Gollard R, Weber R, Kosty MP, Greenway HT, Massullo V, Humberson C. Merkel cell carcinoma: review of 22 cases with surgical, pathologic, and therapeutic considerations. Cancer. 2000;88(8):1842–51.
38. Zeitouni NC, Cheney RT, Delacure MD. Lymphoscintigraphy, sentinel lymph node biopsy, and Mohs micrographic surgery in the treatment of Merkel cell carcinoma. Dermatol Surg. 2000;26(1):12–8.
39. Snow SN, Larson PO, Hardy S, Bentz M, Madjar D, Landeck A, et al. Merkel cell carcinoma of the skin and mucosa: report of 12 cutaneous cases with 2 cases arising from the nasal mucosa. Dermatol Surg. 2001;27(2):165–70.
40. Boyer JD, Zitelli JA, Brodland DG, D'Angelo G. Local control of primary Merkel cell carcinoma: review of 45 cases treated with Mohs micrographic surgery with and without adjuvant radiation. J Am Acad Dermatol. 2002;47(6):885–92.
41. Pathai S, Barlow R, Williams G, Olver J. Mohs' micrographic surgery for Merkel cell carcinomas of the eyelid. Orbit. 2005;24(4):273–5.
42. Mojica P, Smith D, Ellenhorn JD. Adjuvant radiation therapy is associated with improved survival in Merkel cell carcinoma of the skin. J Clin Oncol. 2007;25(9):1043–7.
43. Eng TY, Boersma MG, Fuller CD, Goytia V, Jones III WE, Joyner M, et al. A comprehensive review of the treatment of Merkel cell carcinoma. Am J Clin Oncol. 2007;30(6):624–36.
44. Grobmyer SR, Copeland III EM, Hochwald SN. Treatment of in-transit metastases from Merkel cell carcinoma with isolated hyperthermic limb infusion. Am Surg. 2008;74(12): 1222–3.
45. Zeitouni NC, Giordano CN, Kane JM 3rd. In-transit merkel cell carcinoma treated with isolated limb perfusion or isolated limb infusion: A case series of 12 patients. Dermatol Surg. 2011;37(3):357–64.

Index

J.C. Yao et al. (eds.), *Neuroendocrine Tumors*, Current Clinical Oncology,
DOI 10.1007/978-1-60327-997-0, © Springer Science+Business Media, LLC 2011

R

MIX
Papier aus verantwortungsvollen Quellen
Paper from responsible sources
FSC® C105338

If you have any concerns about our products,
you can contact us on
ProductSafety@springernature.com

In case Publisher is established outside the EU,
the EU authorized representative is:
Springer Nature Customer Service Center GmbH
Europaplatz 3, 69115 Heidelberg, Germany

Printed by Libri Plureos GmbH
in Hamburg, Germany